RadCases

All the key Radiology cases for you rotations, and exams—in print and online!

Simply visit http://RadCases.thieme.com and, when prompted during the registration process, enter the scratch-off code below to get started today.

This book can no longer be returned once this panel is scratched off.

ccess and search 250 nust-know cases online!

ch book in the RadCases series contains 100 cases plus a scratch-f code that allows 12 months of online access to all of the cases m the book plus 150 additional cases—250 cases in all—related that book's subspecialty via **RadCases.thieme.com.**

atures of RadCases online include:

- A user-friendly way to study the most commonly encountered cases in each subspecialty
- Diagnostic videos and color images enhance selected subspecialties
- A flexible search function that lets you locate specific cases by age, differential diagnosis, modality, and more
- The ability to bookmark cases you want to return to and to 'hide' the cases you've already learned
- The same user-friendly organization as your ***RadCases*** book
- Clearly labeled, high-quality radiographs to help you absorb key findings at-a-glance

System requirements for optimal use of RadCases online

	WINDOWS	MAC
Recommended Browser(s)**	Microsoft Internet Explorer 7.0 or later, Firefox 2.x, Firefox 3.x *** all browsers should have JavaScript enabled*	Firefox 2.x, Firefox 3.x, Safari 3.x, Safari 4.x
Flash Player Plug-in	Flash Player 8 or Higher* ** Mac users: ATI Rage 128 GPU does not support full-screen mode with hardware scaling*	
Minimum Hardware Configurations	Intel® Pentium® II 450 MHz, AMD Athlon™ 600 MHz or faster processor (or equivalent) 128 MB of RAM	PowerPC® G3 500 MHz or faster processor Intel Core™ Duo 1.33 GHz or faster processor 128 MB of RAM
Recommended for optimal usage experience	Monitor resolutions: • Normal (4:3) 1024×768 or Higher • Widescreen (16:9) 1280×720 or Higher • Widescreen (16:10) 1440×900 or Higher DSL/Cable internet connection at a minimum speed of 384.0 Kbps or faster	

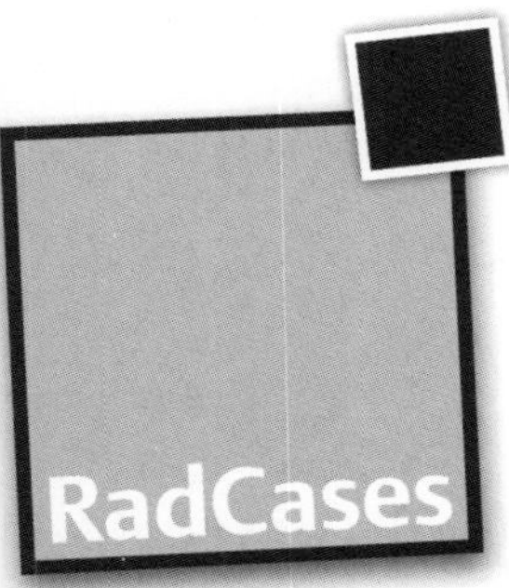

RadCases Nuclear Medicine

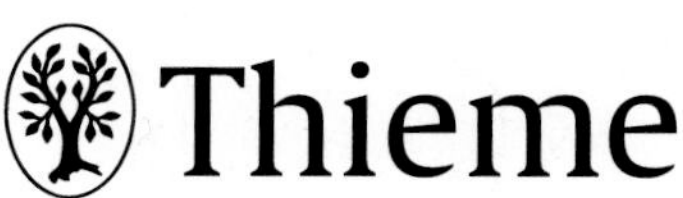

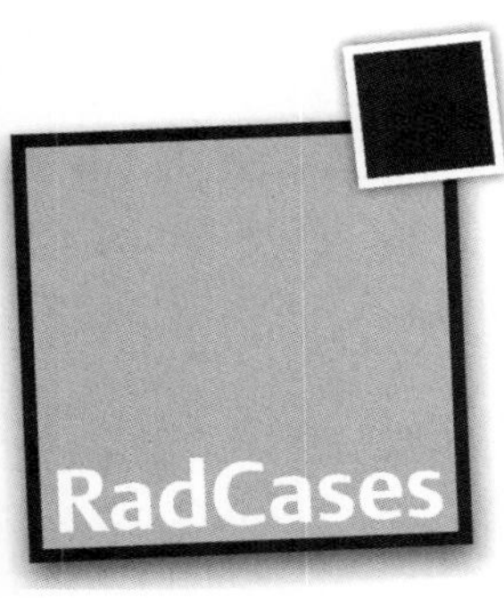

RadCases Nuclear Medicine

Edited by

Daniel Appelbaum, MD
Director of Nuclear Medicine and PET Imaging
Associate Investigator, Comprehensive Cancer Center
Associate Professor of Radiology
The University of Chicago
Chicago, Illinois

John Miliziano, MD
Director of Nuclear Medicine
Morton Plant Mease Healthcare
Clearwater, Florida

Sundeep Nayak, MD
Imaging Department
Kaiser Permanente GSAA Hayward Medical Center
Hayward, California
Associate Clinical Professor
Department of Radiology and Biomedical Imaging
University of California, San Francisco School of Medicine
San Francisco, California

Yong Bradley, MD
Associate Professor of Radiology
Medical Director of Molecular Imaging
Department of Radiology
The University of Tennessee Medical Center
Knoxville, Tennessee

Series Editors

Jonathan Lorenz, MD
Associate Professor of Radiology
Department of Radiology
The University of Chicago
Chicago, Illinois

Hector Ferral, MD
Professor of Radiology
Section Chief, Interventional Radiology
Rush University Medical Center, Chicago
Chicago, Illinois

Thieme
New York • Stuttgart

Thieme Medical Publishers, Inc.
333 Seventh Ave.
New York, NY 10001

Executive Editor: Timothy Hiscock
Editorial Assistant: Adriana di Giorgio, Michael Rowley
Editorial Director: Michael Wachinger
Production Editor: Katy Whipple, Maryland Composition
International Production Director: Andreas Schabert
Vice President, International Marketing and Sales: Cornelia Schulze
Chief Financial Officer: Sarah Vanderbilt
President: Brian D. Scanlan
Compositor: MPS Limited, a Macmillan Company
Printer: Everbest

Library of Congress Cataloging-in-Publication Data

Nuclear medicine / Edited by Daniel Appelbaum, MD, Director of Nuclear Medicine and PET Imaging, Associate Investigator, Comprehensive Cancer Center, Associate Professor of Radiology, The University of Chicago, Chicago, Illinois, John Miliziano, MD, Director of Nuclear Medicine, Morton Plant Mease Healthcare, Clearwater, Florida, Sundeep Nayak, MD, Imaging Department, Kaiser Permanente GSAA Hayward Medical Center, Hayward, California, Associate Clinical Professor, Department of Radiology and Biomedical Imaging, University of California-San Francisco School of Medicine, San Francisco, California, Yong Bradley, MD, Associate Professor of Radiology, Medical Director of Molecular Imaging, Department of Radiology, University of Tennessee Medical Center, Knoxville, Tennessee.
p. ; cm. — (RadCases)
Includes bibliographical references.
ISBN 978-1-60406-230-4 (pbk.)
1. Diagnostic imaging—Case studies. I. Appelbaum, Daniel, editor. II. Miliziano, John, editor.
III. Nayak, Sundeep, editor. IV. Bradley, Yong, editor. V. Series: RadCases.
[DNLM: 1. Diagnostic Imaging—Case Reports. WN 180]
RC78.7.D53N82 2011
616.07'54—dc22

2010053193

Important note: Medical knowledge is ever-changing. As new research and clinical experience broaden our knowledge, changes in treatment and drug therapy may be required. The authors and editors of the material herein have consulted sources believed to be reliable in their efforts to provide information that is complete and in accord with the standards accepted at the time of publication. However, in view of the possibility of human error by the authors, editors, or publisher of the work herein or changes in medical knowledge, neither the authors, editors, nor publisher, nor any other party who has been involved in the preparation of this work, warrants that the information contained herein is in every respect accurate or complete, and they are not responsible for any errors or omissions or for the results obtained from use of such information. Readers are encouraged to confirm the information contained herein with other sources. For example, readers are advised to check the product information sheet included in the package of each drug they plan to administer to be certain that the information contained in this publication is accurate and that changes have not been made in the recommended dose or in the contraindications for administration. This recommendation is of particular importance in connection with new or infrequently used drugs.

Some of the product names, patents, and registered designs referred to in this book are in fact registered trademarks or proprietary names even though specific reference to this fact is not always made in the text. Theref ore, the appearance of a name without designation as proprietary is not to be construed as a representation by the publisher that it is in the public domain.

Printed in China

ISBN 978-1-60406-230-4

Dedication

To my wonderfully silly, inquisitive, dashing, and energetic littlest "residents" Nathan, Noa, Tess, and Mabel, for making it all worthwhile. But mostly for my beautiful brilliant Karin, my precious wife, best friend, and biggest fan (as I am hers). Your support, love, and laughter are everything to me.

–DA

This book is dedicated to my wife Brandi and boys, Zackary, Dominic, and Giovanni. Thank you for all the love and support.

–JM

To Marsha.

–SN

To the loves of my life: my wife, Dawn, and my sons, Caleb and Josiah, for all your support, patience, and love.

–YB

RadCases Series Preface

The ability to assimilate detailed information across the entire spectrum of radiology is the Holy Grail sought by those preparing for the American Board of Radiology examination. As enthusiastic partners in the Thieme RadCases Series who formerly took the examination, we understand the exhaustion and frustration shared by residents and the families of residents engaged in this quest. It has been our observation that despite ongoing efforts to improve Web-based interactive databases, residents still find themselves searching for material they can review while preparing for the radiology board examinations and remain frustrated by the fact that only a few printed guidebooks are available, which are limited in both format and image quality. Perhaps their greatest source of frustration is the inability to easily locate groups of cases across all subspecialties of radiology that are organized and tailored for their immediate study needs. Imagine being able to immediately access groups of high-quality cases to arrange study sessions, quickly extract and master information, and prepare for theme-based radiology conferences. Our goal in creating the RadCases Series was to combine the popularity and portability of printed books with the adaptability, exceptional quality, and interactive features of an electronic case-based format.

The intent of the printed book is to encourage repeated priming in the use of critical information by providing a portable group of exceptional core cases that the resident can master. The best way to determine the format for these cases was to ask residents from around the country to weigh in. Overwhelmingly, the residents said that they would prefer a concise, point-by-point presentation of the Essential Facts of each case in an easy-to-read, bulleted format. This approach is easy on exhausted eyes and provides a quick review of Pearls and Pitfalls as information is absorbed during repeated study sessions. We worked hard to choose cases that could be presented well in this format, recognizing the limitations inherent in reproducing high-quality images in print. Unlike the authors of other case-based radiology review books, we removed the guesswork by providing clear annotations and descriptions for all images. In our opinion, there is nothing worse than being unable to locate a subtle finding on a poorly reproduced image even after one knows the final diagnosis.

The electronic cases expand on the printed book and provide a comprehensive review of the entire subspecialty. Thousands of cases are strategically designed to increase the resident's knowledge by providing exposure to additional case examples—from basic to advanced—and by exploring "Aunt Minnie's," unusual diagnoses, and variability within a single diagnosis. The search engine gives the resident a fighting chance to find the Holy Grail by creating individualized, daily study lists that are not limited by factors such as a radiology subsection. For example, tailor today's study list to cases involving tuberculosis and include cases in every subspecialty and every system of the body. Or study only thoracic cases, including those with links to cardiology, nuclear medicine, and pediatrics. Or study only musculoskeletal cases. The choice is yours.

As enthusiastic partners in this project, we started small and, with the encouragement, talent, and guidance of Tim Hiscock at Thieme, continued to raise the bar in our effort to assist residents in tackling the daunting task of assimilating massive amounts of information. We are passionate about continuing this journey, hoping to expand the cases in our electronic series, adapt cases based on direct feedback from residents, and increase the features intended for board review and self-assessment. As the American Board of Radiology converts its certifying examinations to an electronic format, our series will be the one best suited to meet the needs of the next generation of overworked and exhausted residents in radiology.

Jonathan Lorenz, MD
Hector Ferral, MD
Chicago, IL

Preface

Excepting the authors' families, we do not think anybody reads prefaces any more. Whereas the obvious choice is simply to not put forth a preface, we wish to share why we chose to answer the question "Is there space on my shelf for yet another radiology book?" with a resounding, "Oh yes, please!"

"Unclear medicine" no more, this is not your grandfather's nuclear medicine. Written for the time-starved and information-hungry among us, this compendium (with both paper and electronic iterations) parses critical bits and bytes of scintillating facts and trivia to easily digestible nuggets. In an age of true detail hyperload, only those items absolutely relevant to clinical patient management and compliant with updated society-specific guidelines have been culled over years of nuclear medicine practice in the authors' disparate settings—university and community, hospital and outclinic, urgent and elective, critical and mundane. We have incorporated unique features that are rather hard to find elsewhere, such as discussing key Nuclear Regulatory Commission policy and procedure issues. We have debuted an easy flow chart to help you instantly decipher which wily unknown whole-body scan has come your way. The electronic format permits cinematic display to simulate everyday interpretation and will improve your skills of rapid recognition and response.

Collectively, we have persisted in combining systematic analysis, factual and experiential expertise, and typical illustrative examples to highlight the gamut of clinical scenarios that you, dear reader, would face. It might be on that one day of your qualifying examination. It might be just another day in your busy clinical practice of clinical nuclear medicine.

We simply want to make nuclear medicine a little less mysterious and a lot more lucid by organizing our thoughts for you with our best wishes. However, we are in astonishment that you have read this entire preface to the bitter end!

Acknowledgments

There are many, many individuals to whom I owe a profound debt of gratitude, for without them, this volume would not exist, at least not with my authorship. While most are still with us, a few unfortunately are not, and I would have liked to thank them personally one last time.

To start, thank you to my first nuclear medicine attendings at the University of Chicago, Richard Reba, Malcolm Cooper, and James Ryan for helping me discover, amidst all the other facets of a radiology residency clamoring for attention, the powerful wonders and rewards of nuclear molecular imaging. And many thanks to all those amazing nuclear physicians I had the subsequent honor of learning from at Mallinckrodt—brilliantly colorful characters all—Barry Siegel, Farrokh Dehdashti, Henry Royal, Rob Gropler, Keith Fisher, Jerry Wallis, Mark Mintun, and Tom Miller, who created the strong foundation during my fellowship from which all my subsequent knowledge and understanding in the field has arisen. A particular thanks tinged with sadness for Tom Miller whose guidance and friendship were so important to me, up to the very end.

Acknowledgement is also owed my current nuclear medicine colleagues at the University of Chicago, Yonglin Pu, Bill O'Brien-Penney, and Chris Straus, whose perpetual and tireless assistance and collaboration is so critical to my career and the continued success of our section and department. In addition, I owe not a small amount of gratitude to my recent department chairs, Richard Baron and David Paushter, under whose strong and yet caring leadership I am but one of many to flourish. And of course thank you to all my insightful, delightful University of Chicago residents, past, present and future, who keep me honest (and always on the lookout for great cases).

While the cases contained herein come from far and wide, the majority hail from the University of Chicago Medical Center. And so I would be remiss if I did not acknowledge those that actually created these superb images—Javid Ali, Lindy Arend, Alan Balinao, Julie Adamson-Bell, Jesse Castaneda, Jason Daniel, Anthony Defily, Lashonda Gardner, Merlin James, Alberto Jimenez, Grover Lamb, and James Philips. A finer group of technologists, nuclear or otherwise, you will not find, as the extremely high-quality scintigrams found within these pages will attest.

A much deserved thank you to Thieme executive editor Tim Hiscock as well as Katy Whipple for their tireless and talented efforts on our behalf. Their forbearance for deadlines made and missed was matched only by their tolerance for my idiosyncrasies. I would also like to thank and acknowledge Jonathan Lorenz for graciously including me in his inspired RadCases series.

And finally, a special thanks to my parents, Barbara and David Appelbaum, who have taught me the value of hard work and curiosity, shown me limitless love and affection, all while keeping me on the straight and narrow, or very close to it.

–Daniel Appelbaum

To Daniel Appelbaum for graciously including me in his projects, to George Segall for his exemplary and continuous mentorship, to certified nuclear medicine technologists everywhere whose tireless work and attention to detail make me seem clever and, most of all, to my requesting physicians and their patients who are instrumental in keeping me enthusiastic yet humble, I thank you now and forever.

–Sundeep Nayak

Abbreviations and Trade Name Information

AIDS	acquired immune deficiency syndrome
CT	computed tomography
CTA	computed tomographic angiography
DMSA	dimercaptosuccinic acid
DOPA	dihydroxyphenylalanine
DTPA	diethylene triamine pentaacetic acid
ECD	ethyl cysteinate dimer
ERCP	endoscopic retrograde cholangiopancreatography
FDG	fluorodeoxyglucose
HDP	hydroxymethane diphosphonate
HIDA	hepatobiliary iminodiacetic acid
HMPAO	hexamethylpropyleneamine oxime
MAA	macro aggregated albumin
MAG3	mercaptoacetyltriglycine
MDP	methylene diphosphonate
MIBG	metaiodobenzylguanidine
MIBI	sestamibi
MIP	maximum intensity projection
MRA	magnetic resonance angiography
MRCP	magnetic resonance cholangiopancreatography
MRI	magnetic resonance imaging
MUGA	multi gated acquisition
PET	positron emission tomography
PIOPED	prospective investigation of pulmonary embolism diagnosis
RBC	red blood cell
SCOL	sulfur colloid
SPECT	single photon emission computed tomography
SUV	standardized uptake value
SUV_{max}	maximum standardized uptake value
Tc99m	technetium 99m
TETRO	tetrofosmin
US	ultrasound
WBC	white blood cell

Bexxar (tositumomab I131), GlaxoSmithKline, Research Triangle Park, NC
Ceretec (Tc99m exametazime, formerly known as HMPAO), GE Healthcare, Waukesha, WI
Cardiolite (Tc99m sestamibi), Bristol-Myers Squibb, Princeton, NJ
DaTSCAN (ioflupane I123 injection), GE Healthcare, Princeton, NJ
Metastron (strontium 89 chloride), GE Healthcare, Princeton, NJ
Myoview (Tc99m tetrofosmin), GE Healthcare, Waukesha, WI
Neurolite (Tc99m bicisate, formerly known as ECD), Bristol-Myers Squibb Medical Imaging, N. Billerica, MA
OctreoScan (In111 pentetreotide), Mallinckrodt Inc., St Louis, MO
ProstaScint (In111 capromab pendetide), EUSA Pharma, Langhorne, PA
Quadramet (samarium 153 lexidronam), EUSA Pharma, Langhorne, PA
Thyrogen (thyrotropin alfa), Genzyme, Cambridge, MA
UltraTag kit, Mallinckrodt, Inc. St. Louis, MO
Zevalin (ibritumomab Y90), Spectrum Pharmaceuticals, Irvine, CA

Case 1

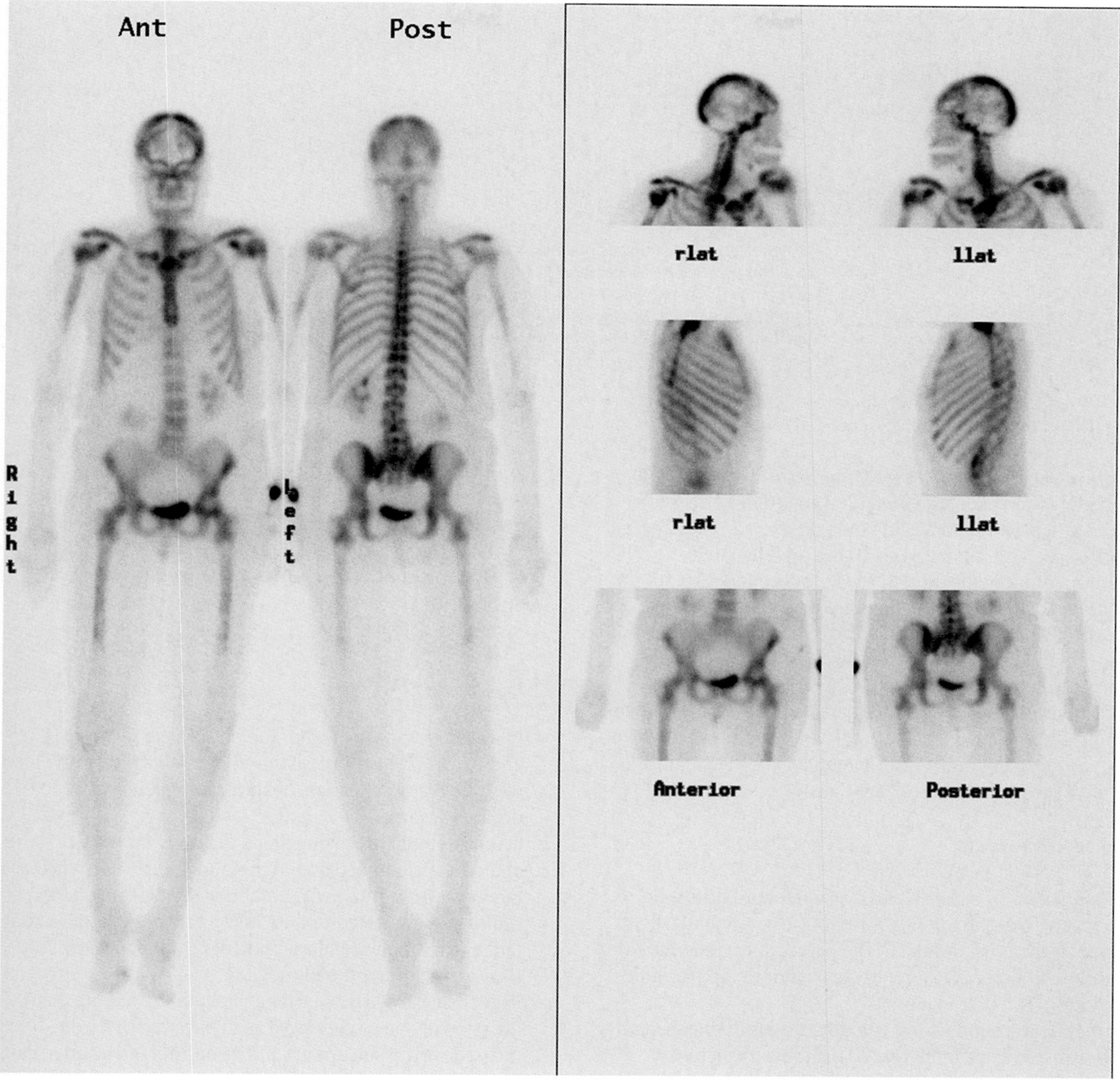

Clinical Presentation

A woman with a history of breast cancer presents for re-evaluation of disease status.

Imaging Findings

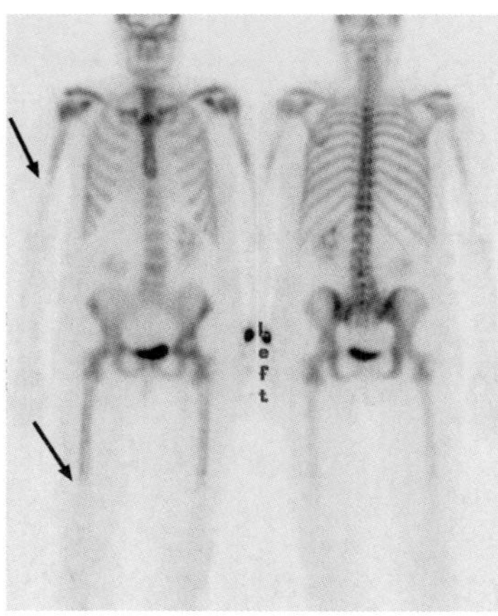

Tc99m HDP bone scintigraphy demonstrates uniformly increased radiotracer throughout the entire axial and proximal appendicular skeleton, with a sharp cutoff in uptake distal to the mid humeri and femora symmetrically (*arrows*). There is also an increase in the ratio of uptake in the visualized skeleton to uptake in the soft tissues, including the kidneys. Subtly decreased right breast uptake suggests a prior mastectomy. Note that the right kidney is located slightly more inferiorly in this patient than is typical.

Differential Diagnosis

- ***Diffuse skeletal metastases ("metastatic superscan"):*** Diffusely increased osseous uptake involving the entire axial and proximal appendicular skeleton and decreased soft-tissue and renal uptake make this the correct, pathognomonic diagnosis.
- *Metabolic bone disease ("metabolic superscan"):* This would also have decreased soft-tissue/renal activity, but the skeletal uptake would be increased throughout the *entire* skeleton (head to toe).
- *Multifocal Paget disease:* This can also be so extensive as to have relatively decreased soft-tissue activity. However, there would be multifocal skeletal lesions, each with typical pagetoid features (see Case 17).

Essential Facts

- "Superscan" on bone scintigraphy refers to diffusely increased skeletal uptake of radiotracer, particularly in comparison with uptake in the soft tissues, including the kidneys, which may show decreased or no appreciable uptake.
- In metastatic superscans, the diffuse, confluent skeletal metastases result in increased osteoblastic activity throughout the involved skeleton. The axial and proximal appendicular skeleton is exclusively affected because typical skeletal metastases localize initially to the hematopoietic (red) marrow. Red marrow is rarely found distal to the mid humeri or femora in a normal adult.
- A metastatic superscan appearance is most commonly seen in prostate cancer in men and breast cancer in women.
- Patients may present with clinical worsening of symptoms and elevated tumor markers.

Other Imaging Findings

- Plain radiographs may be unremarkable, or they may demonstrate multiple sclerotic lesions or diffusely increased density.
- CT can show relatively unremarkable bones or diffuse, multifocal lesions.
- FDG-PET can show diffusely increased uptake in the same red marrow distribution for FDG-avid metastatic disease like breast cancer. The tumor foci themselves are visualized (as opposed to the skeletal remodeling from an adjacent lesion as visualized on bone scintigraphy).

✓ Pearls & × Pitfalls

✓ In a metastatic superscan, the entire visualized axial and proximal appendicular skeleton is diffusely involved with metastatic disease, despite the absence of a focal discrete lesion.

✓ Unlike a metastatic superscan, diffusely increased osteoblastic activity due to metabolic disorders such as hyperparathyroidism (a metabolic superscan) shows uniformly increased uptake in the entire skeleton—axial and entire appendicular—relative to uptake in the soft tissues, including the kidneys.

✓ Paget disease, with its other characteristic features, can occasionally be so extensive as to have relatively decreased soft-tissue uptake and be considered a superscan.

✓ More focal lesions can be superimposed on an otherwise uniform metastatic superscan appearance. This can indicate complication with pathologic fracture, superimposed degenerative joint disease, or more complexity to that particular lesion.

✓ A metastatic superscan in young children (e.g., with neuroblastoma) may involve the entire skeleton (head to toe), as red marrow is still present in their distal extremities.

× The metastatic superscan appearance with its characteristically increased uptake of the axial skeleton and cold, more distal appendicular skeleton should be confidently called even in the absence of a significantly appreciable decrease in soft-tissue/renal radiotracer uptake (unlike a metabolic superscan, which should be considered only with a decrease in soft tissues).

Case 2

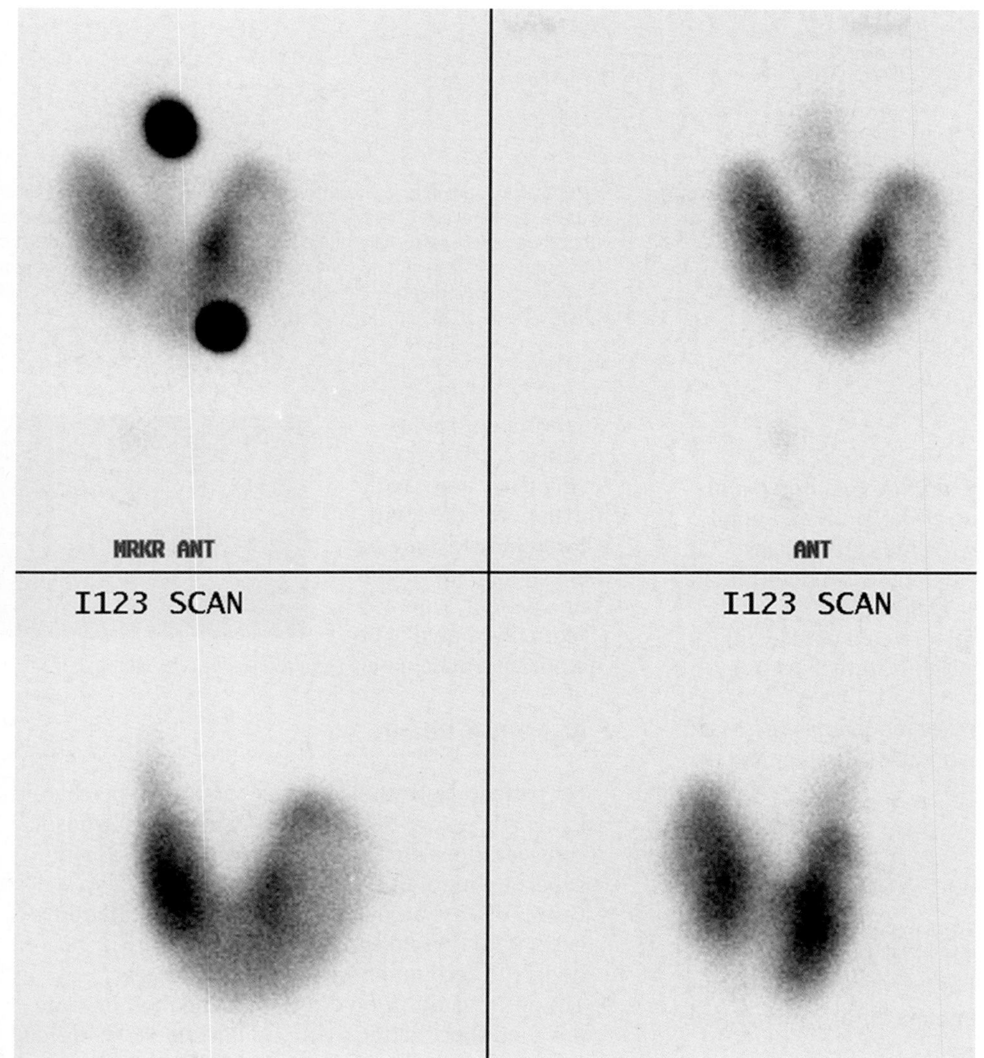

A

Uptake At 5 Hours

Uptake Time: 12/11/2006 15:12
Patient Background:
Patient Thyroid:
Patient Net Counts:

Current Capsule Counts:
Uptake = 59.9 %

Uptake At 24 Hours

Uptake Time: 12/12/2006 09:51
Patient Background:
Patient Thyroid:
Patient Net Counts:

Current Capsule Counts:
Uptake = 69.9 %

B

Clinical Presentation

A 28-year-old woman presents with weight loss and a palpable neck nodule on the left.

Imaging Findings

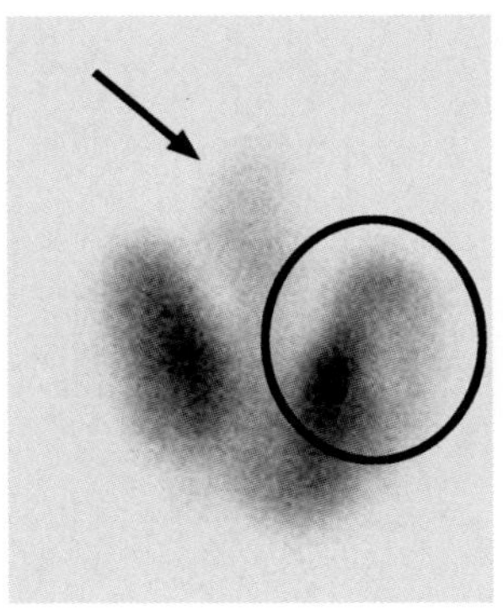

A

Uptake At 5 Hours
Uptake Time: 12/11/2006 15:12
Patient Background:
Patient Thyroid:
Patient Net Counts:

Current Capsule Counts:
Uptake = 59.9 %

Uptake At 24 Hours
Uptake Time: 12/12/2006 09:51
Patient Background:
Patient Thyroid:
Patient Net Counts:

Current Capsule Counts:
Uptake = 69.9 %

B

(A) Anterior and oblique views from an iodine 123 thyroid scan demonstrate a cold focus at the left mid-to-upper lobe (*circle*) with otherwise homogeneous uptake. A linear focus extending superiorly from the midline represents a pyramidal lobe (*arrow*). **(B)** Early and 24-hour thyroid radioactive iodine uptake (RAIU) values are significantly elevated (normal, 10–30% at 24 hours).

Differential Diagnosis

- ***Graves disease plus an indeterminate cold nodule:*** In the setting of hyperthyroidism, elevated thyroid uptake in a diffuse pattern almost always indicates Graves disease. The superimposed cold nodule is indeterminate and carries a 15 to 20% risk for malignancy.
- *Focal thyroiditis:* This can simulate a cold nodule on thyroid scan but will not have significantly increased thyroid uptake values.
- *Toxic nodular goiter:* This can have moderately increased thyroid uptake values, but the nodule(s) are hot and the rest of the gland is suppressed.

Essential Facts

- Graves disease is the most common cause of hyperthyroidism (75%) and is more commonly seen in women.
- Autoimmune antibodies bind to thyroid-stimulating hormone (TSH) receptors and stimulate diffuse autonomous thyroid hyperfunction.
- It typically presents with elevated triiodothyronine (T_3)/thyroxine (T_4) levels, suppressed TSH levels, clinical hyperthyroidism (e.g., weight loss, nervousness, heat intolerance, palpitations), a uniformly enlarged gland, and occasionally exophthalmos.
- Diagnosis is confirmed with diffuse, markedly elevated RAIU (often 60–80%), which distinguishes the condition from subacute thyroiditis.
- Temporary therapies include propylthiouracil (PTU) and methimazole (to block organification/thyroid hormone production) and β-blockers (to relieve symptoms). Radioiodine ablation provides definitive treatment. Surgery is an uncommon option.

Other Imaging Findings

- No imaging is useful in the diagnosis of Graves disease except for thyroid uptake and scanning, typically with I123. Tc99m pertechnetate is occasionally used, but uptake values are less well standardized.
- Superimposed cold nodules carry a risk for malignancy and can be further evaluated with US and biopsy. Shown here is the US from the same patient, who was eventually shown to be harboring a malignancy (as well as Graves disease):

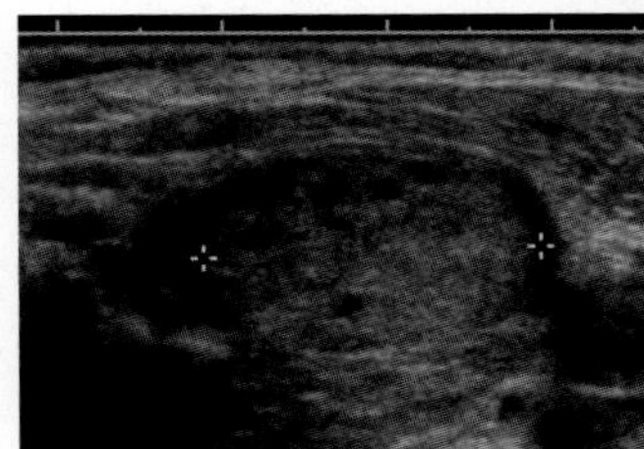

✓ Pearls & × Pitfalls

✓ For patients with clinical and laboratory hyperthyroidism (high T_4, low TSH), the most common diagnostic considerations are Graves disease (high RAIU) and subacute thyroiditis (very low RAIU: < 3%).

✓ Graves disease accounts for 70% of cases of thyrotoxicosis, with thyroiditis representing 20%. Toxic (hot) nodule(s) account for most of the remainder.

✓ The antiorganification drugs, PTU and methimazole, are good short-acting therapies but should be avoided long term to avoid significant side effects, including agranulocytosis.

✓ Doses for I131 therapy typically range from 6 to 30 mCi but can be customized based on gland weight in grams and the 24-hour RAIU. I131 dose = (weight × 100 μCi)/RAIU. Gland weight is estimated from palpation or image-based measurements (e.g., US).

✓ Most treated patients eventually become permanently hypothyroid, requiring levothyroxine months or decades after I131 ablation. Lifelong medical monitoring is therefore required.

✓ Occasionally, Hashimoto disease, which typically manifests as hypothyroidism, can be complicated by a transient Graves disease–like hyperthyroidism with elevated RAIU ("Hashitoxicosis"), which can be also be treated with I131 therapy.

✓ Visualization of the linear pyramidal lobe, an embryologic remnant, increases the likelihood the thyroid scan represents diffuse toxic goiter, *but elevated uptake values must be confirmed with the RAIU.*

Case 3

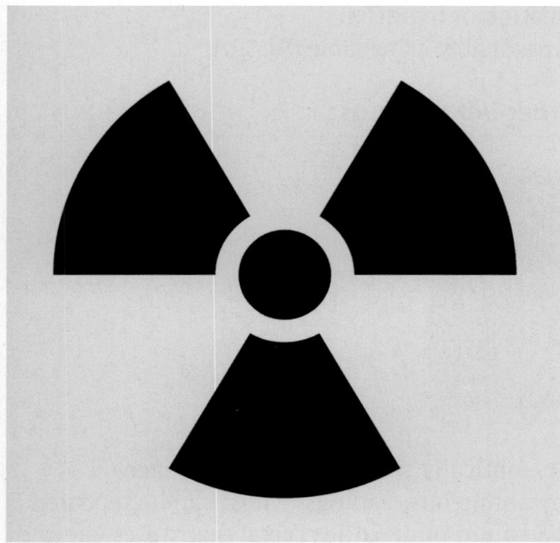

Clinical Presentation

A new part-time technologist arrives in June; he was previously employed as a nuclear medicine technologist at another hospital.

Further Work-up

His exposure report from the current year shows 2 rem (20 mSv) thus far. Is he allowed to begin working at your institution now?

Differential Diagnosis

- This technologist is permitted to work and must be monitored. The annual total effective dose limit for a radiation worker is 5 rem (50 mSv); therefore, he is allowed an additional 3 rem (30 mSv) for the remainder of the calendar year.

Essential Facts

- Even though working only part time, this technologist will require monitoring as is required for any adult likely to receive > 10% of the annual limits. The annual occupational dose limit for an adult radiation worker is 5 rem (50 mSv) total effective dose equivalent (TEDE).
- Organ-specific annual exposure limits also apply:
  - 50 rem (500 mSv) to any organ except the lens of the eye: deep dose equivalent (DDE) + committed dose equivalent (CDE)
  - 15 rem (150 mSv) to the lens of the eye: lens dose equivalent (LDE)
  - 50 rem (500 mSv) to the extremities: shallow dose equivalent (SDE)
- Regulations require that individuals be informed at least annually of their cumulative radiation exposure.
- The dose limit per year for members of the general public is < 0.1 rem (1 mSv) TEDE. Not counted or included are background radiation, medical administration, exposure from released patients, voluntary participation in medical research programs, and licensee's disposal of radioactive materials into the sewer.
- Dose limits are based on the concern for genetic damage from ionizing radiation resulting in increased cancer risk. The Nuclear Regulatory Commission uses a linear no-threshold model, which is considered conservative. This model describes a direct relationship between radiation dose and genetic damage.
- Monitoring is also required in the following cases:
  - Any minor likely to receive an annual external dose > 0.1 rem (1 mSv), a lens dose > 0.15 rem (1.5 mSv), or an extremity dose > 0.5 rem (5 mSv)
  - Any declared pregnant woman likely to receive > 0.1 rem (1 mSv) during the entire pregnancy
  - Any individual entering a high-radiation area (possible exposure of > 0.1 rem/h [1 mSv/h] at 30 cm)
- The occupational dose limit for minors (< 18 years of age) is 10% of adult doses.

Definitions

- TEDE: represents total risk from external and internal exposures (DDE + CEDE)
- DDE: external whole-body exposure at a tissue depth of 1.0 cm
- SDE: external exposure to the skin or extremity at a tissue depth of 0.007 cm
- LDE: external exposure to the lens of the eye at a tissue depth of 0.3 cm
- CDE: the dose equivalent to organs or tissues that will be received from an intake of radioactive material by an individual during the 50-year period following the intake
- Committed effective dose equivalent (CEDE): provides an estimate of the lifetime radiation dose to an individual from radioactive material taken into the body through either inhalation or ingestion
- As low as reasonably achievable (ALARA)

Other Imaging Findings

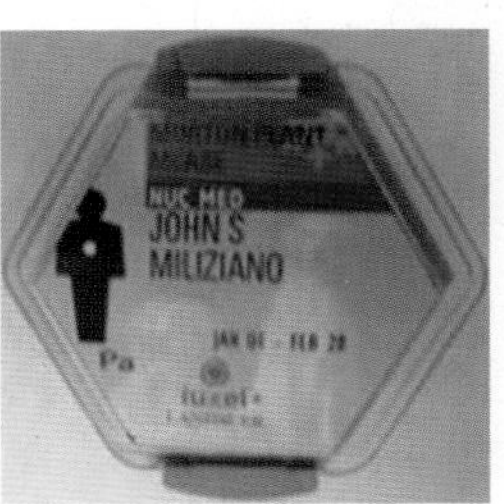

- Body badge—optically stimulated luminescence
  - Allows instantaneous readings, which can be repeated
  - Contains an aluminum oxide crystal that stores energy from ionizing radiation
  - A laser is used to stimulate the crystal and energy is released as blue light. Light intensity is directly related to exposure.

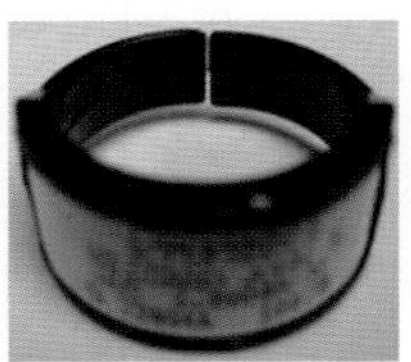

- Ring badge—thermoluminescent display
  - Can be read only once
  - Contains chemicals that retain energy from radiation exposure
  - When heated, energy is released in the form of light in proportion to exposure.

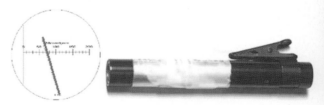

- Pocket ion chamber—real-time reading
  - Sealed cylindric chamber filled with air and a charged quartz fiber

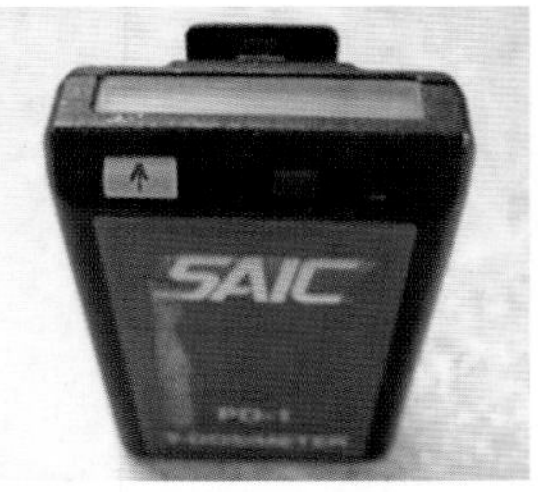

- Electronic dosimeter—real-time reading
  - Uses an energy-compensated Geiger-Müller tube or solid-state electronics

Case 4

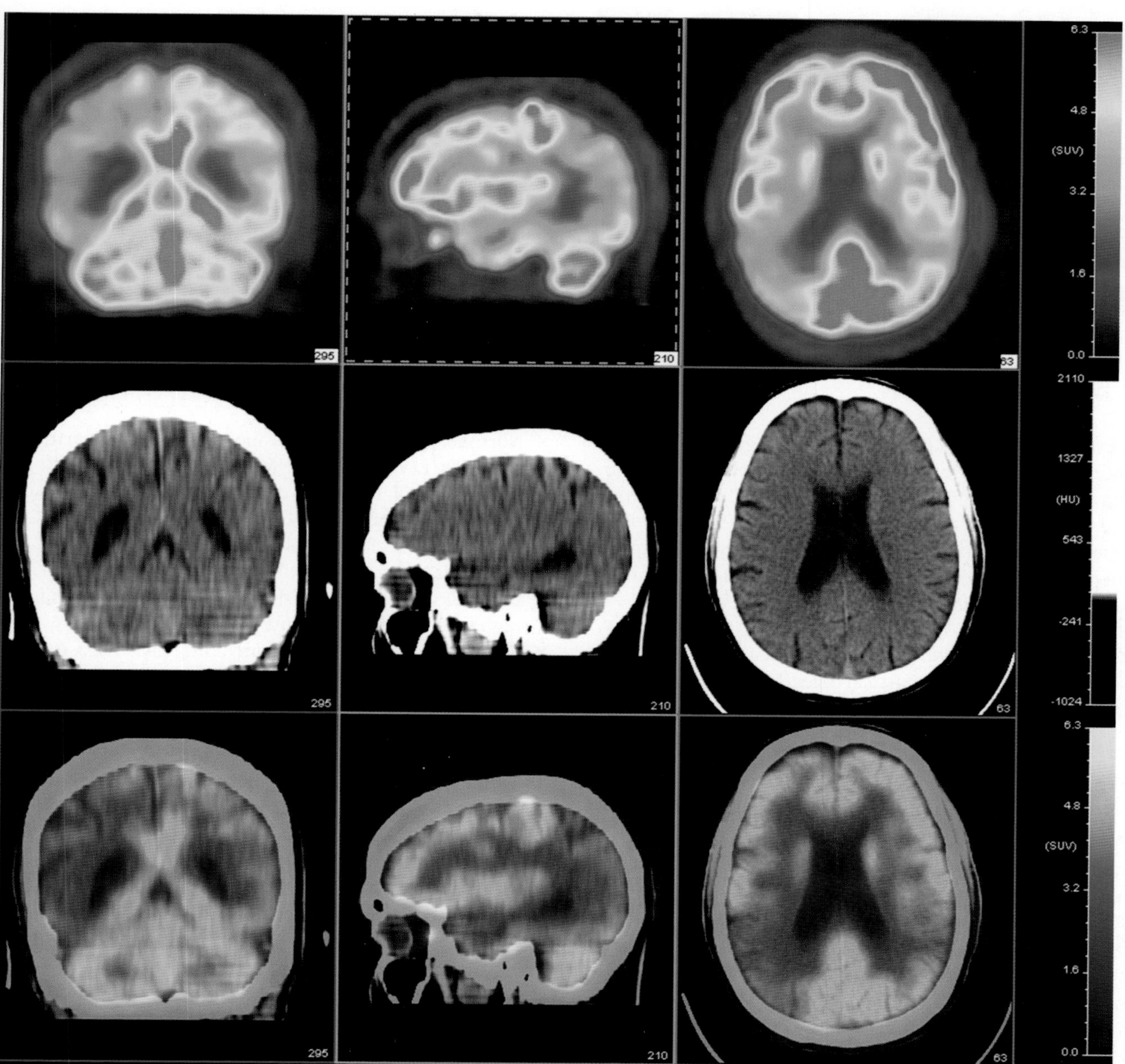

Clinical Presentation

A 63-year-old woman with memory loss.

Imaging Findings

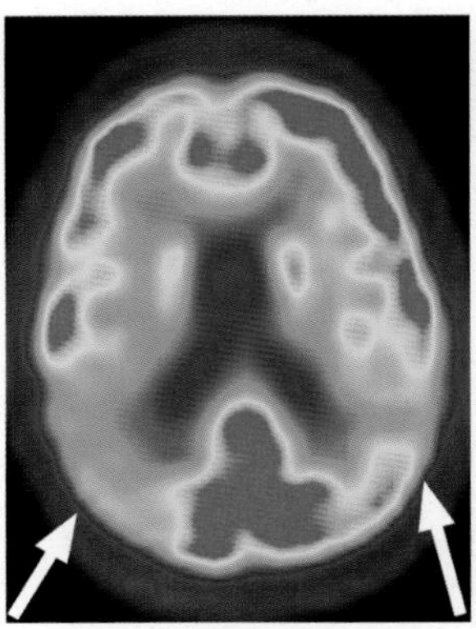

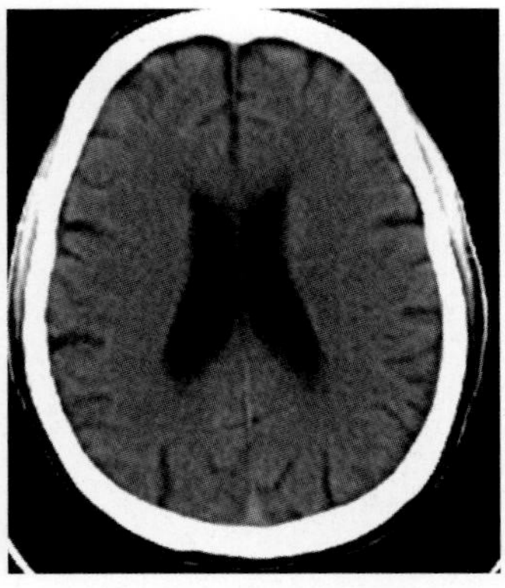

Selected axial, sagittal, and coronal images from an FDG-PET/CT of the brain demonstrate nearly symmetric, markedly decreased glucose metabolism of the posterior temporal and parietal lobes (*arrows*). CT shows mildly prominent ventricles for age, but findings are otherwise normal.

Differential Diagnosis

- ***Alzheimer dementia (AD):*** Nearly symmetric involvement of the posterior temporoparietal cortices with sparing of the occipital lobes, basal ganglia, and cerebellum is the typical appearance of this diagnosis, as shown here.
- *Lewy body dementia (DLB):* This is the second most common degenerative dementia after AD. It can look similar to AD but typically has more pronounced occipital involvement.
- *Multi-infarct dementia (MID):* MID appears as multiple scattered, asymmetric cortical defects that can also involve the basal ganglia.

Essential Facts

- AD is the most common dementia, estimated to affect more than half of the population older than 85 years of age and increasing in prevalence in younger patients.
- AD can present with memory loss, personality changes, and dysfunction of higher cortical activities.
- Pathology demonstrates amyloid plaques and fibrillary tangles.
- The rising prevalence of AD and the emergence of more effective drugs make the accurate and early detection of the disease increasingly important.

Other Imaging Findings

- CT and MRI can be useful to evaluate MID and exclude other intracranial pathologies but are otherwise insensitive in the diagnosis of neurodegenerative dementias. They may show nonspecific atrophy.
- Newer SPECT and PET agents in development, such as florbetapir, image the amyloid plaques directly and may be more accurate in diagnosing AD in the future.

✓ Pearls & × Pitfalls

✓ Normal FDG-PET brain metabolism and brain perfusion SPECT (with Tc99m HMPAO or ECD) examinations can look similar; normal cerebellar activity tends to be relatively higher in SPECT than in PET.

✓ Many nonvascular neurologic diseases, including dementias, will have similar abnormalities on metabolic FDG-PET and perfusion SPECT. PET tends to have a higher sensitivity for many.

✓ Frontotemporal dementias, including Pick disease, typically have anterior frontal and temporal hypoperfusion/hypometabolism, and they tend to spare the occipital regions.

✓ DLB can be associated with dementia (like AD), Parkinsonian symptoms, or both. Scintigraphy of the dopaminergic system (e.g., ^{18}F-DOPA PET, DaTSCAN SPECT) can distinguish DLB from AD (decreased basal ganglia uptake in DLB).

✓ AIDS-associated dementia can look similar to MID, with scattered cortical, subcortical, and basal ganglia defects on PET or SPECT, but the patient history and a relatively normal MRI can be highly suggestive.

✓ Involvement of the posterior cingulate cortex is common in AD (in addition to temporoparietal involvement).

× AD may be asymmetric in the early stages and involve the frontal lobes in advanced disease (but generally still less than temporoparietal involvement).

Case 5

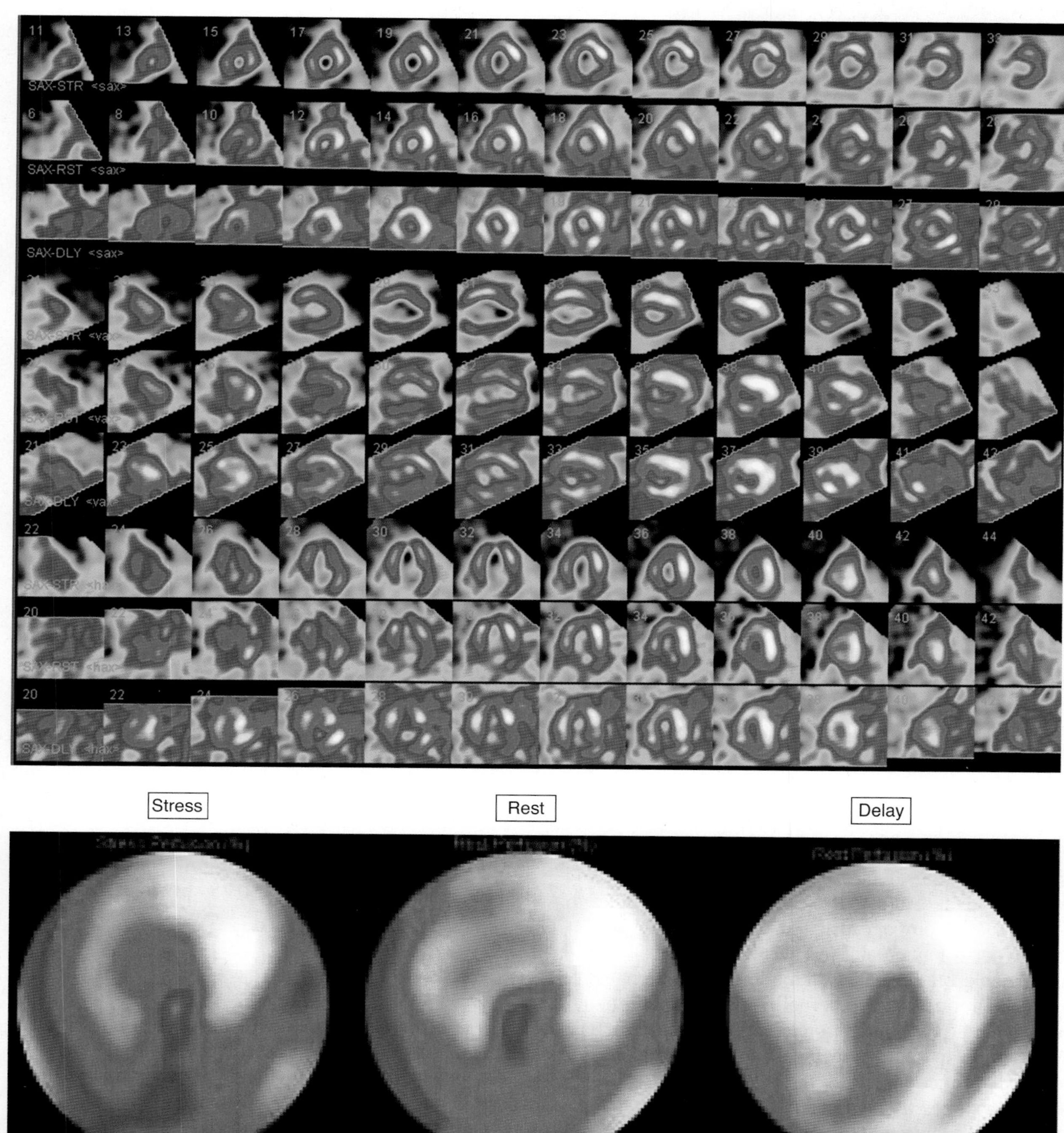

Clinical Presentation

A 48-year-old woman presents with shortness of breath and chest discomfort. The top two rows are standard stress and rest imaging obtained with Tc99m MIBI and thallium 201, respectively; the bottom row of each axis is 24-hour-delay imaging of the Tl201 energy window.

Imaging Findings

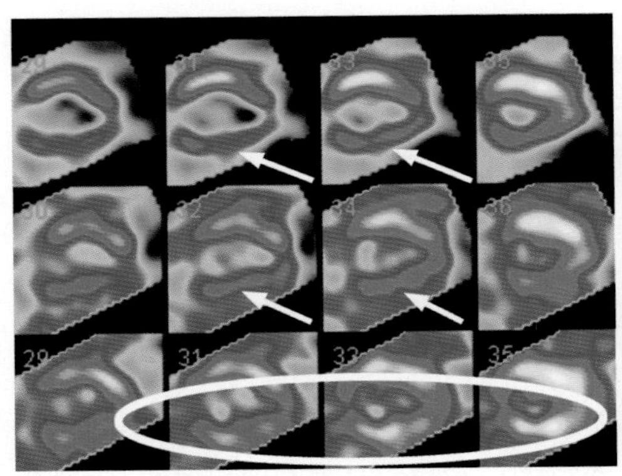

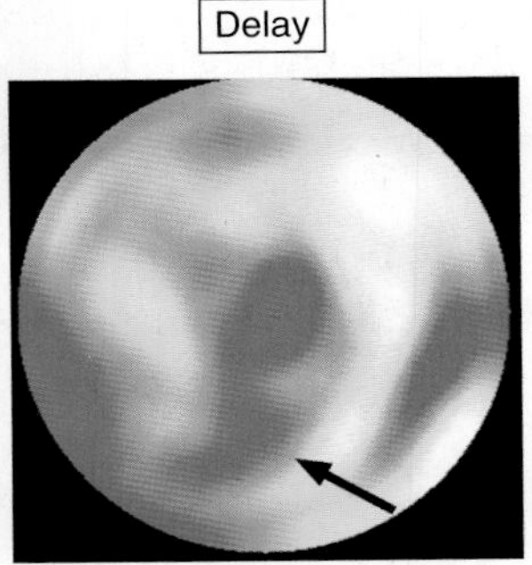

A B

(A) Standard initial stress and rest myocardial perfusion scintigraphy (top two rows) demonstrates a predominantly fixed (only slightly reversible) inferolateral perfusion defect (*arrows*). However, there is normalization of tracer on the delayed redistribution images (*circle*, third row). **(B)** These findings are confirmed on the polar maps (*arrow*).

Differential Diagnosis

- ***Hibernating myocardium:*** A defect at rest that resolves/redistributes on delayed thallium imaging indicates hibernating myocardium.
- *Myocardial infarction:* This will also have a resting perfusion defect but will not redistribute on delayed imaging.
- *Stress-induced reversible ischemia:* This will also have a perfusion defect on stress images but will normalize on the initial same-day resting images (no redistribution imaging required).

Essential Facts

- Hibernating myocardium (also known as resting ischemia) results when coronary perfusion is severely decreased even at rest (as opposed to being stress-induced), but not to the point of causing infarction.
- Enough perfusion remains (e.g., via collaterals) to keep the tissue viable, but regional wall motion dysfunction results.
- Unlike infarction (scar), hibernating tissue is potentially amenable to revascularization (stents or coronary artery bypass graft) to improve regional and resulting global left ventricular function.
- Following successful revascularization, perfusion imaging will normalize immediately, but a return of normal function may require several months.
- An initial resting perfusion defect (regardless of additional stress-induced ischemia) may represent infarct or hibernating tissue. Both typically have wall motion abnormalities on gated imaging but may be distinguished by redistribution imaging.
- Redistribution imaging on SPECT may be performed *only with thallium 201* (a potassium channel analogue), which redistributes to intact cell membranes (not to scar).
- MIBI/TETRO *cannot* be used for redistribution imaging (both are mitochondrial binding agents that do not redistribute).

Other Imaging Findings

- Cardiac FDG-PET will show significant metabolic activity in hibernating tissue and can be used to distinguish it from infarct. (Cardiac perfusion PET, such as with rubidium 82, will show a resting defect for both infarcted and hibernating tissue.)
- Dobutamine infusion will transiently improve the wall motion of hibernating tissue and so can be used in conjunction with echocardiography, MUGA scan, or gated SPECT to assess for functional improvement.
- Contrast cardiac MRI can also identify infarcted tissue.

✓ Pearls & × Pitfalls

✓ Infarct and hibernation will look identical on initial rest/stress SPECT. Delayed imaging (with thallium) is needed to distinguish. No reinjection of thallium is necessary.

✓ Delayed imaging can be performed up to 96 hours later because of the 3-day half-life of Tl201.

✓ Infarct and resting ischemia will both have a resting wall motion abnormality. Completely reversible stress-induced ischemia should have normal resting wall motion (unless there is stunning). Attenuation defects also have normal wall motion.

× Although both infarct and hibernating tissue will have a perfusion defect at rest, either can have superimposed stress-induced reversible ischemia (i.e., either can look worse at stress).

Case 6

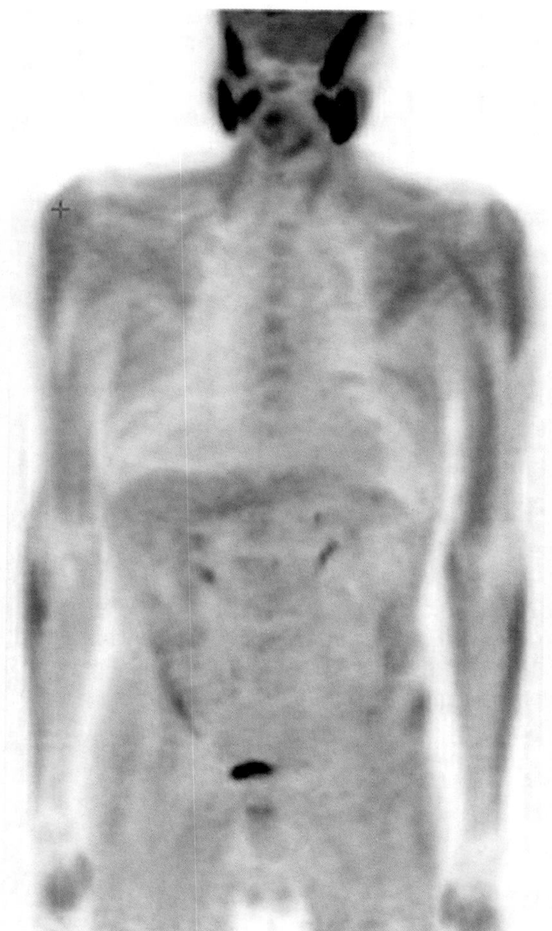

A

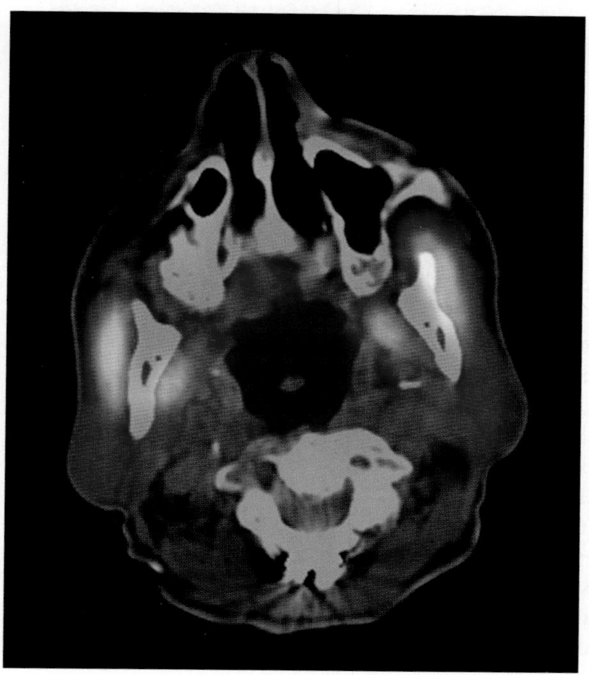

B

Clinical Presentation

An 80-year-old man with weight loss, back pain, and a history of prostate cancer.

Imaging Findings

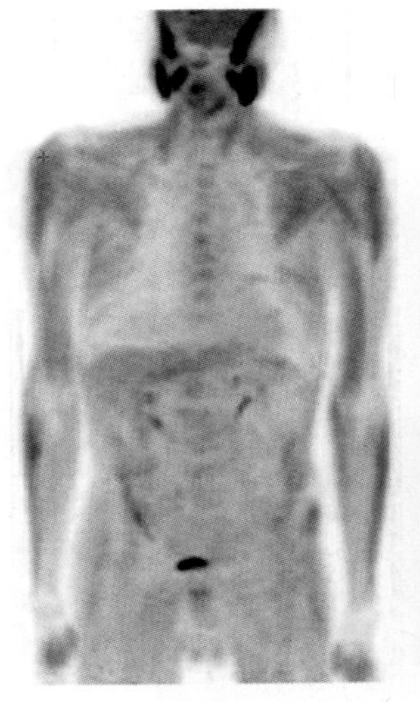

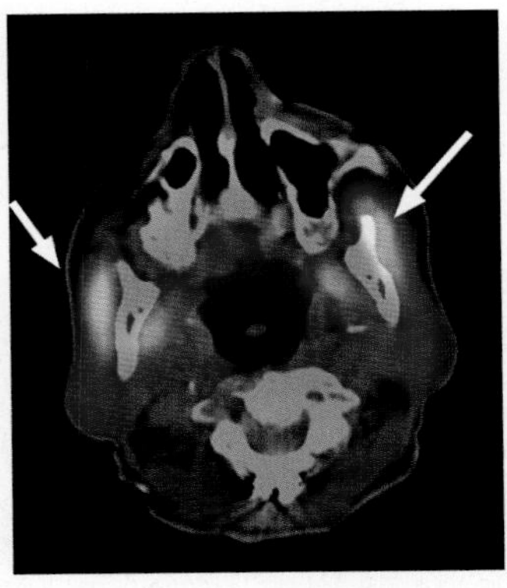

(A) MIP image from whole-body FDG-PET demonstrates a diffuse shift in moderate radiotracer uptake to skeletal musculature. **(B)** Fused PET-CT axial slice from the same patient demonstrates marked uptake in the muscles of mastication (*arrows*).

Differential Diagnosis

- ***Altered biodistribution from hyperinsulinemia:*** Diffusely increased activity throughout the skeletal musculature makes this the most likely diagnosis.
- *Brown fat hypermetabolism:* This can also cause symmetric linear uptake near muscles, but the activity localizes to fat—typically only in the neck, shoulders, mediastinum, and/or spine, not the extremities (see Case 58).
- *Myositis/recent exercise:* This will also show increased linear muscle uptake but not involve all muscle groups diffusely. The uptake in this patient's mastication muscles is from exercise (chewing).

Essential Facts

- FDG is a glucose analogue, and its biodistribution is mediated by insulin.
- Elevated *insulin* levels from a recent meal (even if measured serum *glucose* is low) or a recent insulin injection will drive FDG into skeletal muscle and decrease tumor uptake.
- Elevated *glucose* levels above 150 to 200 mg/dL (even with low or normal endogenous insulin levels) can compete with FDG and also cause decreased tumor uptake via competitive inhibition, although with generally less muscle uptake than in hyperinsulinemia.

Other Imaging Findings

- CT from the PET-CT can confirm muscle as the location of increased uptake, although this is rarely necessary as the FDG-PET pattern is usually pathognomonic.

✓ Pearls & × Pitfalls

✓ Patient preparation is critical to ensure the normal background biodistribution necessary to achieve high-quality FDG-PET images. For comparison, here is a normal biodistribution of FDG-PET in a different patient:

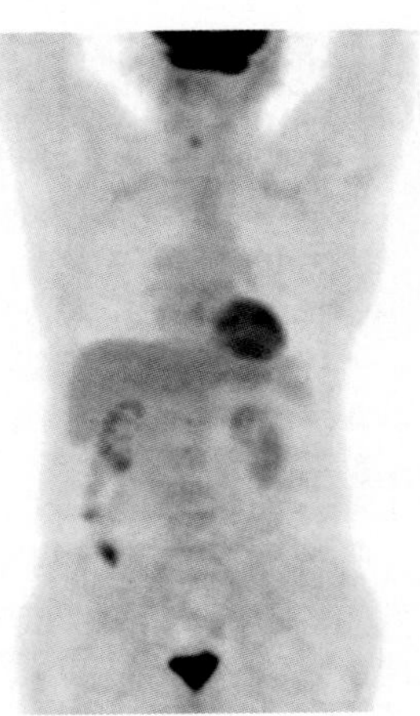

✓ Patients should fast for at least 4 to 6 hours before FDG injection.

✓ Some centers recommend a low-carbohydrate diet for 24 hours before the FDG-PET to further decrease insulin levels and decrease cardiac uptake (which will shift to fatty acid metabolism).

✓ Diabetic patients should have no recent short-acting insulin injection (within 2–4 hours).

× Patients should perform no strenuous exercise shortly before the PET and lie calmly and quietly (to decrease laryngeal uptake) during the uptake phase following FDG injection; in this patient, all muscles of mastication have intense uptake—another clue to a recent meal, possibly consumed right *after* FDG injection.

× Poor patient preparation can significantly alter SUV calculations, rendering them inaccurate.

Case 7

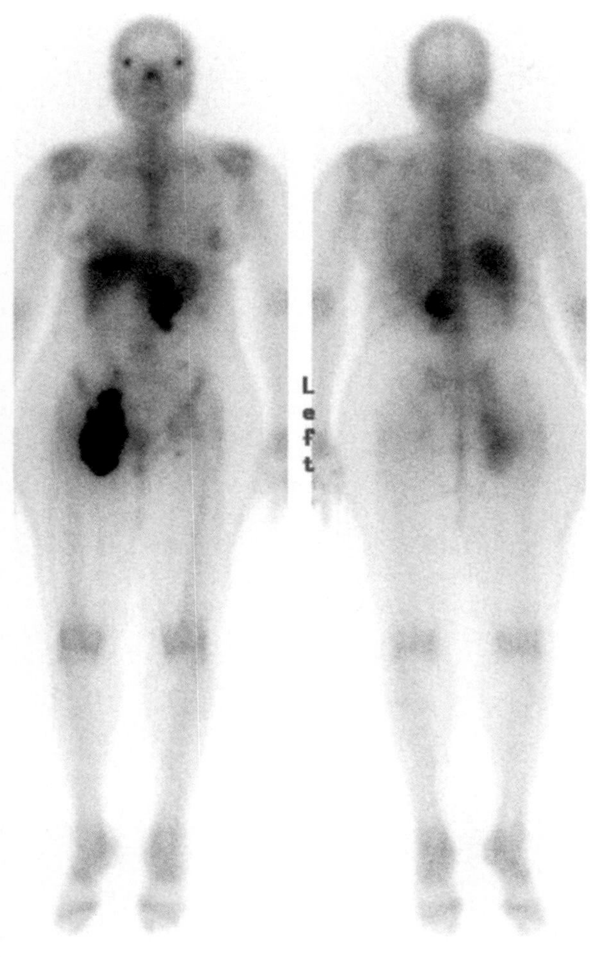

Clinical Presentation

A 33-year-old woman with a history of malignancy presents for restaging.

Further Work-up

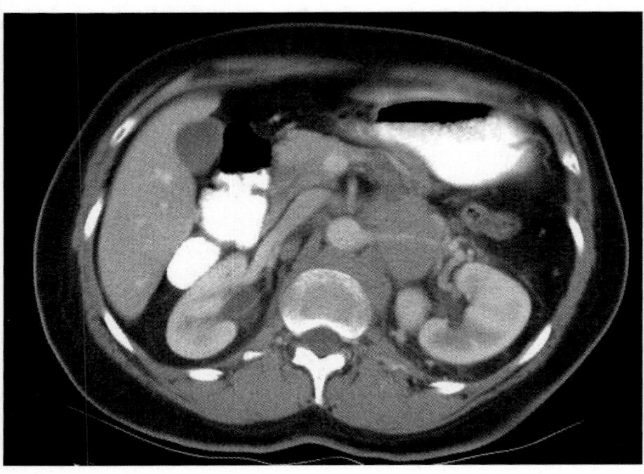

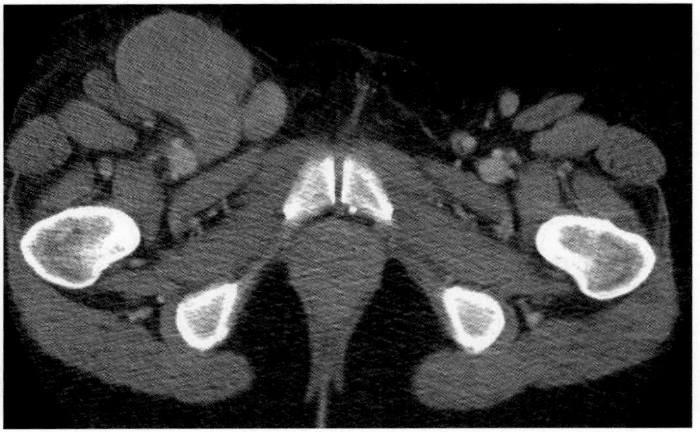

c

Imaging Findings

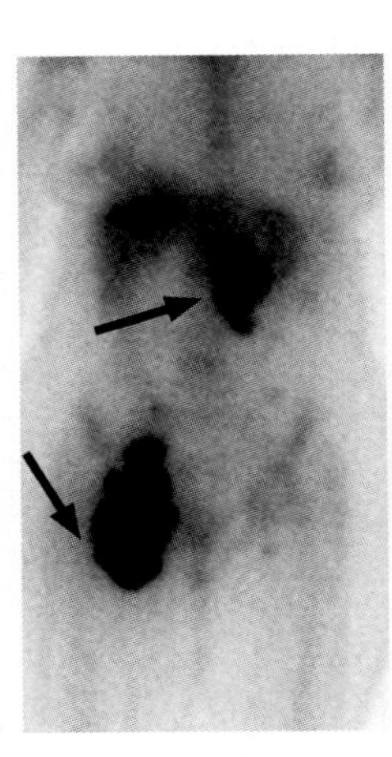

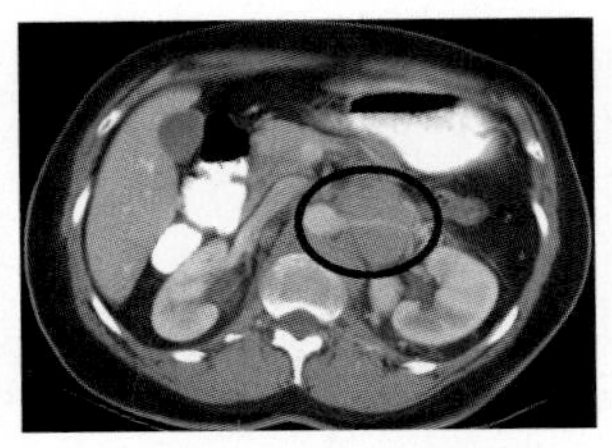

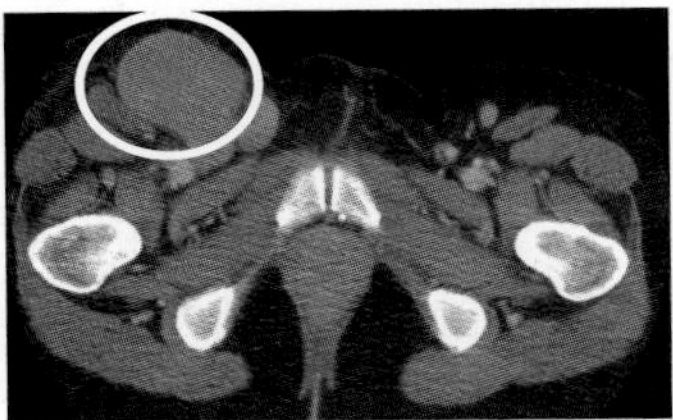

(A) Anterior and posterior whole-body views from a whole-body scan demonstrate abnormal uptake in the right anterior pelvis and left mid abdomen (*arrows*). Physiologic lacrimal, hepatic, splenic, osseous, and bowel activity is seen. **(B,C)** Contrast-enhanced CT axial images demonstrate soft-tissue masses encasing the left renal artery and in the right inguinal region (*circles*).

Differential Diagnosis

- ***Gallium scan showing lymphoma:*** The presence of physiologic liver, spleen, colon, bone, and lacrimal gland uptake makes Ga67 the most likely scan; lymphoma is a common gallium-avid tumor, with masses demonstrated on the accompanying CT.
- *Gallium scan showing sarcoid:* Sarcoid is commonly gallium-avid, although the distribution and size of the soft-tissue masses would be atypical.
- *WBC scan showing areas of active infection:* This can also show liver, spleen, and bone marrow with normal uptake, but splenic uptake tends to be > liver uptake, and there would be no lacrimal uptake. Normal colonic uptake may be seen only if the WBCs are labeled with Tc99m (not with indium 111).

Essential Facts

- Ga67 is a nonspecific neoplasm and infection/inflammation imaging agent.
- Ga67 is an iron analogue with uptake mediated by transferrin receptors.
- Gallium-avid tumors include Hodgkin disease (HD), non-Hodgkin lymphoma (NHL), melanoma, sarcoma, hepatoma, and lung tumor.
- The most common use of Ga67 has been for HD and NHL staging and for assessing response to therapy (scar vs. residual tumor) with planar and SPECT imaging.
- Gallium is also used to assess for sarcoid, pulmonary infections (including *Pneumocystis carinii/jiroveci* pneumonia), fever of unknown origin, and diskitis/spinal osteomyelitis.

Other Imaging Findings

- For lymphoma, CT is typically used in conjunction with scintigraphy to identify and localize enlarged lymph nodes, soft-tissue masses, and other abnormalities, such as splenic lesions or enlargement.
- FDG-PET has replaced gallium for evaluating most tumors, including lymphoma. PET may also replace gallium for inflammation/infection imaging in the near future.
- MRI is uncommonly used for lymphoma, except to occasionally evaluate for central nervous system or skeletal involvement.

✓ Pearls & ✗ Pitfalls

- ✓ If liver, spleen, and bone marrow uptake is present on an unknown whole-body scan, consider gallium or WBC; if lacrimal uptake is present, it must be gallium (see "Interpreting Whole-Body Scans").
- ✓ If normal growth plates are hot, an unknown study may be a bone or gallium scan (gallium is also a "poor man's bone scan" and will show bone cortical, not just marrow, elements); then if liver, spleen, and colon are apparent, scan = gallium, as in this case from a child:
- ✓ Any osseous focus that is hot on a bone scan can be hot on a gallium scan, even chronic degenerative changes or fractures.
- ✗ Kaposi sarcoma is *not* gallium-avid, although other sarcomas generally are.
- ✗ Although there is significant overlap between labeled WBCs and gallium for infection imaging, spinal osteomyelitis/diskitis and pulmonary inflammation are often better seen on gallium; abdominal processes are often better seen on WBC imaging.

Case 8

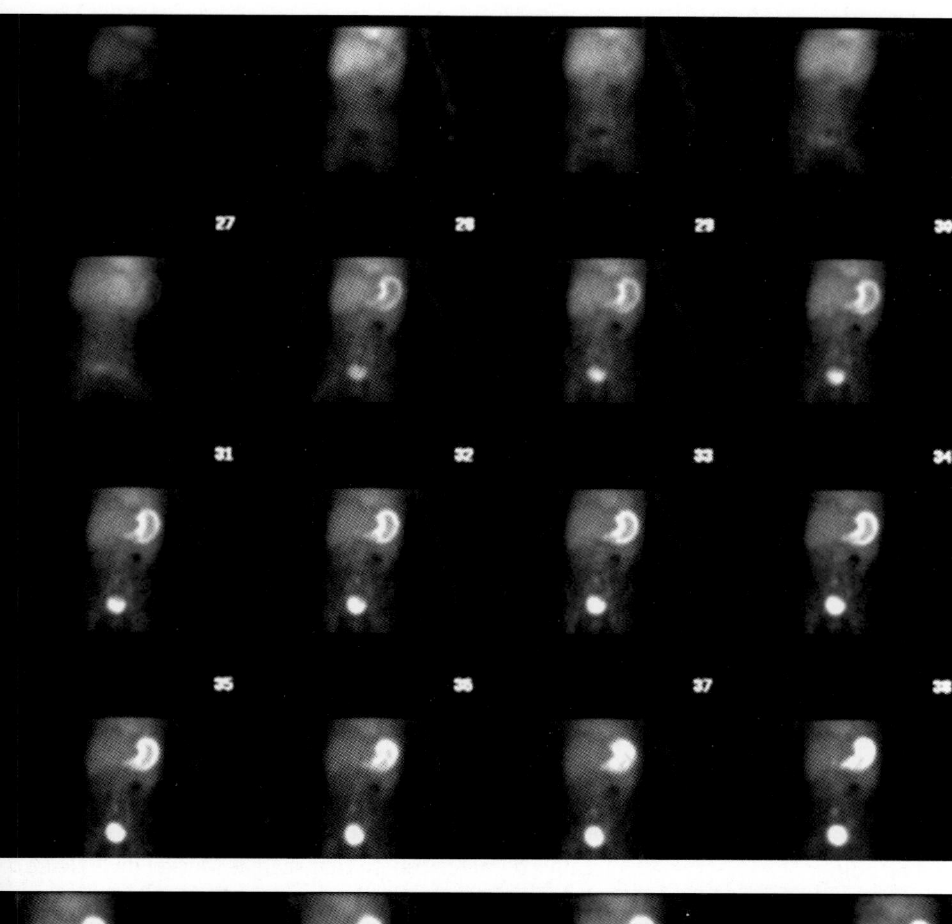

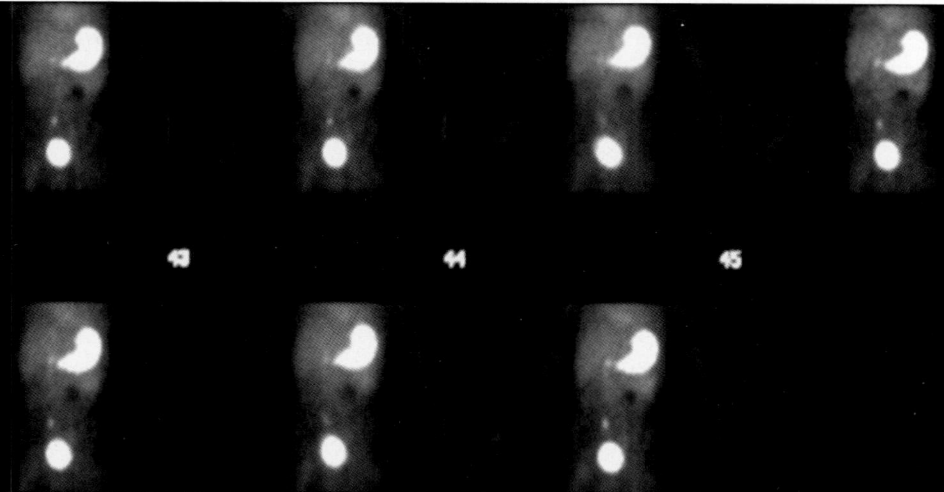

One minute/frame

Clinical Presentation

An 18-month-old boy with painless rectal bleeding.

Imaging Findings

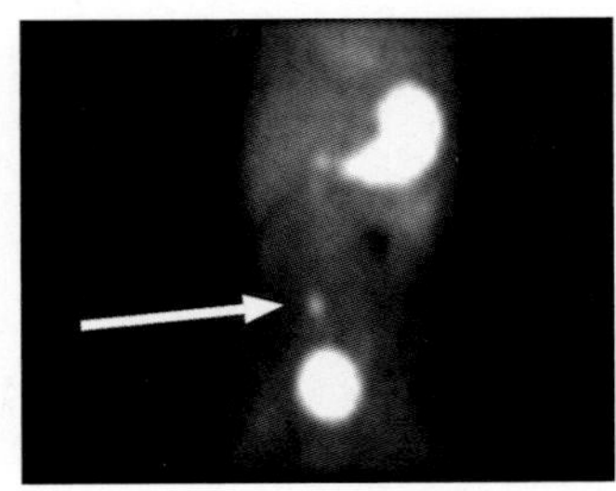

Sequential imaging immediately following intravenous administration of Tc99m pertechnetate ("Meckel scan") demonstrates an abnormal and persistent focus in the right lower quadrant (RLQ), which begins to appear at the same time as normal mucosal activity in the stomach (*arrow*).

Differential Diagnosis

- ***Ectopic gastric mucosa in a Meckel diverticulum:*** A persistent focus in the RLQ whose uptake follows that of the mucosa in the stomach is the most likely etiology, given the history.
- *Ectopic gastric mucosa in a duplication cyst:* A known potential false-positive, this is less likely, given the typical location of a Meckel diverticulum in the RLQ and the history.
- *Ectopic renal pelvis:* Another potential false-positive, this is less likely because the timing of tracer uptake in this lesion follows the stomach, not the urinary system.

Essential Facts

- A Meckel diverticulum is an embryologic remnant of the omphalomesenteric duct
- The vast majority remain asymptomatic; the most common presentation is painless rectal bleeding.
- Follows "rule of 2s":
  - Found in 2% of the population
  - Presents around 2 years of age
  - Is twice as common in males
  - Is 2 inches in size, 2 feet from the ileocecal valve
  - Only 20% contain gastric mucosa.
- Only those that contain gastric mucosa will be seen on a Meckel scan, and only those will typically bleed.
- Other manifestations of a Meckel diverticulum (which may or may not contain gastric mucosa) include pain, perforation, and intussusception/obstruction.
- Treatment is surgery.

Other Imaging Findings

- Small-bowel enteroclysis can be attempted to visualize the diverticulum; standard small-bowel follow-through is less likely to opacify it. Angiography can visualize only an active, rapidly bleeding lesion.

✓ Pearls & × Pitfalls

✓ Premedication has equivocal value with a Meckel scan but can include pentagastrin (increases gastric mucosal tracer uptake), cimetidine (decreases mucosal secretion), and glucagon (decreases bowel motion).

✓ Look for a focus that appears at the same time and increases as mucosa in the stomach.

✓ Postvoid and spot lateral views can increase accuracy: Meckel diverticula are anterior to the urinary collecting system, such as on this lateral view (*arrow*):

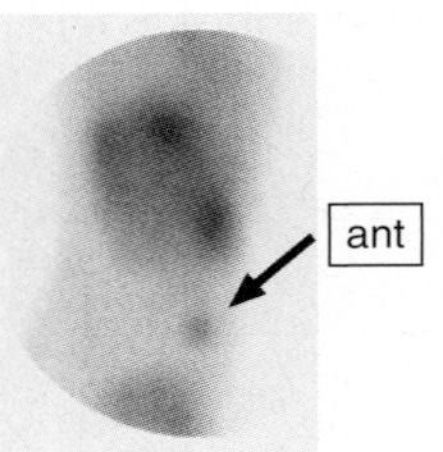

✓ Meckel diverticula do not have to be actively bleeding to be visualized on a Meckel scan (need only to contain gastric mucosa); actively bleeding lesions can also be visualized on a labeled RBC scan (but cannot be specifically characterized on that scan as Meckel diverticula).

× False-positives include other foci of ectopic gastric mucosa (e.g., duplication cysts), intussusception with obstruction, urinary activity in congenital renal anomalies (e.g., ectopic kidney), bowel inflammation (e.g., irritable bowel disease), and vascular anomalies (e.g., arterial aneurysms).

× Another common false-positive can be created from antegrade passage of tracer secreted by the stomach, as in this case from another patient showing a true Meckel diverticulum in the RLQ (*thin arrow*) plus antegrade passage of physiologic gastric secretion of tracer in the small bowel in the LUQ (*thick arrow*):

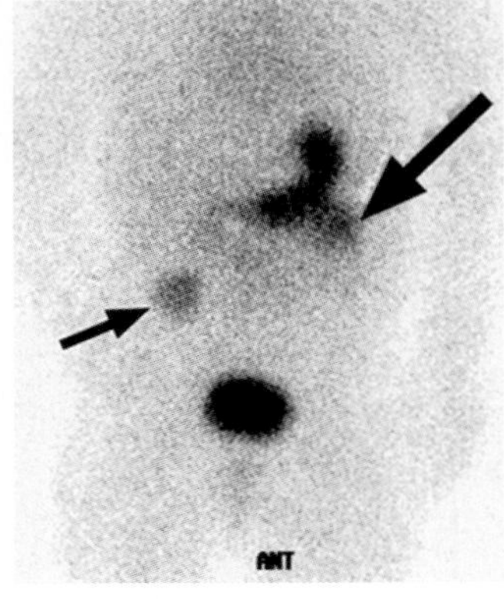

Case 9

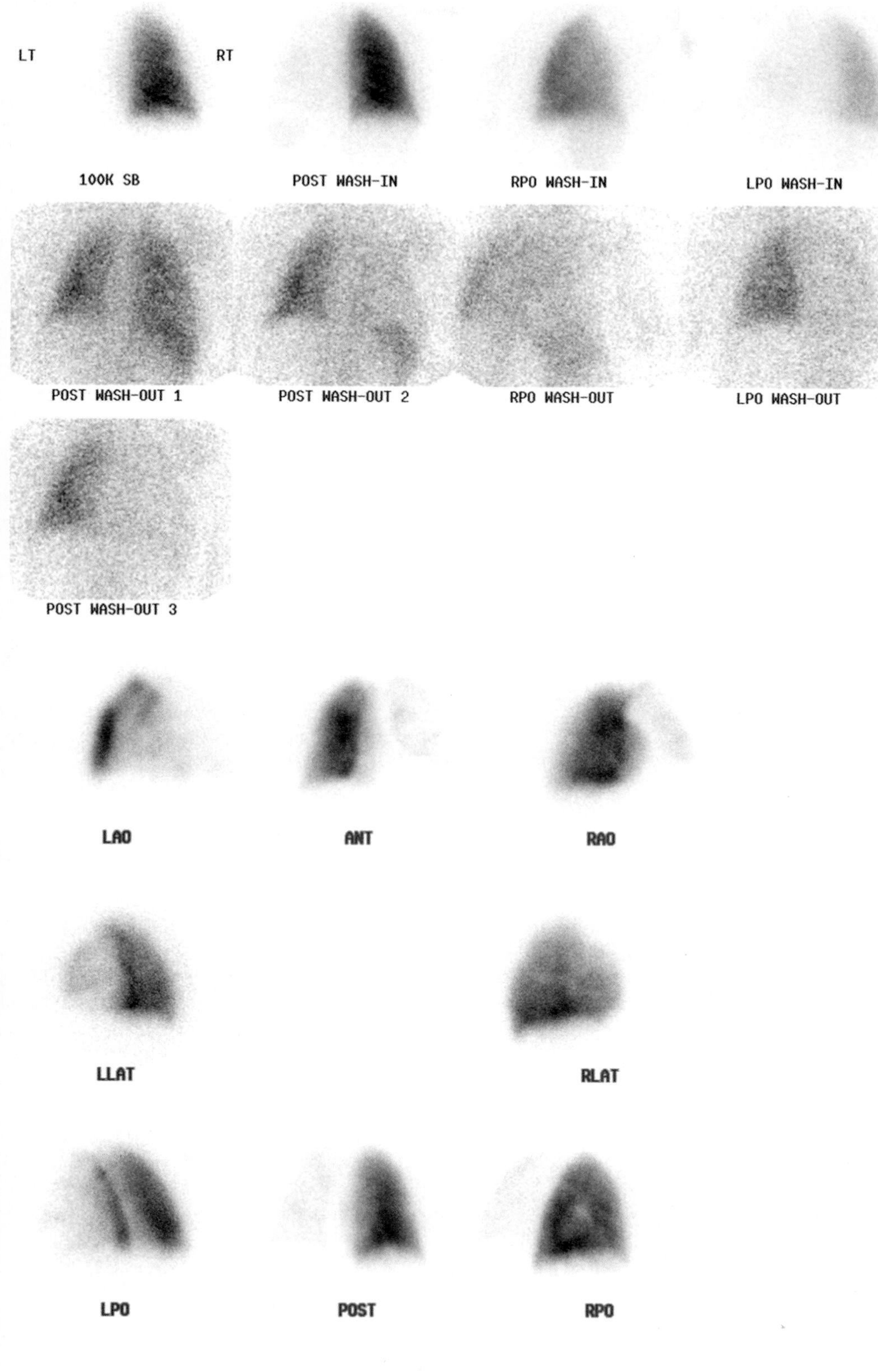

Clinical Presentation

59-year-old woman with shortness of breath. Chest radiographs were unremarkable.

Imaging Findings

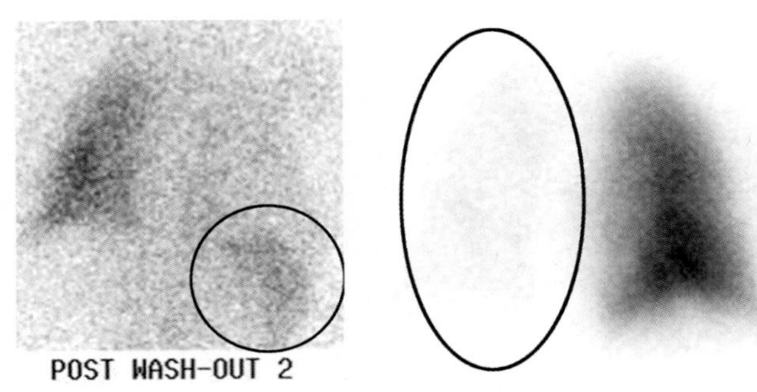

A B

(A) Xenon 133 ventilation scintigraphy demonstrates decreased ventilation to the entire left lung on single breath and wash-in. There is eventual equilibration but then abnormal retention throughout the entire left lung on washout. More focal retention of radiotracer is seen inferiorly on the right (*circle*). **(B)** Tc99m MAA perfusion images demonstrate markedly decreased perfusion to the entire left lung (*circle*).

Differential Diagnosis

- ***Low probability for pulmonary embolism (PE) and xenon retention in a fatty liver:*** Matched perfusion defects, even if large, with normal chest x-ray (CXR) findings are always low (or very low) probability. The right lower Xe133 activity is below the diaphragm and the classic appearance for a fatty liver.
- *Ventilatory retention at the right lung base:* A common mistake. On review of all the images, this activity is below the diaphragm in the right upper quadrant.
- *Intermediate probability for PE:* Lobar or whole-lung perfusion defects (matched or mismatched) are unlikely to be from PE and are classified as low (or very low) probability. These are often from mediastinal masses or fibrosis.

Essential Facts

- Xe133 will cross the alveolar membrane and be distributed by the blood.
- Xenon is lipophilic and will accumulate in the right upper quadrant in patients with fatty liver infiltration. This should be distinguished from true ventilatory retention in the right lower lobe (above the diaphragm).
- PIOPED criteria for low probability include small perfusion defects (matched or mismatched), matched moderate or large perfusion defects (except a lower lobe triple match), lobar or entire-lung perfusion defects (matched or mismatched), and perfusion defects smaller than a corresponding radiographic abnormality.
- A perfusion defect is considered small if 0 to 25% of a segment, medium if 25 to 75%, and large if 75 to 100%.
- A low-probability scan indicates a likelihood ratio of < 20% for PE. The clinician should combine this ratio with the patient's clinical pretest probability to arrive at the final post-test probability for PE.
- Some interpreters use the *very low probability* category (< 10% likelihood for PE), which includes findings such as three or fewer small perfusion defects, stripe sign, or solitary triple match in the middle or upper lung zone.

Other Imaging Findings

- CTA has become the modality of choice for diagnosing PE in most patients with the highest accuracy.
- However, lung ventilation–perfusion (VQ) scintigraphy can be employed for patients who cannot tolerate iodinated contrast or have an equivocal CTA. It can also be used to minimize exposure of the breasts to radiation in younger women.
- Catheter pulmonary angiography was once considered the gold standard in diagnosing PE but is no longer commonly employed with the advent of CTA.

✓ Pearls & × Pitfalls

✓ With the presence one moderately sized (25–75% of a segment) *mismatched* perfusion defect, the study cannot be classified as low probability.

✓ VQ scans should always be interpreted with a recent CXR (one from after the time the symptoms suggesting PE arose). Nonsegmental perfusion defects, including those from cardiomegaly, large hila, and elevated diaphragms, are also generally considered low or very low probability.

× Tc99m DTPA is used for ventilation scans at many institutions. This tracer will demonstrate only single-breath ventilation distribution (not equilibrium or washout) and will not accumulate in a fatty liver.

Case 10

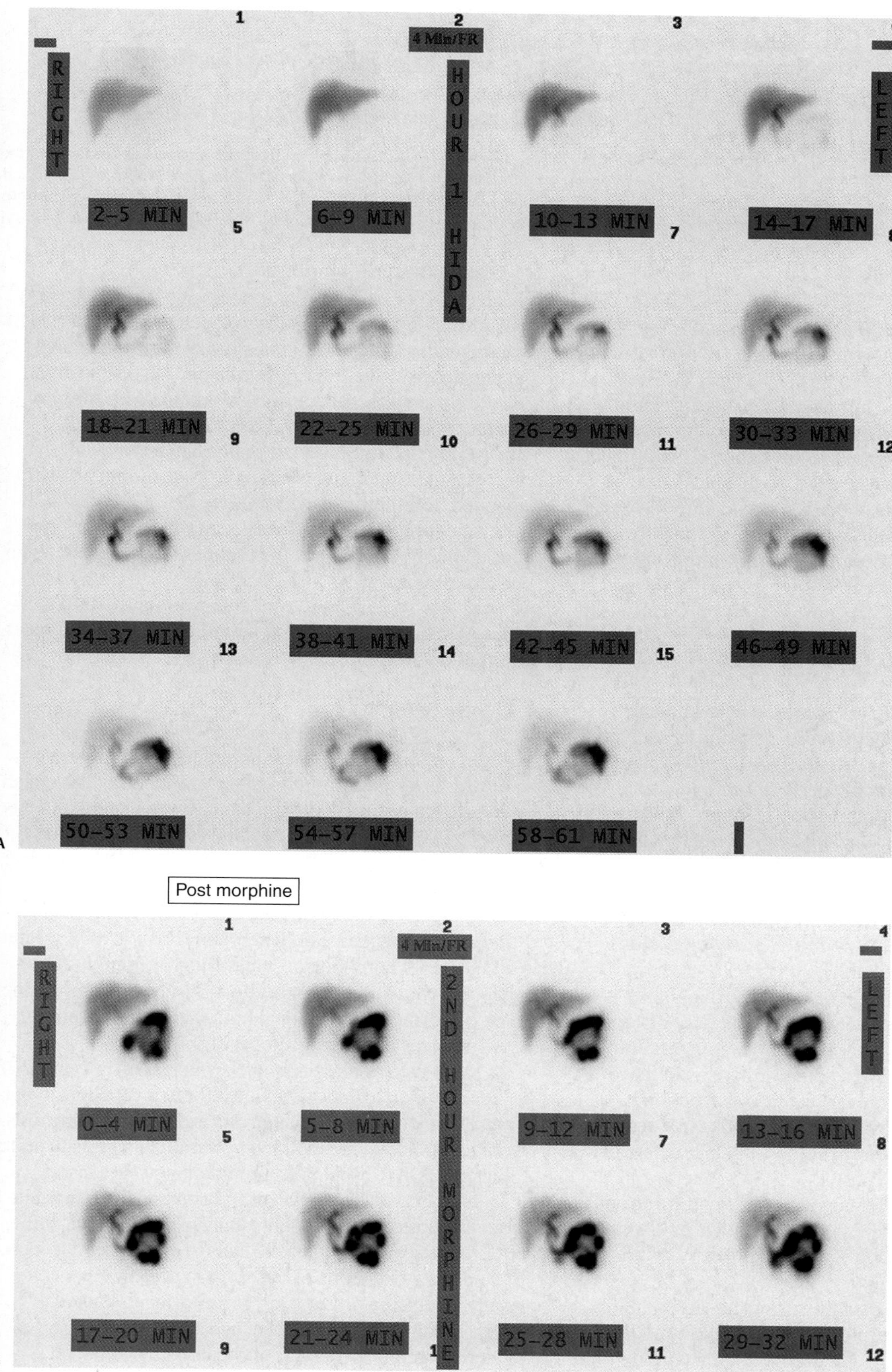

Clinical Presentation

A 40-year-old woman with acute right upper quadrant pain.

Imaging Findings

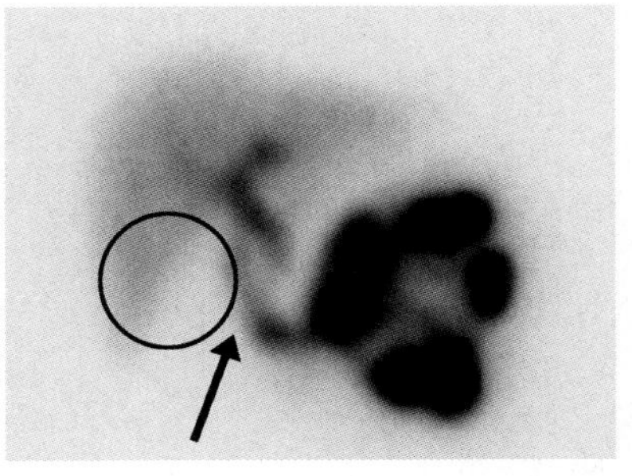

HIDA scan sequential imaging over 60 minutes (A in Clinical Presentation) demonstrates excretion of tracer into the duodenum (*arrow*) but no gallbladder (GB) filling (expected GB location circled). An additional 32 minutes of imaging after morphine administration (B in Clinical Presentation) again fails to demonstrate GB filling.

Differential Diagnosis

- ***Acute cholecystitis:*** Lack of GB filling, even after morphine administration, is highly suggestive of acute calculous cholecystitis.
- *Acalculous cholecystitis:* This most often appears identical to calculous cholecystitis on HIDA (no GB filling even after morphine). However, these are typically critically ill inpatients (e.g., with burns, sepsis, or diabetes).
- *Chronic cholecystitis:* This is usually normal on HIDA scans but may occasionally lack GB filling initially; however, filling will be achieved after morphine or delayed imaging.

Essential Facts

- Acute calculous cholecystitis is caused by a stone impacted in the GB neck or cystic duct, leading to venous and lymphatic congestion, GB mucosal edema, inflammation, necrosis, and eventually perforation.
- It presents with severe right upper quadrant (RUQ) or epigastric pain, nausea, vomiting, and fever. Liver function tests are often normal.
- GB filling, before or after morphine administration, effectively excludes this diagnosis (imaging typically performed 1 hour without and then 30 minutes after morphine if no initial filling).
- Acalculous cholecystitis is acute cholecystitis in the absence of stones, typically in critically ill patients, most commonly with cystic duct obstruction from inflammatory edema and debris; occasionally, there is direct GB infection in the absence of cystic duct obstruction.
- Acute acalculous cholecystitis usually looks like acute calculous cholecystitis on HIDA (no GB filling before or after morphine).
- Chronic cholecystitis: Patients experience intermittent RUQ pain, often with meals, in the setting of gallstones. GB fibrosis and infiltration with inflammatory cells is seen at pathology.
- Chronic cholecystitis is usually normal on HIDA (GB filling by 1 hour before morphine); abnormalities on HIDA are less common and include GB filling only with delayed imaging or morphine, delayed biliary to bowel transit (> 60 minutes), and/or diminished GB ejection fraction (< 35%) with cholecystokinin (CCK).

Other Imaging Findings

- HIDA "rim" sign: More advanced cholecystitis, such as with a gangrenous GB, can result in a rim of increased activity in hepatocytes adjacent to the inflamed GB fossa. This is due to hyperemia (more tracer in) and focal hepatocyte dysfunction with impaired excretion (less tracer out).
- HIDA "nubbin" sign: a cystic duct occluded in acute cholecystitis can dilate proximally (and should be distinguished from filling of a diminutive GB).
- US can demonstrate GB stones, wall thickening, pericholecystic fluid, and the "sonographic Murphy" sign in acute cholecystitis.
- CT can also show stones, wall enhancement with thickening, and surrounding stranding in advanced cases, although US is more sensitive early.

✓ Pearls & ✗ Pitfalls

- ✓ Right lateral and left anterior oblique spot views with HIDA can be performed to more confidently distinguish the GB from the duodenum or common bile duct (GB is typically oriented anteriorly and to the right). Also, duodenal activity will increase and decrease over time; GB activity should only increase.
- ✓ GB filling rules out acute (calculous) cholecystitis; nonfilling is very suggestive of cholecystitis but not 100% specific
- ✓ If initial GB nonfilling occurs through 1 hour and morphine is not an option, additional delayed imaging can be performed (3 additional hours without morphine = 30 minutes of imaging after morphine).
- ✓ CCK can help rule out acalculous cholecystitis in those less common instances in which there is GB filling. A normal GB ejection fraction (> 35%) excludes this diagnosis.
- ✗ Patients should have nothing by mouth for at least 4 hours before HIDA to avoid GB contraction; however, fasting > 24 hours can also yield false-positives due to thick bile concentration. Pretreat these long-fasting patients with CCK (always slowly injected) before HIDA tracer injection.
- ✗ If no biliary excretion of tracer is achieved by 1 hour, further delayed imaging can be performed. However, this usually indicates a global hepatocyte dysfunction (e.g., hepatitis, cirrhosis), *not* cholecystitis (although occasionally seen with CBD obstruction). Another clue to global hepatocyte dysfunction is prolonged radiotracer in the blood pool (past 15 minutes) with poor hepatic uptake

Case 11

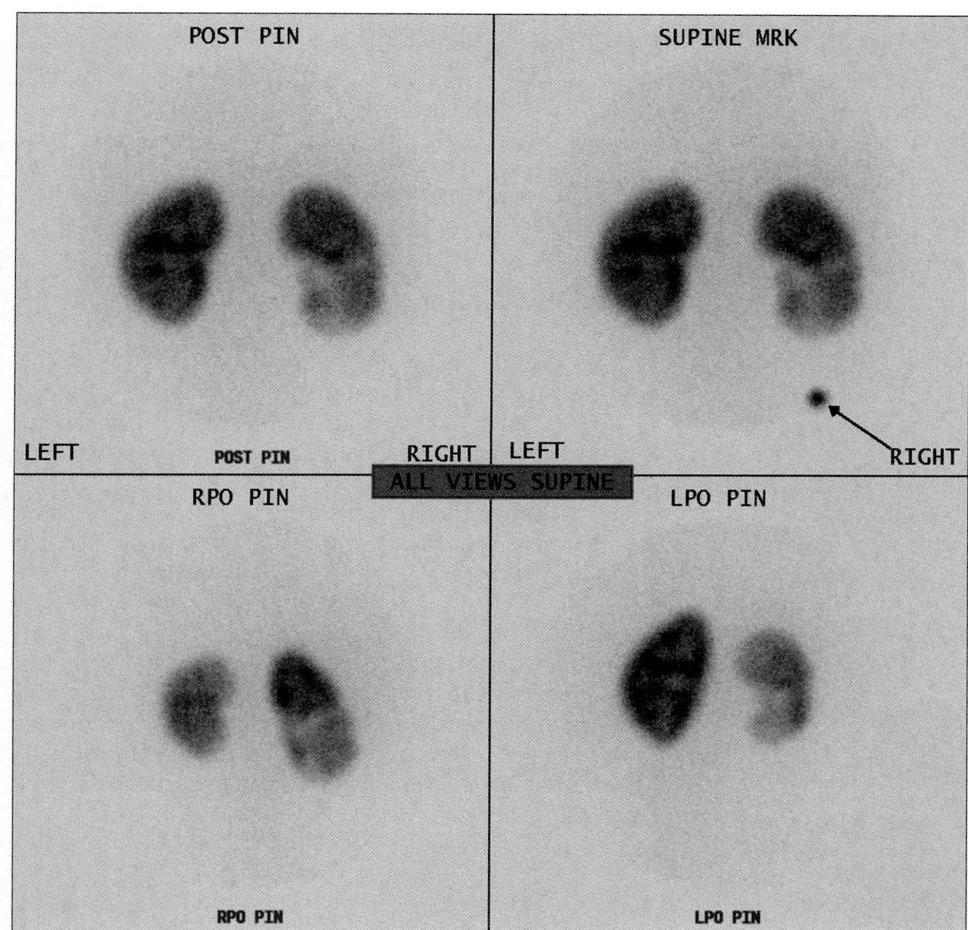

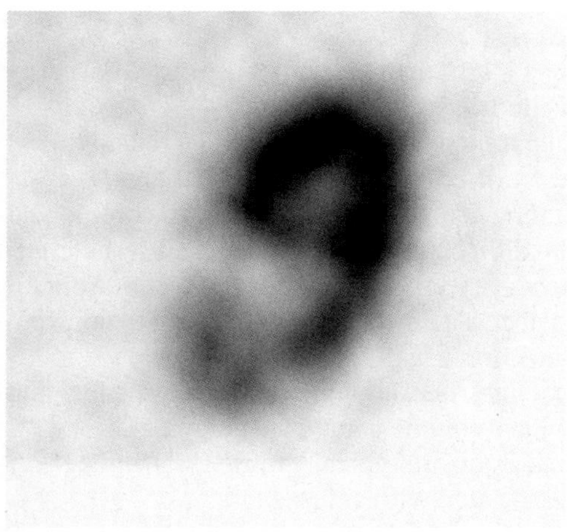

Sagittal SPECT-right kidney

Clinical Presentation

An 8-year-old boy with fever and flank pain.

Imaging Findings

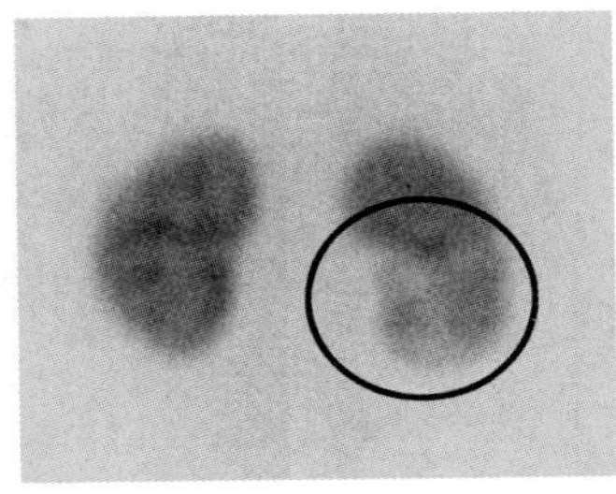

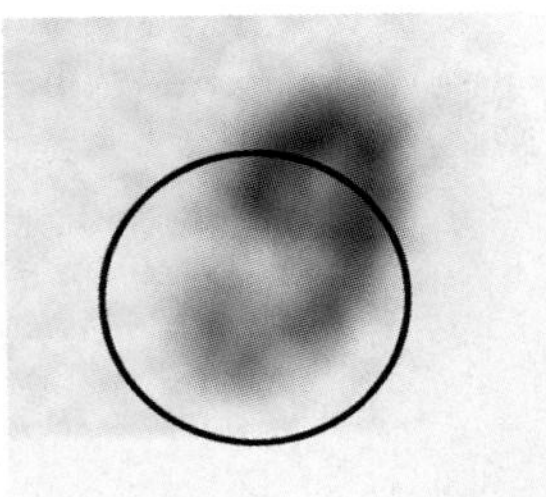

(A) Tc99m DMSA renal cortical pinhole planar views demonstrate decreased activity to the inferior right kidney (*circle*). **(B)** Sagittal SPECT image also shows decreased cortical uptake of the right kidney inferiorly (*circle*).

Differential Diagnosis

- ***Acute pyelonephritis:*** Regional decreased renal parenchymal uptake makes this the most likely diagnosis.
- *Chronic renal scarring:* This will also have regional parenchymal defects, but these tend to be more focal and peripheral, and unlike acute pyelonephritis, chronic renal scarring may have associated volume loss.
- *Renal tumor:* Although any space-occupying lesion, including renal cysts or neoplasm, can have decreased uptake, the appearance is typically more focal and masslike, as seen in this DMSA scan from a different patient:

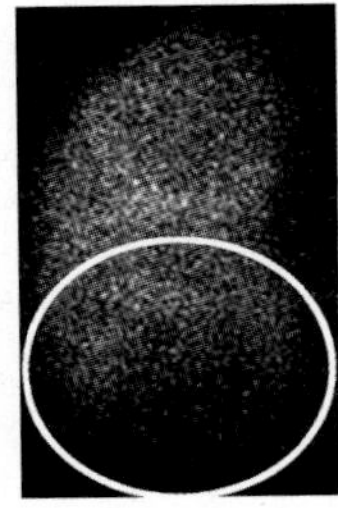

Essential Facts

- Tc99m-DMSA localizes to the kidneys via cortical tubular binding (40%). (Tc99m-glucoheptonate has also been used but has less cortical uptake [20%].)
- DMSA can be used to assess for regional parenchymal dysfunction seen in acute pyelonephritis and resultant scarring. It can also distinguish a pseudomass like a prominent column of Bertin seen on US, which has normal DSMA uptake, from a true space-occupying lesion.
- Clinical signs and symptoms of acute pyelonephritis can be absent in a young child, and DMSA imaging is often considered the gold standard for identifying infection in these patients.
- The extent of renal scarring from reflux/infection can be important to identify, as these patients are at risk for later complications, including hypertension and renal failure.

Other Imaging Findings

- CT or MRI: Pyelonephritis can demonstrate regionally decreased parenchymal perfusion or increased contrast retention with a "striated nephrogram." Renal scarring can appear as a focal peripheral parenchymal defect or lobulation.
- US: acute pyelonephritis can demonstrate abnormalities such as regionally decreased parenchymal perfusion on Doppler, but it is less sensitive than DMSA.
- Dynamic renal flow and function scintigraphy, such as with Tc99m-DTPA, can rarely demonstrate regional parenchymal dysfunction in acute pyelonephritis and a focal parenchymal defect in scarring. However, this is generally considered inferior to a DMSA scan for these indications because rapid renal transit precludes high-resolution scintigraphic planar imaging or SPECT.

✓ Pearls & × Pitfalls

- ✓ A combination of standard planar, pinhole, and/or SPECT imaging can be useful in renal cortical scintigraphy.
- ✓ DMSA binds intensely to the renal parenchymal *cortex*, not the medulla or collecting system.
- ✓ Split renal parenchymal function can be reliably estimated on DMSA scans (as with DTPA and MAG3).
- ✓ Differentiating acute pyelonephritis from chronic scarring can be difficult on a single study, and serial imaging may be necessary to assess for possible resolution. Any residual defect seen on follow-up imaging 6 months after an infection usually indicates a scar.
- ✓ Acute renal *infection* should not have volume loss and may even have volume gain (from edema). Chronic scars of *infarction* are typically more focal and peripheral and associated with volume loss.
- × Both upper renal poles may appear mildly decreased on a normal DMSA scan because of impression or attenuation from the adjacent liver and spleen. This should not be confused with pathology.

Case 12

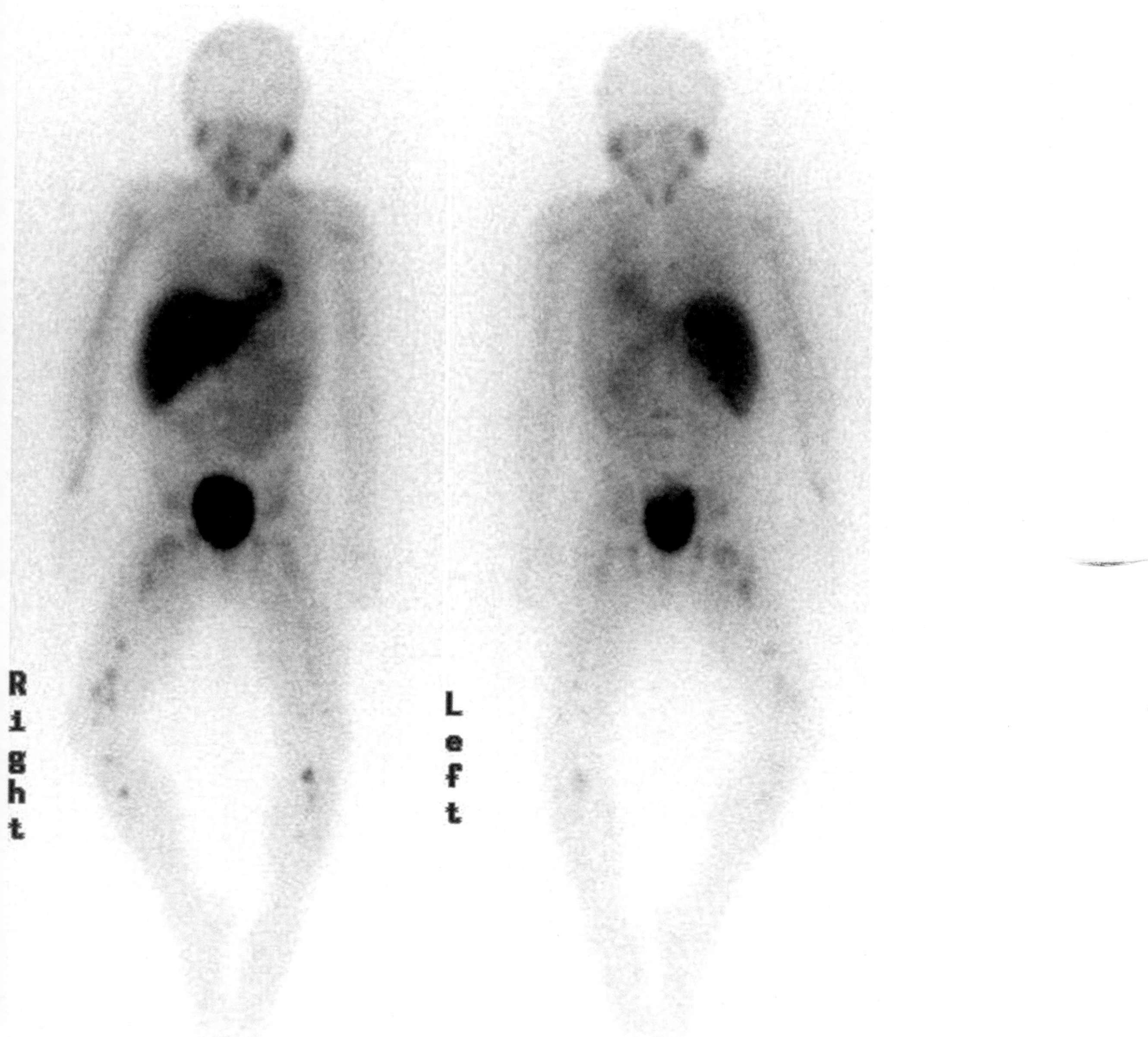

Clinical Presentation

A 5-year-old boy with a history of malignancy presents for restaging.

Imaging Findings

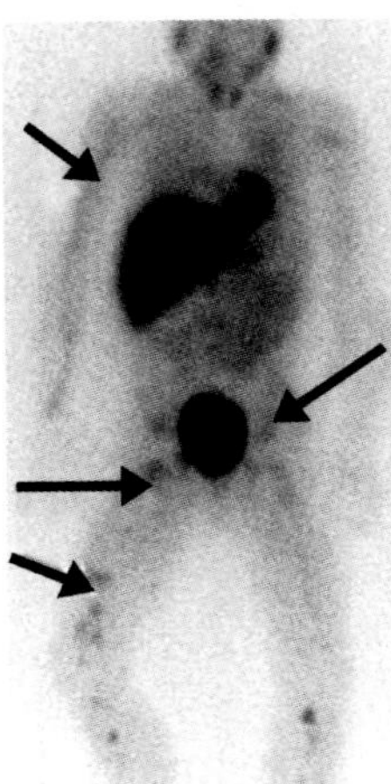

Anterior and posterior whole-body (WB) views demonstrate normal salivary, hepatic, enteric, and myocardial activity with widespread abnormal patchy marrow uptake (*arrows*).

Differential Diagnosis

- ***MIBG scan showing metastatic neuroblastoma (NB):*** The presence of cardiac uptake and the lack of *normal* skeletal uptake make the neuroendocrine-avid MIBG scan most likely. In a young child, NB is most commonly seen. The bone uptake is abnormal.
- *Iodine 131 scan showing metastatic thyroid carcinoma:* This can look similar to an MIBG scan, with no normal marrow uptake. However, normal cardiac activity should not be seen, and recurrence is also typically seen in the neck.
- *Octreotide scan showing metastatic tumor:* This can also be used for neuroendocrine tumor imaging and also does not have normal marrow uptake. However, intense normal spleen and renal cortical uptake is characteristic, and there would be no normal cardiac activity.

Essential Facts

- MIBG is a guanethidine analogue that accumulates in catecholamine-producing neuroendocrine tumors, commonly NB in children and pheochromocytoma in adults.
- NB is a bone-metastasizing neural crest tumor found in young children, typically originating in the retroperitoneum (adrenal or abdominal sympathetic chain) or less commonly the chest (thoracic sympathetics).
- MIBG is more sensitive and specific than bone scintigraphy for differentiating skeletal metastases from NB, but a combination of both studies finds the most lesions.
- MIBG is preferable to octreotide for adrenal neuroendocrine tumors, given the normally intense adjacent renal cortical uptake of the latter.
- Although MIBG can be used for other neuroendocrine tumors, such as islet cell, OctreoScan is generally more sensitive for these.

Other Imaging Findings

- Bone scintigraphy can be used in conjunction with MIBG to assess for skeletal metastases.
- Occasionally, soft-tissue uptake is seen in the primary NB lesion on bone scan (see Case 37).
- CT or MRI can demonstrate soft-tissue findings such as adrenal, central retroperitoneal, or thoracic paraspinal masses, which may be partially calcified.
- FDG-PET can detect primary and metastatic NB and is used at some centers as a complement to MIBG.

✓ Pearls & × Pitfalls

✓ For WB scans, if normal skeletal activity is *absent*, the study is probably an MIBG scan, an I131 WB scan, or OctreoScan (see "Interpreting Whole-Body Scans").

✓ If normal *myocardial* activity (as opposed to blood pool in the cardiac chambers) is present, the study is likely an MIBG or WB MIBI.

✓ MIBG looks similar to a radioiodine WB scan, but abnormal activity is typically below the diaphragm with MIBG.

✓ Block the thyroid (with a cold iodine source, such as potassium iodide) before and after injection for MIBG scans to reduce thyroid radiation because some free iodine breakdown does occur with MIBG. However, one may still see diffuse thyroid uptake faintly.

✓ MIBG may be labeled with I123 or I131. The former is preferable, given the better image quality and lower level of patient radiation.

× Any skeletal uptake on MIBG, I131, or OctreoScan imaging is abnormal and indicates metastatic disease.

× Skeletal metastases can be so diffuse on MIBG that they may, on initial inspection, appear "normal."

Case 13

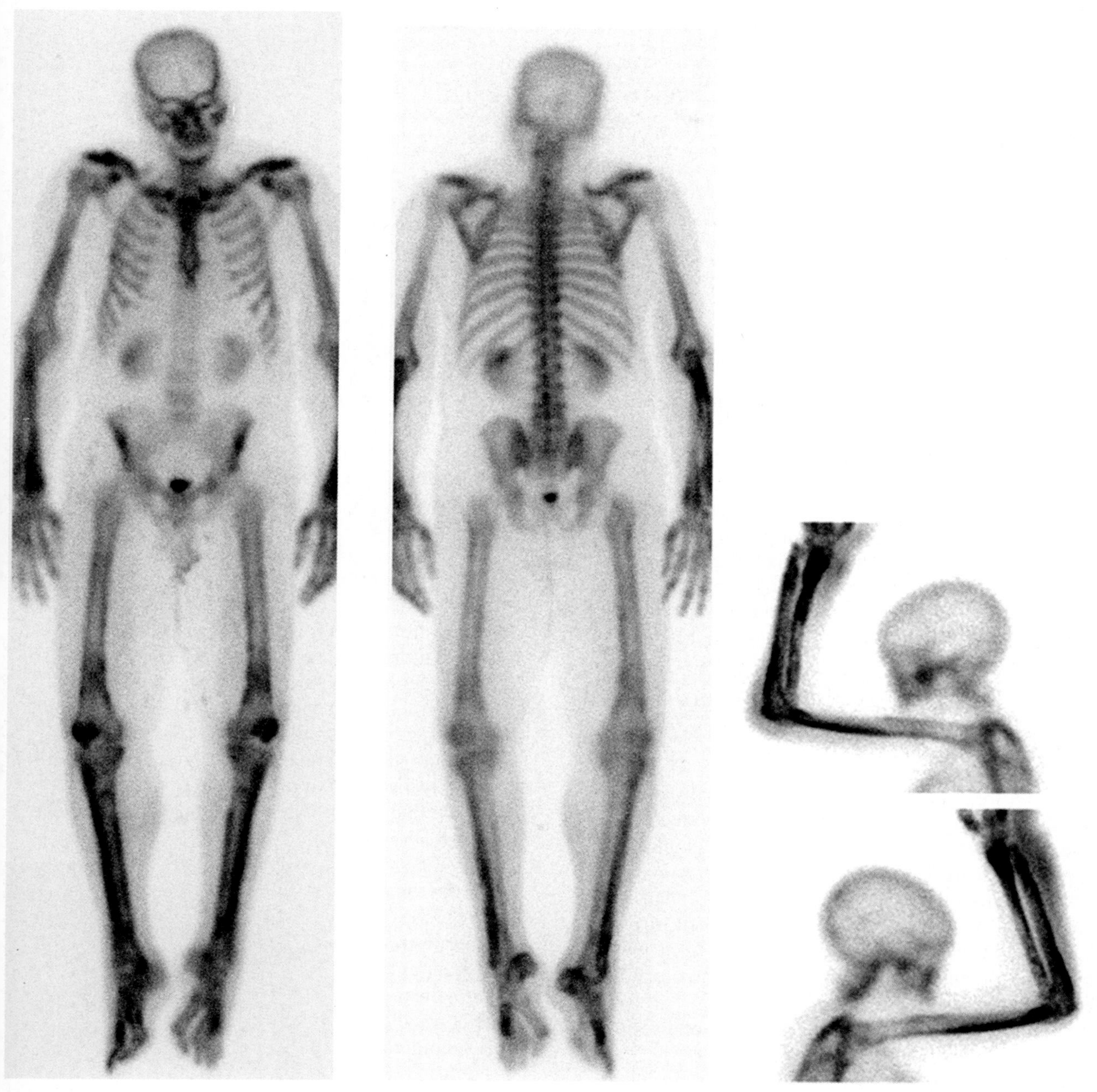

Clinical Presentation

A 53-year-old man with recently diagnosed lung carcinoma.

Imaging Findings

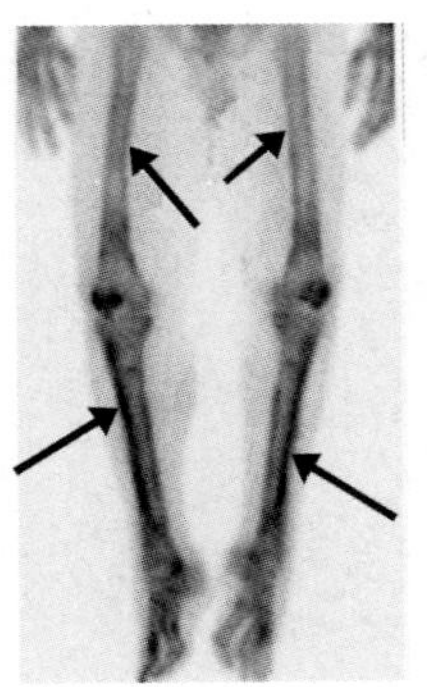
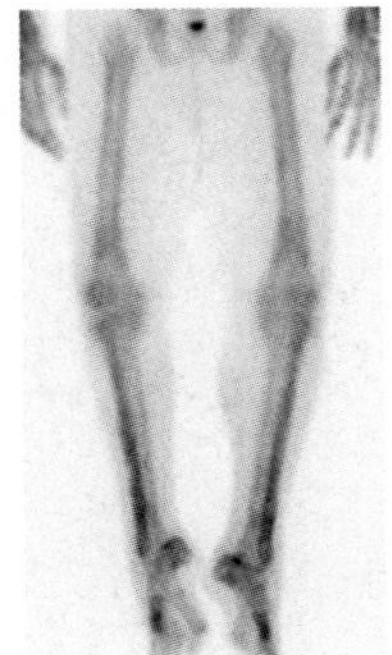
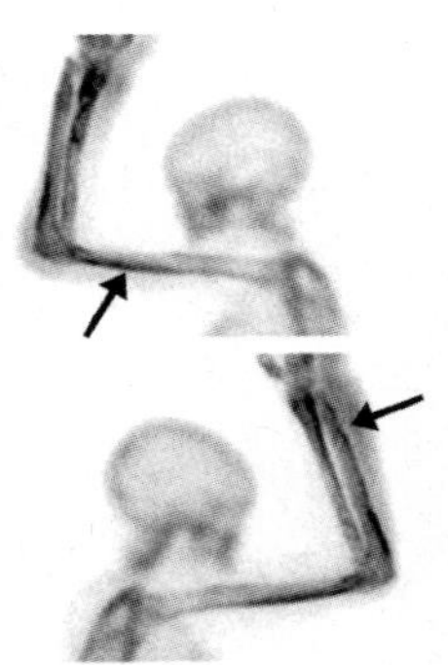

Anterior and posterior whole-body and arm spot views from a bone scan demonstrate diffusely increased cortical/periosteal linear uptake involving the upper and lower extremities symmetrically (*arrows*). The femora, tibiae, fibulae, humeri, radii, ulnae, and metatarsals are all involved.

Differential Diagnosis

- ***Hypertrophic osteoarthropathy (HOA):*** Diffuse, symmetric "tram tracking" appearance along the periosteal surfaces of the extremities makes this the most likely diagnosis.
- *Shin splints:* These will also have linear periosteal uptake of the lower extremities but will be confined to the mid-to-distal tibiae and will not affect the upper extremities.
- *Paget disease:* This can also involve long segments of the peripheral skeleton but will lead to bowing and cortical expansion of the affected bones and would not be this diffuse or symmetric.

Essential Facts

- HOA is a diffuse, symmetric periostitis involving both the lower and upper extremities in association with clubbing of the fingers/toes, skin thickening, and painful joints.
- The exact mechanism is unknown but can be primary (pachydermoperiostosis, which is rare) or secondary (hypertrophic pulmonary osteoarthropathy [HPOA]) in patients with tumors involving the pleura (e.g., lung cancer, mesothelioma) or with benign/inflammatory pleural disease (e.g., fibroma).
- Bone scan is the most sensitive for detection of disease presence and extent.
- Clinical signs of clubbing, painful joints, and skin changes plus imaging features suggest the diagnosis.
- HPOA may regress after the primary underlying disease process is treated.

Other Imaging Findings

- Chest radiographs or CT can demonstrate an underlying causative pulmonary abnormality.
- Plain bone radiographs can demonstrate periosteal changes, but not as sensitively as scintigraphy.
- MRI depiction is uncommon but may show periostitis and edema in the adjacent soft tissues.
- FDG-PET will often show a primary pulmonary lesion but will generally not include the distal extremities in the field of view.

✓ Pearls & ✗ Pitfalls

✓ Although diffuse metadiaphyseal periosteal uptake of the extremities on bone scan is typical, HOA may also appear irregular and periarticular and may involve more central bones, such as the mandible and scapula.

✗ Do not forget to assess the upper extremities for involvement with HOA on bone scintigraphy. These are commonly involved but often suboptimally imaged on whole-body views. Additional spot images may be necessary.

✗ The lateral cortices of the tibiae often demonstrate a prominent symmetric linear appearance normally. This should not be confused with the lateral and medial "tram tracking" seen in HOA. Shin splints may also have an appearance similar to that of HOA, but the distribution is confined to the tibiae.

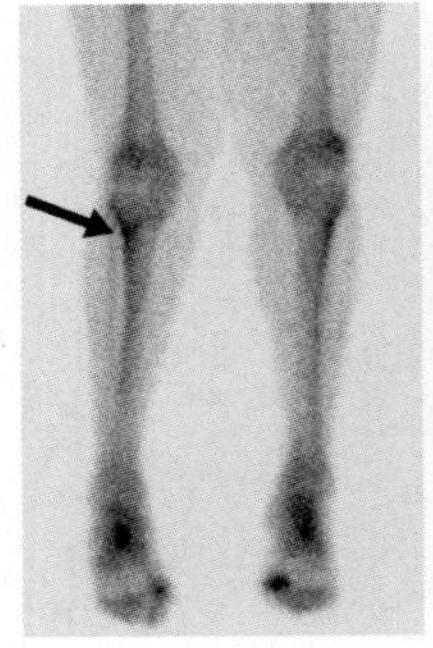

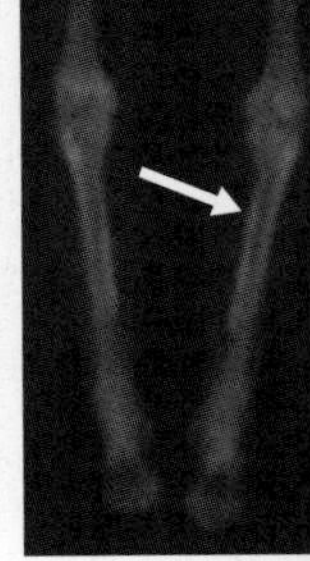

✗ Venous stasis can cause symmetric periosteal uptake, similar to HOA, but is typically confined to the regions below the knees.

Case 14

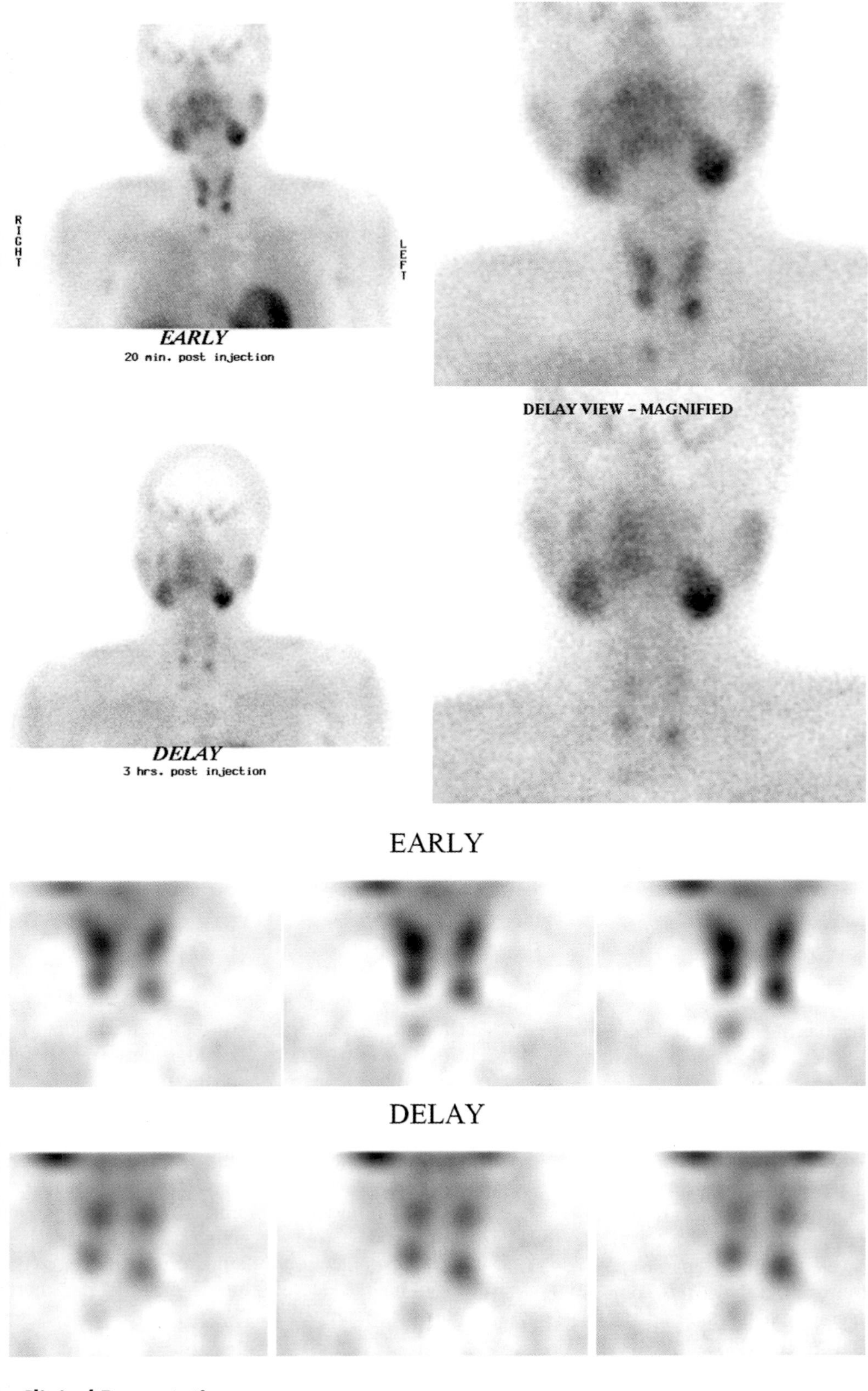

Clinical Presentation

A 42-year-old woman with hypercalcemia.

Imaging Findings

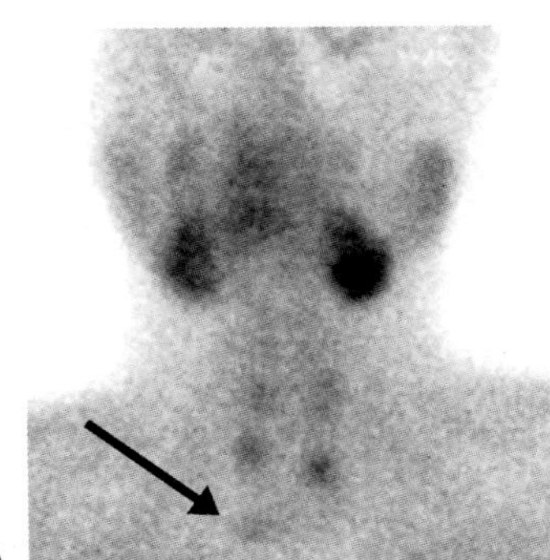

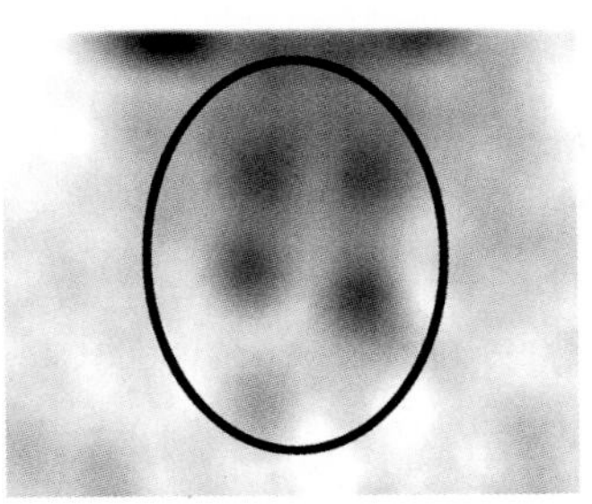

(A) Planar images 20 minutes and 3 hours after Tc99m MIBI injection (parathyroid scan) demonstrate persistent, focally increased activity in the expected locations of the four parathyroid glands as well as a fifth focus inferior to the thyroid on the right (*arrow*). **(B)** Early and delayed SPECT images confirm the planar findings (*circle*).

Differential Diagnosis

- ***Parathyroid hyperplasia with a supernumerary gland:*** The multiple foci in typical locations together with the history make parathyroid hyperplasia the most likely etiology in this patient with five parathyroid glands.
- *Multiple parathyroid adenomas:* These will also appear as persistent increased foci and can be multiple but would be extremely unlikely to present as five adenomas.
- *Multiple thyroid adenomas:* A common false-positive can appear as focal, persistent lesion(s) but would be unlikely to appear in the expected locations of all parathyroid glands and might present with hyperthyroidism, not hyperparathyroidism.

Essential Facts

- Hyperparathyroidism can be primary (autonomous hyperfunction of gland[s]), secondary (physiologic gland hyperfunction to compensate for low calcium with renal failure), or tertiary (also in renal failure but in which a parathyroid gland[s] becomes autonomous).
- Patients with elevated parathyroid hormone (PTH) and elevated serum calcium typically have primary hyperparathyroidism.
- Primary hyperparathyroidism is most commonly due to parathyroid adenoma (85–90%), less often hyperplasia (10%), and rarely parathyroid carcinoma (< 1%).
- Ten percent of people have a fifth gland. Ectopic or supernumerary glands may have normal function or hyperfunction.
- Treatment for parathyroid adenoma is surgical resection of the abnormal gland(s); for hyperplasia, it is resection of three and one-half of four glands.
- Tc99m-MIBI early and delayed imaging is the most common method for parathyroid scintigraphy. Tracer binds to increased mitochondria in abnormal parathyroid glands plus normal thyroid early; it washes out of thyroid late but persists in abnormal parathyroids.
- Scintigraphic preoperative imaging (for diagnosis and localization) has become standard, particularly with minimally invasive techniques, and is often used in conjunction with intraoperative localization with a gamma probe following repeat radiotracer injection.

Other Imaging Findings

- Tc99m-TETRO has a mechanism of uptake very similar to that of MIBI (mitochondrial binding), and early/delayed parathyroid imaging with this tracer is preferred at some institutions.
- Dual-isotope subtraction of a tracer specific for the thyroid gland from a tracer that also binds to abnormal parathyroids is another option. Historically, thallium/pertechnetate was used with mixed results, although today early MIBI/iodine 123 subtraction is possible with higher accuracy.
- US, CT, and MRI can also be performed to look for enlarged parathyroid gland(s) but are nonspecific and may not find smaller or ectopic lesions.

✓ Pearls & × Pitfalls

✓ SPECT increases examination accuracy. If only one SPECT image is acquired, it should be performed *early* to use the normal thyroid as a landmark.

✓ The sensitivity of scintigraphy is much higher for a parathyroid adenoma (90%) than for hyperplasia (50%).

× MIBI and TETRO are nonspecific neoplastic and inflammatory (and myocardial) tracers. Focal uptake can represent parathyroid adenoma, parathyroid carcinoma, thyroid adenoma, thyroid carcinoma, metastasis, lymphoma, or infection/inflammation. However, in the setting of high PTH levels, the specificity for parathyroid adenoma is excellent.

Case 15

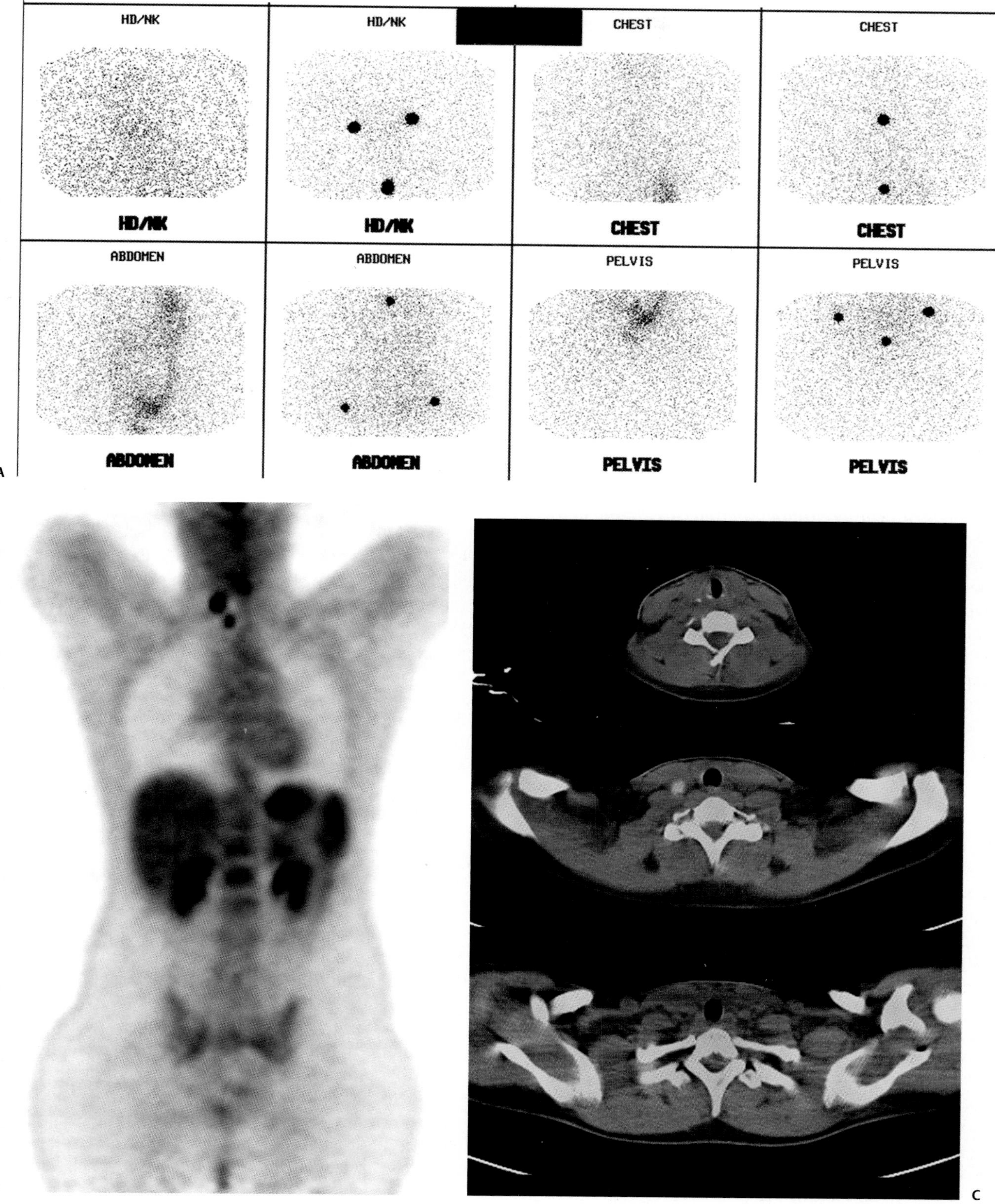

A

B

C

Clinical Presentation

A 40-year-old woman with a history of papillary thyroid carcinoma, 5 years status post thyroidectomy and radioiodine ablation, now presents with rising serum thyroglobulin levels.

Imaging Findings

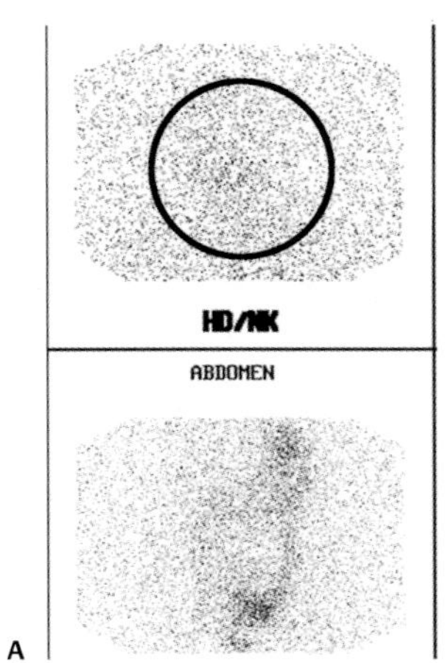

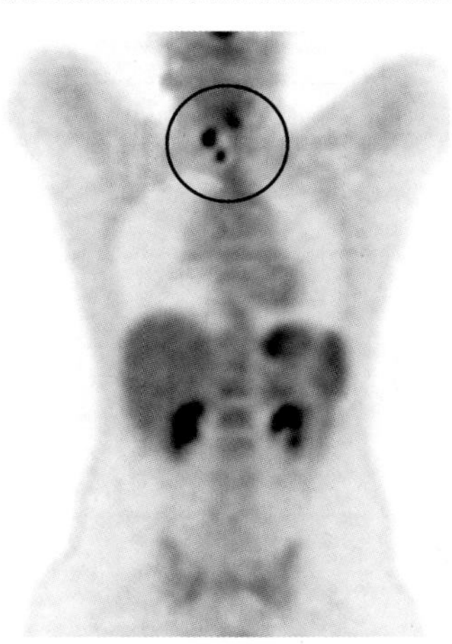

(A) Whole-body iodine 131 scintigraphy demonstrates no abnormal I131-avid lesion. Enteric, urinary, and faint salivary (*circle*) physiologic activity is present. **(B)** PET/CT demonstrates three abnormal FDG-avid lesions in the neck (*circle*).

Differential Diagnosis

All three will be FDG-avid and negative on I131. However, the typical location and history make recurrent thyroid cancer the most likely etiology.

- ***Metastatic dedifferentiated thyroid carcinoma:*** In the setting of a rising serum thyroglobulin (Tg) level after thyroidectomy and radioiodine (RAI) ablation and a negative I131 scan, FDG-avid lesions are most consistent with this diagnosis.
- *Hodgkin lymphoma:* This can look very similar to dedifferentiated thyroid carcinoma on FDG-PET, but the history, including the Tg value, is much more suggestive of recurrent thyroid carcinoma.
- *Head and neck carcinoma:* This can also look very similar to thyroid carcinoma on FDG-PET, but again, the history is much more suggestive of recurrent thyroid carcinoma.

Essential Facts

- Papillary and follicular cancers are the most common thyroid cancers (90%), followed by medullary and anaplastic cancers.
- Papillary and follicular cancers are both typically I131-avid and more common in women, are more likely in patients with a history of prior neck radiotherapy, and appear as cold nodules (relative to normal thyroid) on thyroid bed scan.
- Treatment includes total thyroidectomy (although small, expected thyroid remnant initially remains) followed by RAI ablation; follow-up is with radioiodine scans and serum Tg measurements.
- Rising Tg (> 10 ng/mL) suggests recurrence; negative I131 scan in this setting suggests dedifferentiation of the tumor, which may now be only FDG-avid (or iodine-avid but micrometastatic and below the planar imaging threshold).
- Positive FDG-PET confirms the diagnosis.
- Treatment options in this setting include surgery if recurrence is limited to the regional nodes or an empiric trial of high-dose I131 (despite negative I131 scan); more experimental options include conventional chemotherapeutic agents and external-beam radiation therapy.

Other Imaging Findings

- US, CT, or MRI of the neck can be used to visualize enlarged or enhancing lymph nodes in regional neck recurrence. CT of the chest will detect pulmonary metastases.
- Whole-body bone scintigraphy can identify skeletal metastases. Sensitivity may be decreased, however, for lytic lesions, which are more commonly seen with thyroid cancer.
- Whole-body MIBI scanning has been used to detect dedifferentiated, non–I131-avid thyroid metastases. This use has now been replaced by FDG-PET.
- Neuroendocrine scintigraphic tracers (i.e., octreotide, MIBG) can detect medullary thyroid cancers (which also are not iodine-avid).

✓ Pearls & ✗ Pitfalls

✓ Elevate thyroid-stimulating hormone (TSH) for radioiodine scan, I131 therapy, *and FDG-PET scan* before dosing (and before serum Tg measurement).

✓ Thyroid hormone withdrawal methods to increase TSH levels to > 30 μU/mL are optimal. Pretreatment with synthetic Thyrogen is a slightly less sensitive but acceptable option that avoids the patient discomfort of hypothyroidism.

✗ Incidental focal thyroidal uptake on FDG-PET should have further work-up with US, I123 thyroid bed scanning, and/or biopsy to exclude malignancy, but it may also represent a benign etiology, such as a functioning thyroid adenoma or focal thyroiditis.

✗ *Diffusely* increased thyroidal uptake on FDG-PET is consistent with benign medical thyroid disease.

✗ Low-grade papillary/follicular thyroid cancers will often be *non*–FDG-avid (but radioiodine-avid).

Case 16

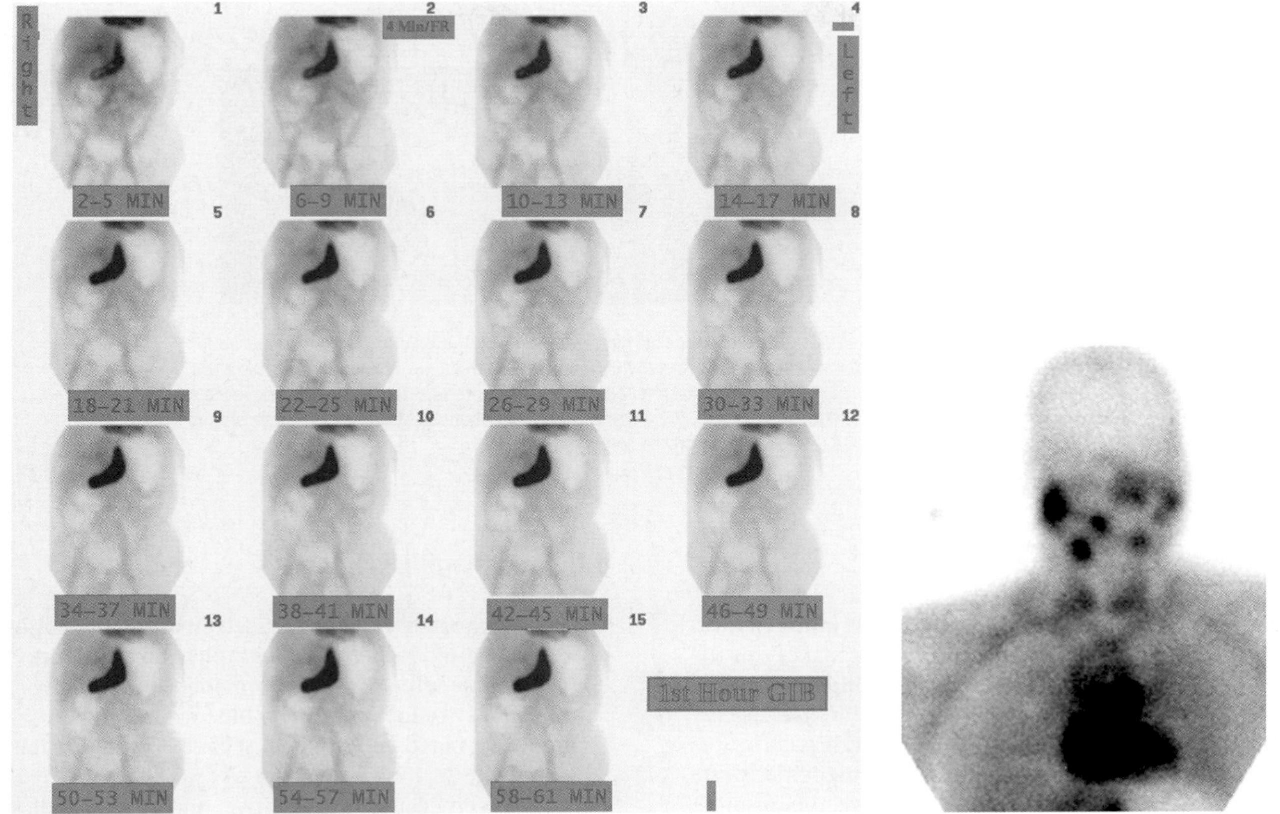

Clinical Presentation

A patient with passage of bright red blood per rectum.

Further Work-up

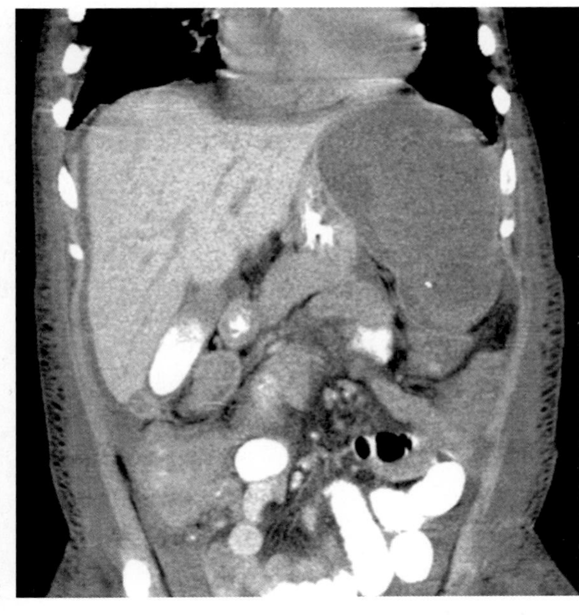

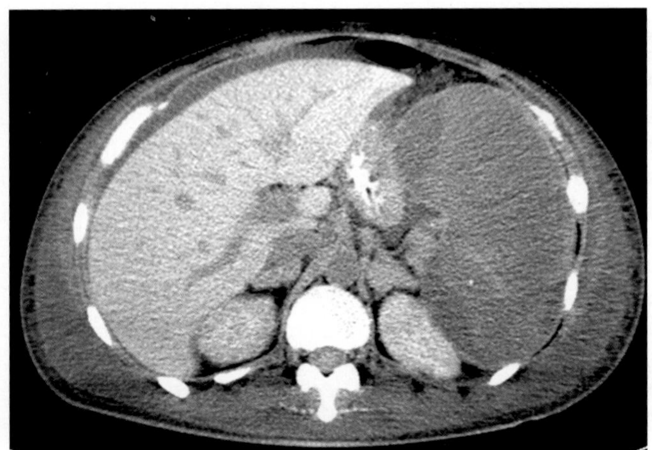

Imaging Findings

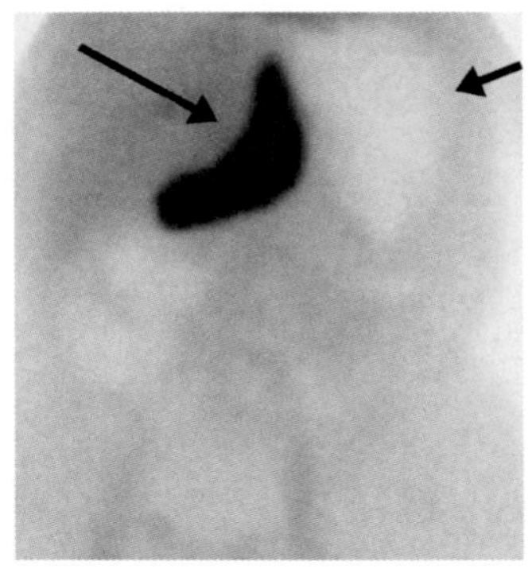

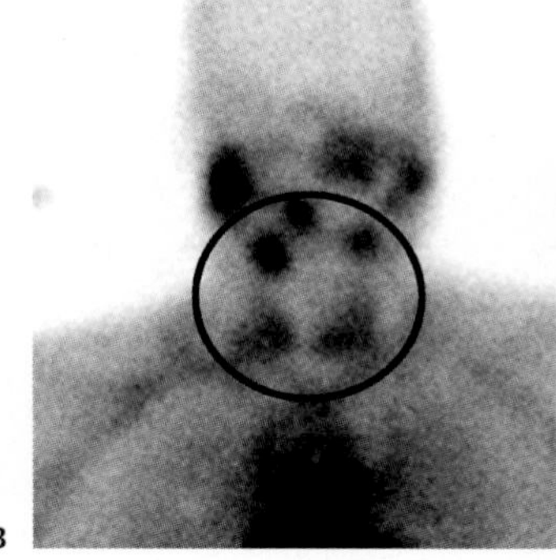

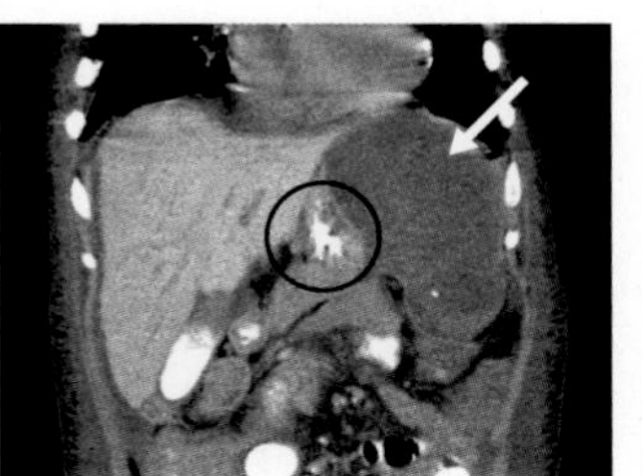

(A) Anterior images from Tc99m-tagged RBC study demonstrate immediate, intense, abnormal uptake in the upper mid abdomen (*long arrow*). After review of the CT scan, this localizes to the stomach, which is displaced medially by an enlarged, infarcted spleen. The infarcted spleen demonstrates no normal RBC accumulation (*short arrow*). **(B)** Anterior image of the neck reveals salivary and thyroid uptake, which is abnormal for an RBC scan (*circle*). **(C)** Coronal and axial enhanced abdominal CT scan shows the stomach (*circle*) displaced medially by an enlarged, hypodense, infarcted spleen (*arrow*).

Differential Diagnosis

- ***Free pertechnetate artifact (and splenic infarct):*** Gastric and thyroid accumulation of radiotracer makes this the correct diagnosis. A photopenic spleen indicates infarction, as splenic RBC uptake is normally intense.
- *Gastric bleed:* This would also demonstrate gastric uptake and is the main differential but would not demonstrate thyroid and salivary uptake. Furthermore, the history suggests a lower gastrointestinal (GI) bleed.
- *Aortic aneurysm:* This can also have focally increased RBC uptake but would be a very atypical configuration (and would also not have thyroid or salivary uptake).

Essential Facts

- Free pertechnetate contamination artifact can occasionally be seen in studies for which Tc99m is used as the radioisotope.
- For red cell labeling, two steps are required: (1) provide an intercellular reducing agent (cold tin is used) so that the (2) subsequently introduced Tc99m will bind to the hemoglobin.
- Both steps can be performed in a test tube (in vitro; e.g., UltraTag kit), both in the patient (in vivo), or one step in each (modified in vivo, or "in vivtro"). The more steps performed in a test tube, the better the labeling efficiency.
- If the Tc99m radiolabeling is poor or if Tc99m dissociates from the pharmaceutical portion of the radiopharmaceutical, free pertechnetate is formed and quickly excreted by the kidneys and stomach.
- Accumulation of free pertechnetate also occurs in the salivary glands, nasopharyngeal mucosa, and thyroid, and a spot image of the head and neck can be used to confirm this artifact.

Other Imaging Findings

- Free pertechnetate is not visualized on other modalities.
- For GI bleeding, catheter angiography can be used to image the bleeding as well as provide therapy. However, sensitivity for detecting a bleed is lower, and the window for bleed activity is in seconds (vs. hours for RBC).
- CTA is also emerging as a sensitive, noninvasive tool, and the bleed need not be active for the source to be seen.

✓ Pearls & × Pitfalls

✓ Gastric lavage via nasogastric tube will exclude most gastric bleeds before an RBC scan is ordered. Patients with positive lavage results then go to upper GI endoscopy for confirmation and often treatment. For this reason, true upper GI bleeds are less commonly encountered on RBC scans.

✓ Any Tc99m-labeled study can have free pertechnetate artifact (e.g., bone scans with gastric uptake). Always check for thyroid/salivary uptake if this is a concern.

× Both a true gastric bleed and gastric excretion of artifactual free pertechnetate can move antegrade through bowel, and therefore this is not a reliable distinguishing feature.

× Other recent Tc99m studies performed within 24 hours can cause free pertechnetate artifact (e.g., MUGA scan followed by bone scan).

Case 17

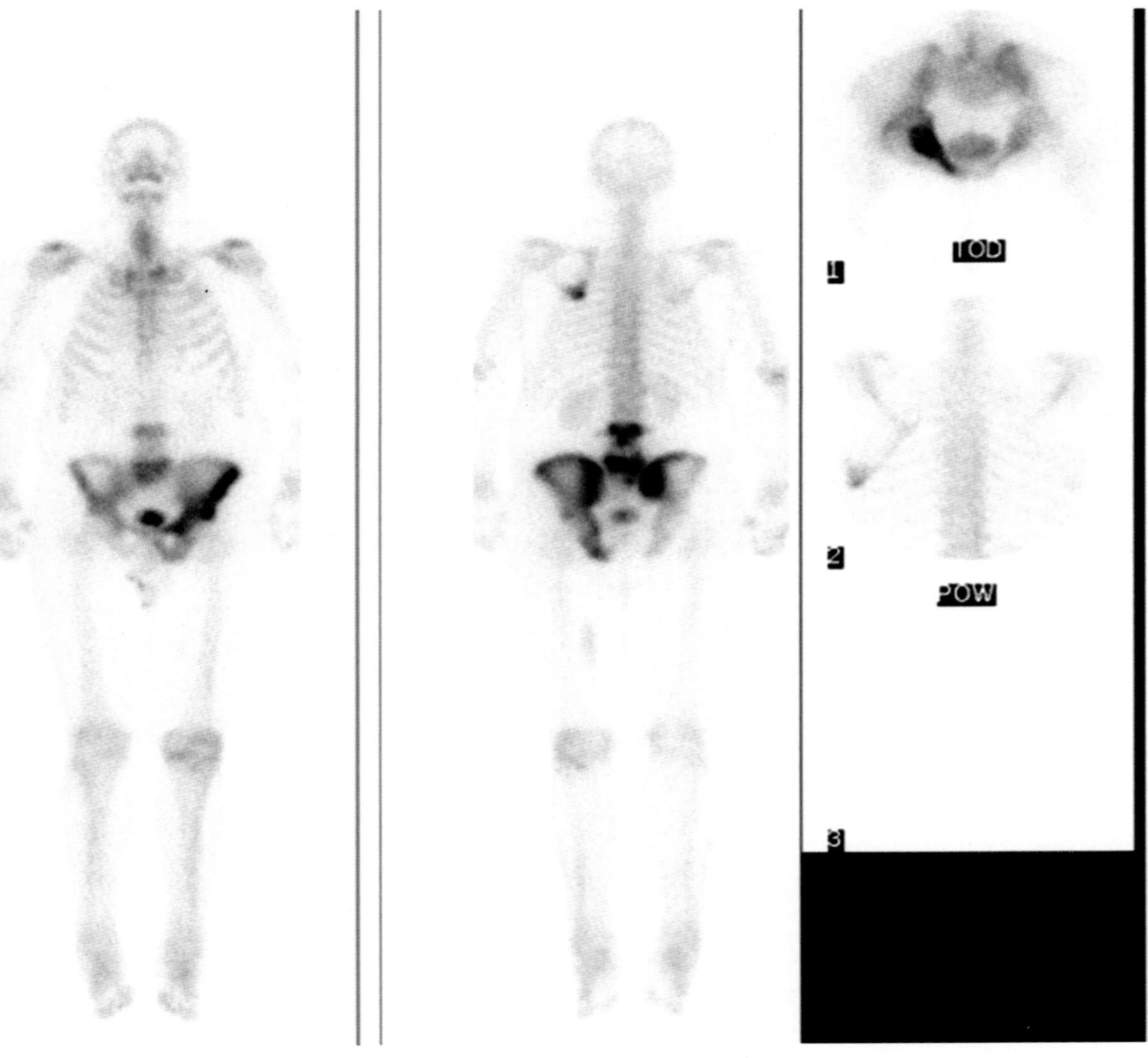

Clinical Presentation

A patient with newly diagnosed prostate cancer and elevated alkaline phosphatase.

Imaging Findings

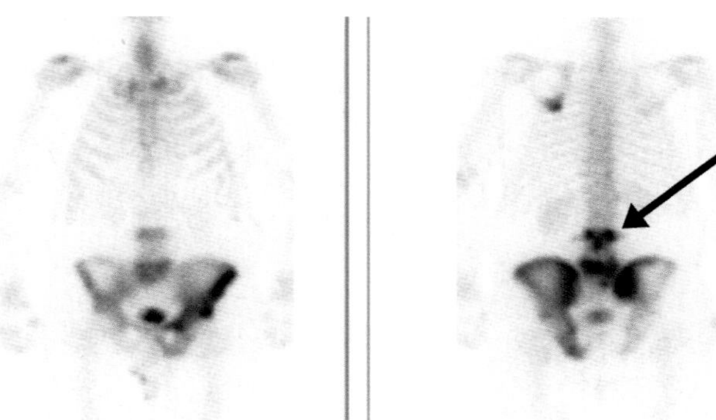

Tc99m MDP bone scintigraphy including whole-body and spot "tail on detector" views demonstrates multiple skeletal lesions of increased activity that generally involve large segments of bone with associated cortical expansion. Long-segment lesions with cortical thickening are seen involving the pelvis. Another lesion starts at the extreme scapular tip. An entire lumbar vertebral level (anterior and posterior elements) is involved diffusely ("Mickey Mouse" sign; *arrow*).

Differential Diagnosis

- ***Paget disease (PD):*** Multiple bone lesions, many with long segments and starting at the bone end or involving entire bones and with cortical expansion, make PD the most likely diagnosis.
- *Skeletal metastatic disease:* This can look superficially similar to PD with multiple lesions. However, the lesions are usually more focal and do not cause cortical thickening. They are most commonly confined to the red marrow (i.e., more central) skeletal distribution, as (incidentally) seen in this case.
- *Hyperparathyroidism:* This typically involves the entire skeleton fairly uniformly, although it may be most severe in the skull and around large joints. It often occurs with an associated decrease in soft-tissue and renal uptake ("metabolic superscan").

Essential Facts

- PD is a common disorder most frequently affecting middle-aged or elderly persons, men > women.
- The cause is likely a slow virus, but there may also be a hereditary susceptibility (e.g., Anglo-Saxon descent).
- Symptoms may be absent or include bone pain or the effects of hyperemia, such as high-output congestive heart failure; skull involvement may lead to headaches, increasing head size, hearing loss, and cranial nerve palsies; alkaline phosphatase is usually elevated.
- Bisphosphonate class drugs are often effective therapy.
- Phases of PD: early: osteolytic (decreased density on radiograph, intense on bone scan); mixed phase; then late: osteoblastic (sclerotic on radiograph, mildly increased on bone scan).
- PD is more commonly polyostotic; a small percentage of cases undergo sarcomatous degeneration.

Other Imaging Findings

- Bone scintigraphy: cortical involvement with expansion predominates, long segments start at the bone end with sharp cutoffs or involve the entire bone, pelvis and skull (round or diffuse) commonly involved, "Mickey Mouse" sign in the spine (entire vertebral level).
- Because PD lesions originate in the cortical bone, they are not confined to a red marrow distribution (unlike typical metastases) and may appear in the distal appendicular skeleton, as seen in this other patient:

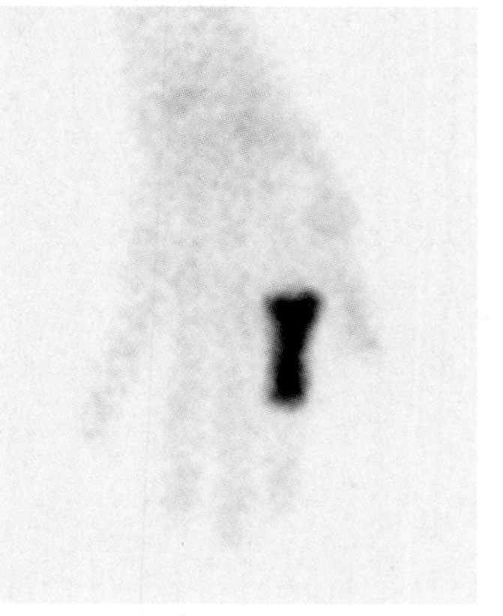

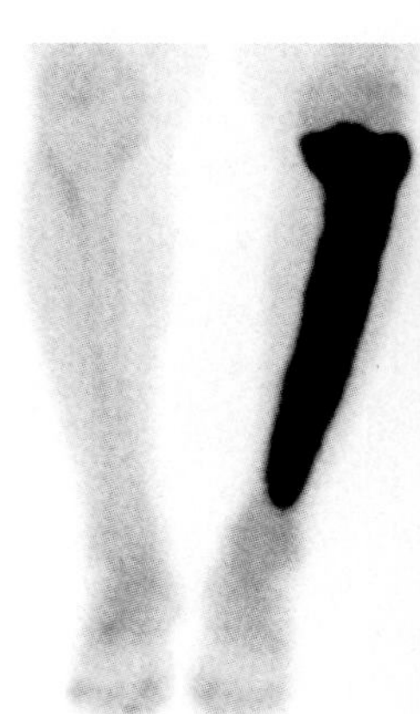

- Plain radiographs: increased density with cortical and trabecular thickening; skull: cotton wool, osteoporosis circumscripta; "picture frame" spine; long bones: "blade of grass" sharp cutoff; may cause bowing.
- CT: cortical and trabecular thickening
- MRI: cortical and trabecular thickening; can enhance
- FDG-PET: PD can be hot if in its earlier phases.

✓ Pearls & ✗ Pitfalls

✓ PD is not uncommon; before giving a patient with multiple bone lesions a diagnosis of metastatic disease, be sure the appearance is not more consistent with PD.

✓ Unlike metastases, PD is *not* red marrow–based and thus can often involve the more distal appendicular skeleton.

✓ PD can occasionally be so extensive that it results in a "superscan" appearance with a relative decrease in soft tissues (see Case 1).

✗ PD can coexist with skeletal metastases, and it can occasionally be very difficult to differentiate all lesions on any modality. Follow-up or bone biopsy may become necessary.

Case 18

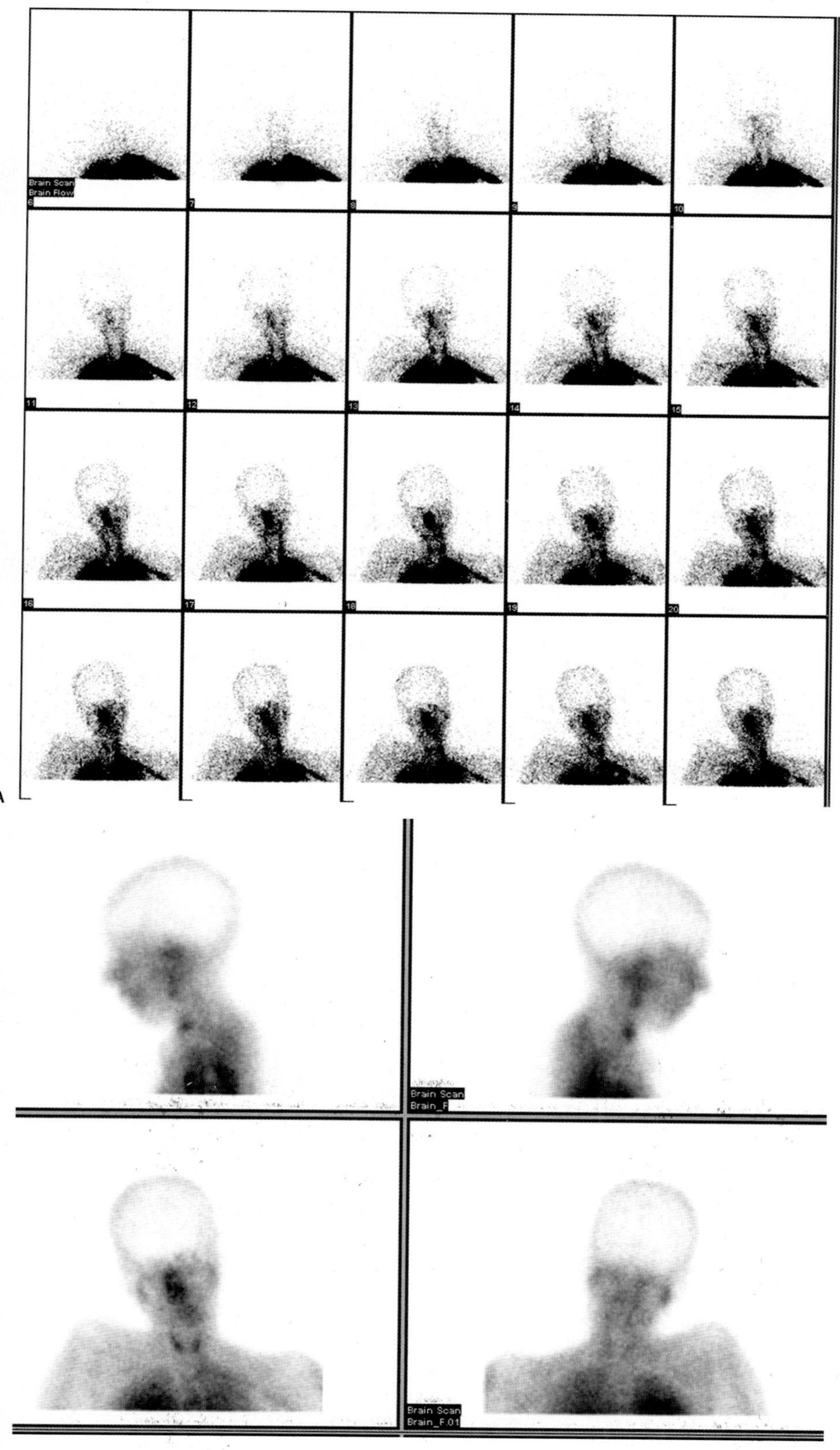

Clinical Presentation

History withheld.

Imaging Findings

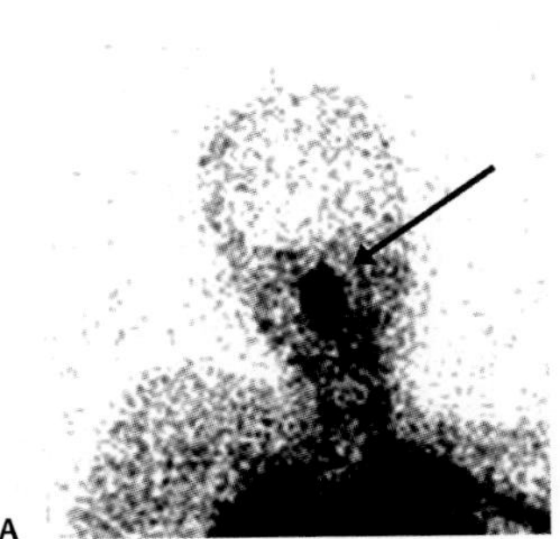

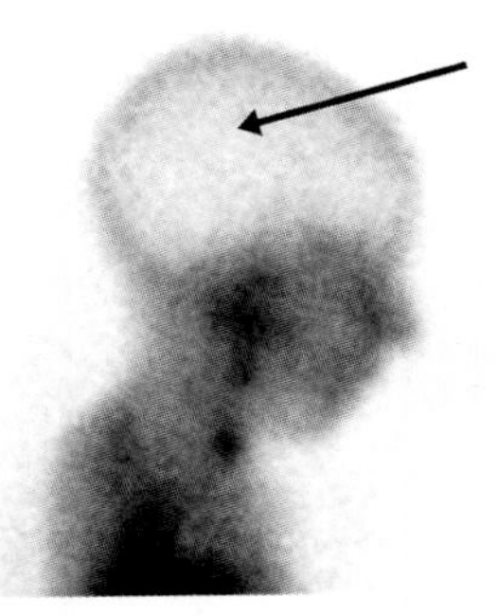

(A) Anterior radionuclide angiographic images with Tc99m HMPAO reveal radiotracer at the common carotid level bilaterally. However, no arterial flow (internal carotid artery [ICA]) is seen above the skull base. Activity is seen in the scalp. Intense activity is also seen in the nasal region ("hot nose" sign; *arrow*). **(B)** Delayed lateral, anterior, and posterior spot images of the head reveal no cerebral cortical activity (*arrow*).

Differential Diagnosis

- ***Brain death:*** The lack of intracranial blood flow is compatible with brain death.
- *Infiltrated radiotracer dose:* An injected dose that does not enter the vascular system at all or with a very poor bolus can demonstrate a similar radionuclide angiogram. In this case, good blood pool activity is seen in the left arm and chest, indicating a good injection. If some infiltrated tracer eventually enters the vascular system, delayed images *should* demonstrate intracranial activity.
- *Cerebrovascular disease:* Severe bilateral carotid artery disease may cause decreased or delayed perfusion of the brain on angiographic images. However, significant cerebral activity would be seen on delayed images (with HMPAO or ECD).

Essential Facts

- Brain death is caused by a catastrophic cerebral anoxia leading to cerebral edema, elevated intracranial pressures, and lack of intracranial blood flow.
- The diagnosis can be established with a combination of clinical features (e.g., no cranial nerve reflexes or pain response), electroencephalography (EEG), and scintigraphy. Reversible causes (hypothermia, drugs) must be excluded.
- Almost any radiotracer can be used as the early dynamic angiographic agent. The typical ones are all Tc99m-labeled and include pertechnetate, DTPA, glucoheptonate, HMPAO (Ceretec), and ECD (Neurolite). Tc99m agents are best because of the higher count rate and ideal dynamic imaging characteristics.

Other Imaging Findings

- The hot nose sign seen in Figure A is due to preferential flow to the external carotid circulation, given the lack of ICA perfusion.
- Scalp activity is normally seen because of flow through the external carotid arteries. A tourniquet can be used to avoid this occasionally confusing appearance in adults.
- Catheter cerebral angiography will also demonstrate no intracranial blood flow from any artery but is invasive.
- CT and MRI can demonstrate diffuse cerebral edema ± infarcts with brain death but are not specific.

✓ Pearls & × Pitfalls

✓ The use of a brain-specific agent such as HMPAO or ECD allows delayed imaging and therefore does not completely require a good bolus. In fact, no angiographic imaging is necessary with these agents. (They are more expensive and not as readily available as the blood flow–only tracers, however). Here are delayed HMPAO spot planar images in a different normal patient for comparison (SPECT not required):

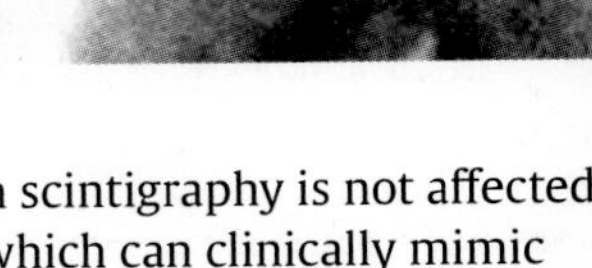

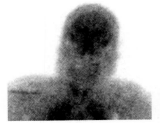

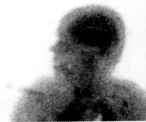

✓ Unlike EEG, brain perfusion scintigraphy is not affected by drugs or hypothermia, which can clinically mimic brain death (perfusion scan will be normal).

× Venous activity in the transverse or sagittal sinus may be seen even in the setting of no ICA perfusion (brain death) because of scalp collaterals. A scalp tourniquet can be applied, or repeat imaging can be performed in 24 to 48 hours.

× A scalp tourniquet is contraindicated in children as this may raise intracranial pressure, or the tourniquet may exacerbate a traumatic brain injury.

× A tightly injected radiotracer bolus is critical for diagnostic angiographic images.

Case 19

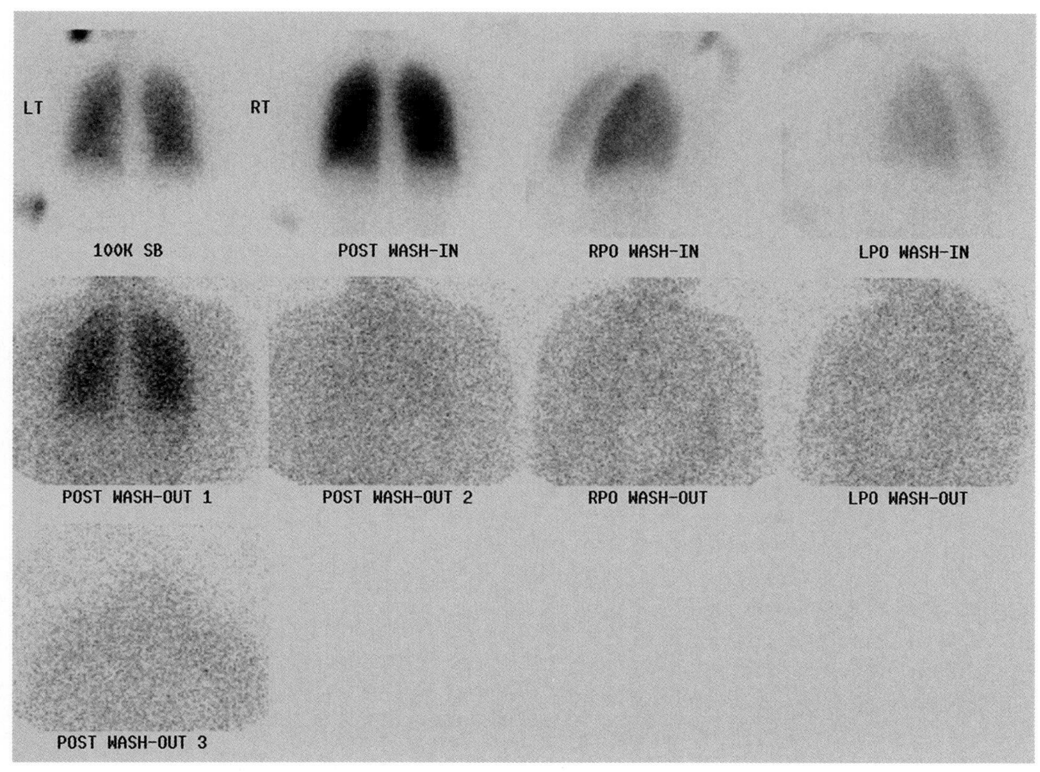

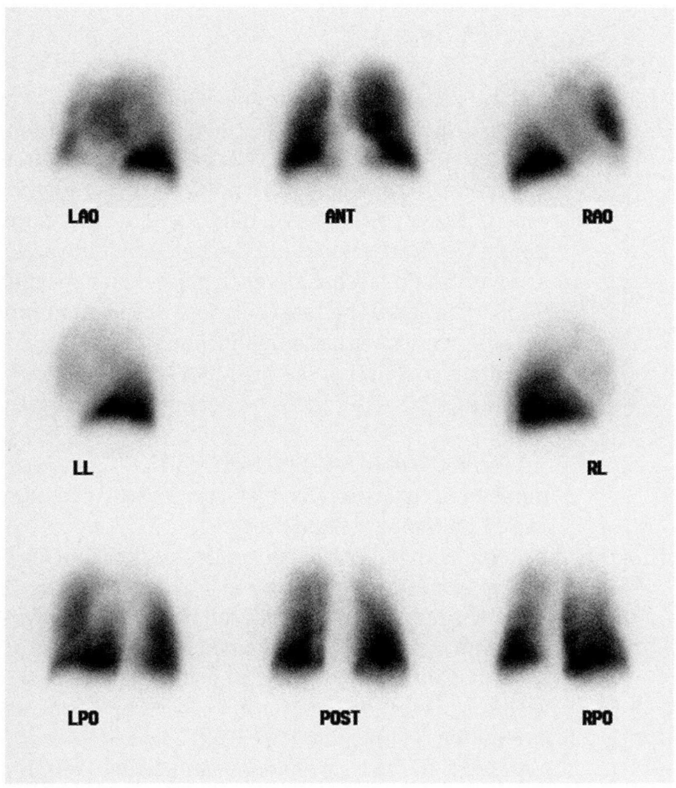

Clinical Presentation

A 35-year-old woman with recent shortness of breath. Chest radiographs were unremarkable.

Imaging Findings

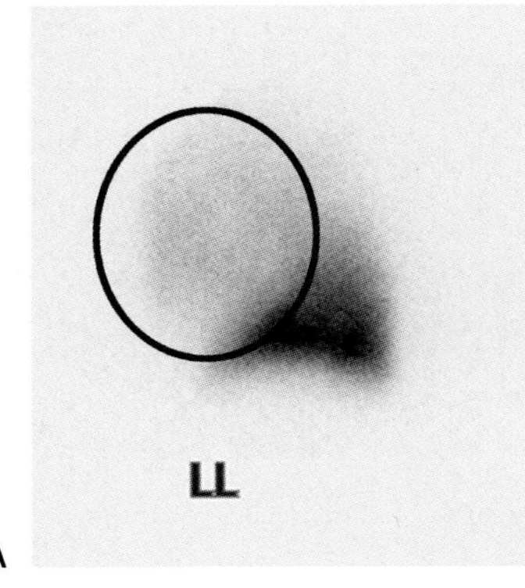

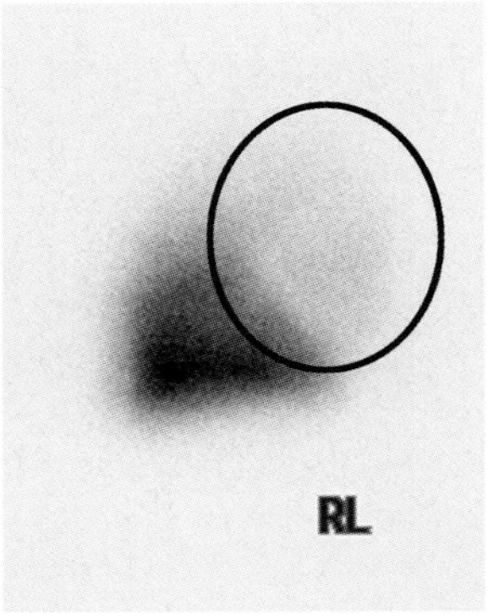

A B **(A,B)** Tc99m MAA perfusion images demonstrate significantly decreased perfusion to the upper lobes bilaterally, most dramatically on the lateral views (*circles*). Xenon 133 ventilation images are normal, so these are mismatched perfusion abnormalities.

Differential Diagnosis

- ***Artifact of upright Tc99m-MAA injection:*** Uniform, symmetric, markedly decreased perfusion to the upper lobes with normal ventilation makes this the most likely diagnosis.
- *High probability for pulmonary embolism (PE):* This also appears as large, mismatched perfusion defects. However, the defects are rarely this symmetric and most commonly include the lower lobes as well (lower lobes receive the most blood flow).
- *Asthma/chronic obstructive pulmonary disease:* This can commonly demonstrate symmetric upper lobe perfusion abnormalities. However, these will be secondary to *matched* upper lobe ventilation abnormalities.

Essential Facts

- Technical considerations are particularly important for proper lung ventilation–perfusion imaging.
- MAA injection should be performed over several respiratory cycles with the patient supine to properly visualize the entire (nonoccluded) pulmonary arterial bed. Compare with the normal appearance in this different patient properly injected with MAA while supine:

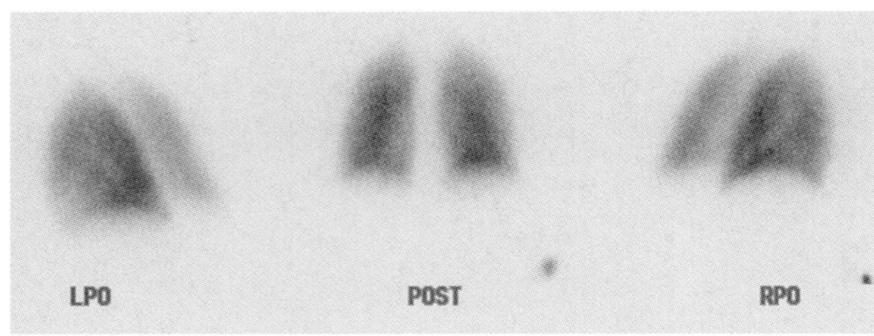

- Technologists are trained not to draw blood back into the MAA syringe before injection so as to avoid clumping and reinjection of "hot clots," which will also degrade image quality.
- Following MAA injection, perfusion imaging can be performed with the patient supine or upright (particles are fixed in place).
- Ventilation imaging (with Xe133 gas or Tc99m-DTPA aerosol) can also be performed with the patient supine or upright.

Other Imaging Findings

- CTA is commonly employed to detect PE and is not subject to these types of artifacts (the patient is always supine). However, CTA studies may be degraded by other factors, including improper contrast bolus timing or patient motion.

✓ Pearls & ✗ Pitfalls

✓ Red blood cells and capillaries have diameters of ~7 µm.

✓ MAA particles range from 5 to 100 µm, with most in the range of 10 to 30 µm. By U.S. Pharmacopeia regulation, 90% must be 10 to 90 µm, with no particle > 150 µm.

✓ For the injected Tc99m-MAA, radiation dose and number of particles are related but are independent variables that should be considered separately for specific patient conditions. The ratio between dose and number of particles varies with the freshness of the MAA kit.

✓ For adults, 3 to 5 mCi of Tc99m-MAA is administered. The *dose* of radioactivity can be decreased for pregnant women.

✓ A total of 200,000 to 600,000 MAA particles is typically administered to an adult (which temporarily occlude ~0.1% of pulmonary capillaries).

✓ In patients with pulmonary arterial hypertension (fewer capillaries) or known right-to-left shunts and in pregnant women, the number of *particles* can be reduced. However, a minimum of 100,000 is recommended to avoid the possibility of quantum mottle and an inadequate study.

✗ Regardless of method, ventilation should be performed *before* perfusion imaging. This avoids downscatter from Tc99m-MAA in the case of xenon ventilation (xenon has lower-energy photons) and prevents overwhelming the lower radioactivity in the case of aerosolized DTPA (because only ~1 mCi of DTPA makes it to the lungs vs. the ~4 mCi of MAA perfusion activity).

Case 20

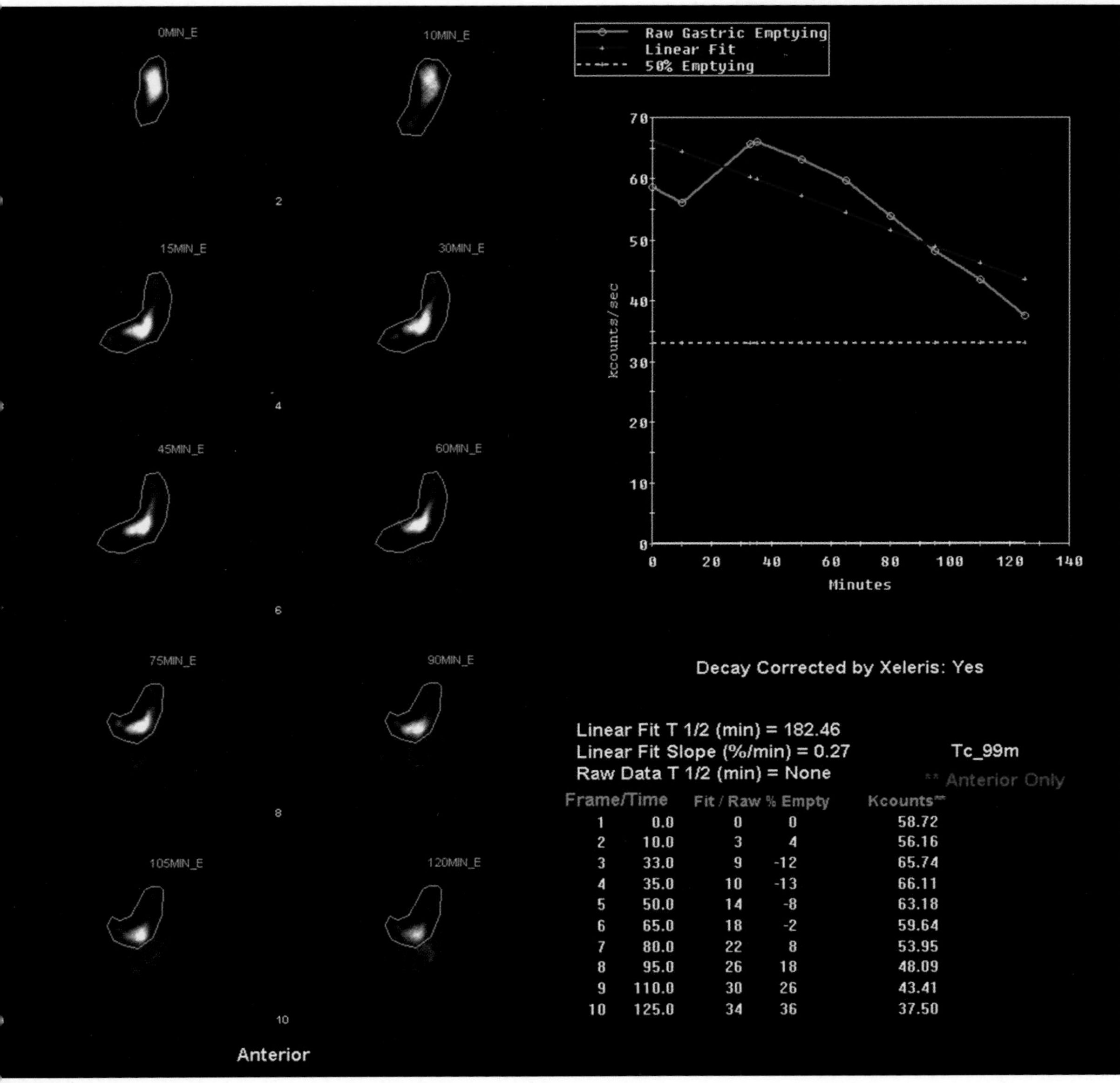

Clinical Presentation

A 49-year-old woman with nausea and early satiety.

Imaging Findings

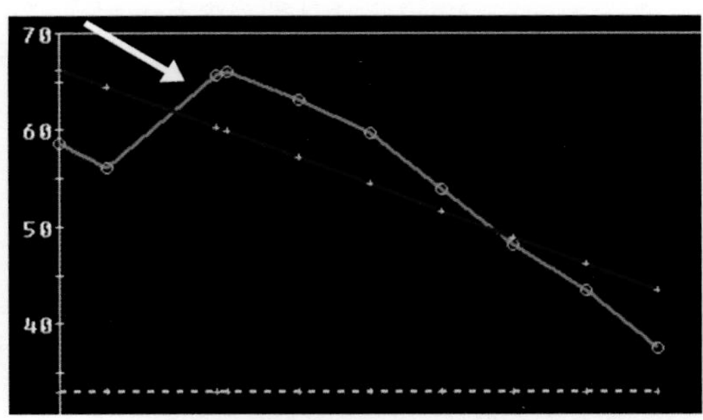

Anterior planar images from a solid-phase (scrambled eggs and toast) Tc99m SCOL gastric emptying study reveal a prolonged lag phase (*arrow*) and delayed tracer movement into the small bowel. The half-emptying time is > 120 minutes, and only 36% emptying is seen at 125 minutes.

Differential Diagnosis

Delayed transit of radiotracer into the small bowel has numerous causes, which cannot be differentiated by scintigraphy.

- ***Delayed gastric emptying:*** For a solid-phase meal, the half-emptying time is typically used as a measure to differentiate normal form abnormal. This time is highly variable and differs based on the various meals offered at different institutions.
- *Causes of delayed gastric emptying are numerous:* Some causes include diabetic gastroparesis, peptic ulcer disease, medications, prior surgery, obstruction, and hypothyroidism.

Essential Facts

- Gastric emptying is a complex process that depends on many variables, most importantly the content of the meal. Fat, protein, and carbohydrate all empty at different rates.
- Factors such as the time of day, size of the meal, gender, and patient position also affect emptying.
- Standardization of the test has been one of the most problematic aspects of the study, and each clinic should determine normal values based on its protocol and meal.
- Recently, a new protocol based on a standardized egg meal and using measurement of gastric retention (anterior/posterior geometric means) at 0, 1, 2, and 4 hours has gained acceptance, with normal gastric emptying > 90% at 4 hours.
- The gastric emptying curve for solids is biphasic. An initial lag phase is seen without any emptying, during which food is emulsified into particles small enough to exit the pylorus. This is followed by the linear emptying phase.
- Liquid emptying does not have a lag phase. It is also volume-dependent, slowing as volume decreases, so the curve is exponential, not linear. It is generally considered not as accurate an assessment of gastroparesis.
- Some of the more common causes of delayed gastric emptying include diabetic gastroparesis, peptic ulcer disease, and medications.

Other Imaging Findings

- Esophagogastroduodenoscopy or upper gastrointestinal studies can help exclude an anatomic abnormality such as ulcer disease, obstruction, or tumor.

✓ Pearls & ✗ Pitfalls

✓ This examination may be performed before and after the use of prokinetic agents to evaluate response to treatment.

✓ Anterior/posterior imaging with geometric mean analysis eliminates apparent increased gastric activity over time due to movement of radiotracer from the fundus to the antrum (posterior to anterior) seen in the anterior-only study.

✓ Rapid gastric emptying can be seen with hyperthyroidism, Zollinger–Ellison syndrome, and gastric surgery.

✗ Pay close attention to the first image to ensure that the region of interest includes all activity in the field of view, within the stomach, esophagus, and more distal bowel. In cases of rapid gastric emptying, tracer may already be in the bowel. Retention or reflux may be seen in the esophagus, which may give the appearance of delayed gastric emptying.

✗ Subsequent regions of interest must be evaluated to ensure that duodenal and bowel activity is excluded. Overlap of bowel and gastric activity will affect emptying calculations.

Case 21

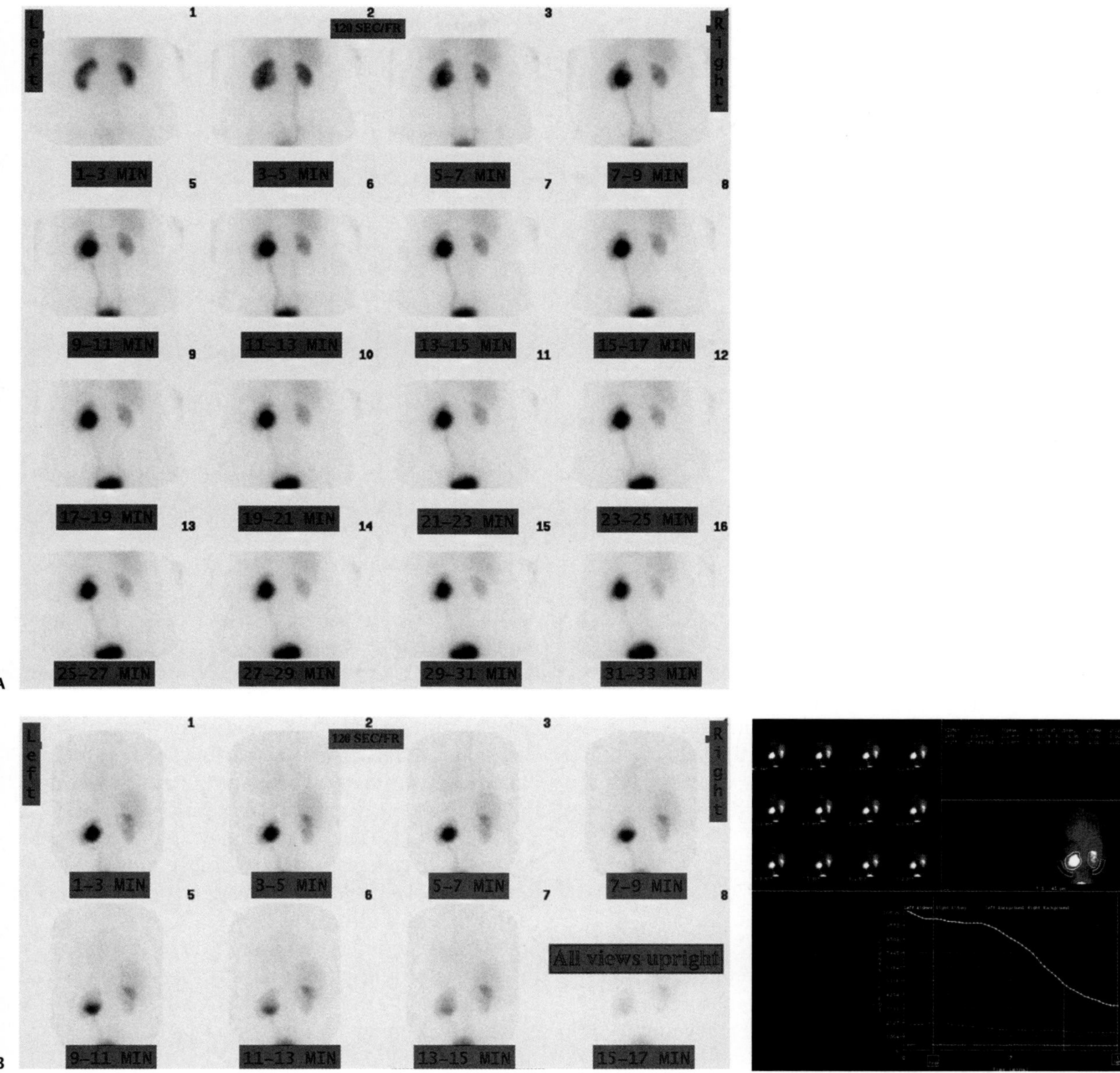

Furosemide administered at 3 minutes

Clinical Presentation

A 23-year-old woman with hydronephrosis detected on abdominal US.

Imaging Findings

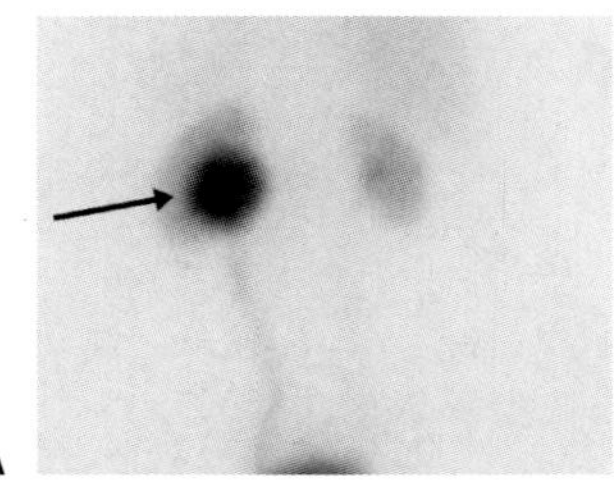
A

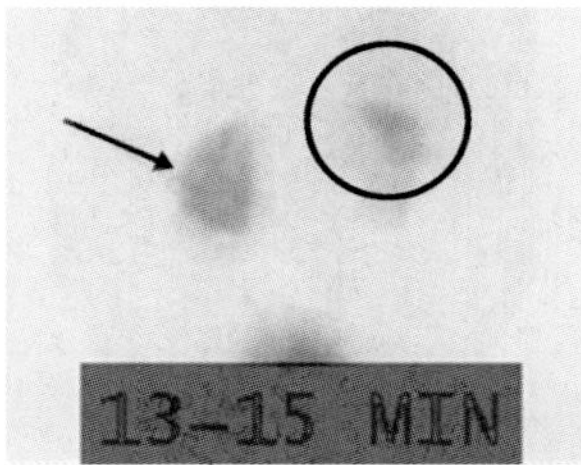

B

(A) Tc99m MAG3 renal scintigraphy demonstrates nearly symmetric renal parenchymal function (similar parenchymal counts at 1–3 minutes) but progressive radiotracer accumulation into a dilated renal pelvis on the left (*arrow*). Both ureters are seen and do not appear significantly dilated. **(B)** Following furosemide, there is rapid washout from the left collecting system (*arrow*) with a half-time of 9 minutes. Progressive physiologic excretion is seen in the gallbladder (*circle*), which can be seen with MAG3 (but not DTPA).

Differential Diagnosis

- ***Dilated but nonobstructed upper renal collecting system:*** Renal pelvocaliceal dilatation but with rapid washout into the bladder after diuretic makes this the most likely diagnosis.
- *Chronic reflux:* This can also have renal pelvic dilatation and rapid washout. However, some degree of ureteral dilatation can usually be appreciated as well.
- *Current renal obstruction:* This will also have pelvocaliceal dilatation but will demonstrate poor washout after diuretic.

Essential Facts

- A dilated renal collecting system may be caused by current obstruction, prior corrected obstruction, chronic reflux, or congenital syndromes (e.g., megaureter).
- Collecting system obstruction (current or previous) has several potential etiologies, including stones, congenital ureteropelvic junction atresia, acquired strictures, tumor, fungus ball, and blood clot.
- Current obstruction needs to be distinguished from mere dilatation and treated (relieved) to avoid complications, including renal parenchymal dysfunction. A dilated but nonobstructed system may be followed.
- Following the initial renal scintigram, a diuretic need be administered only in the presence of persistent tracer in a (usually dilated) collecting system. However, in young children, who may be sedated, the diuretic is often given as a default ("well tempered") before the prediuretic images are reviewed.
- Following diuretic, a half-time renal pelvic washout of < 10 minutes is considered normal, > 20 minutes obstructed, and 10 to 20 minutes indeterminate. A qualitative review of the images is also important, however.

Other Imaging Findings

- CT, MRI, and US will accurately demonstrate collecting system dilatation but are less reliable for determining current obstruction. Here is the CT scan of this same patient showing the dilated right upper system (*arrow*). It is uncertain if there is current obstruction based on this CT scan:

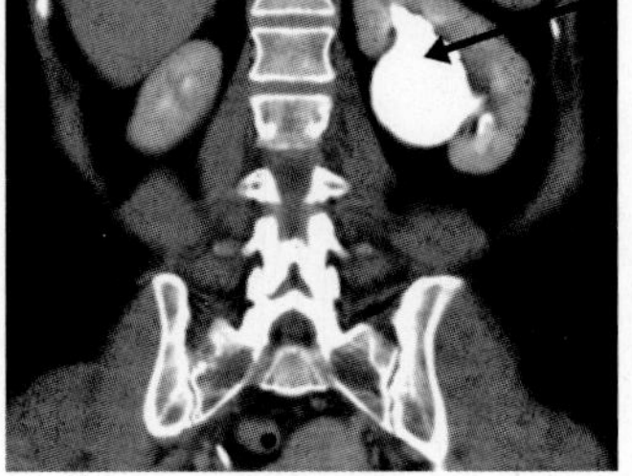

✓ Pearls & ✗ Pitfalls

- ✓ A well-hydrated patient is essential for accurate diuretic renal scintigraphy.
- ✓ Both Tc99m-DTPA and -MAG3 can be used for dynamic renal scintigraphy, including with diuretic. However, MAG3 can demonstrate better collecting system accumulation, particularly as renal parenchymal function becomes impaired, owing to its unique excretion pathway (active tubular secretion vs. glomerular filtration with DTPA).
- ✓ Unlike DTPA, MAG3 can accumulate in the gallbladder as well (as in this case) and even move subsequently into small bowel on delayed images. This should not be confused with a urinary leak.
- ✓ Split renal function is determined by relative counts in the renal *parenchyma* (typically assessed on images between 1 and 3 minutes and before diuretic). Washout curves are generated from regions of interest around the *collecting systems*.
- ✗ The role of a diuretic is to "wash" tracer from the upper collecting system into the bladder, not from the renal parenchyma into the collecting system. If initial imaging demonstrates persistent renal parenchymal retention and little collecting system activity, then additional delayed imaging should be performed before a diuretic is considered.
- ✗ Diuretic renal scintigraphy assumes sufficient renal parenchymal function to generate increased urinary washout flow. However, if there is significant parenchymal impairment from any cause, the scan may be falsely positive for obstruction or indeterminate.
- ✗ A nonobstructed but severely dilated pelvocaliceal collecting system may also have a false-positive result for obstruction because of pooling of tracer in the very large volume system, causing the appearance of slow washout.

Case 22

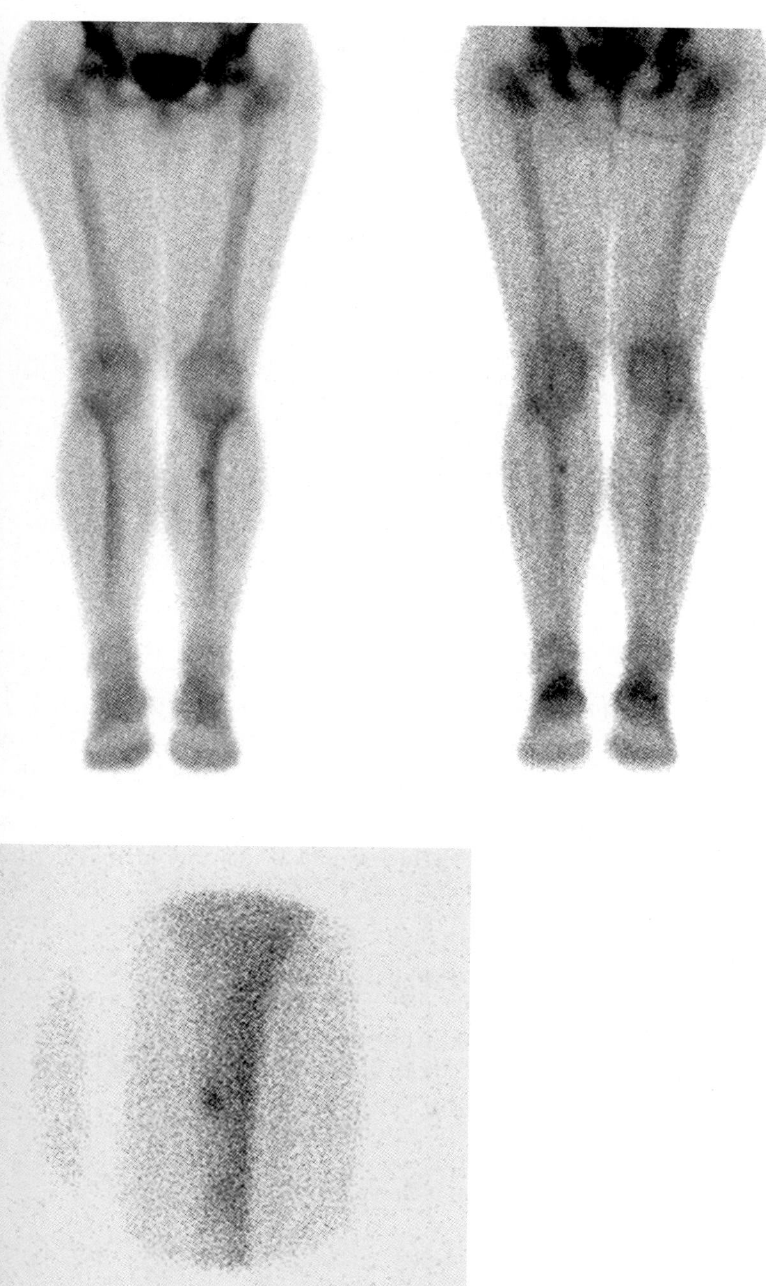

Clinical Presentation

A 23-year-old woman who is a runner presents with left leg pain.

Imaging Findings

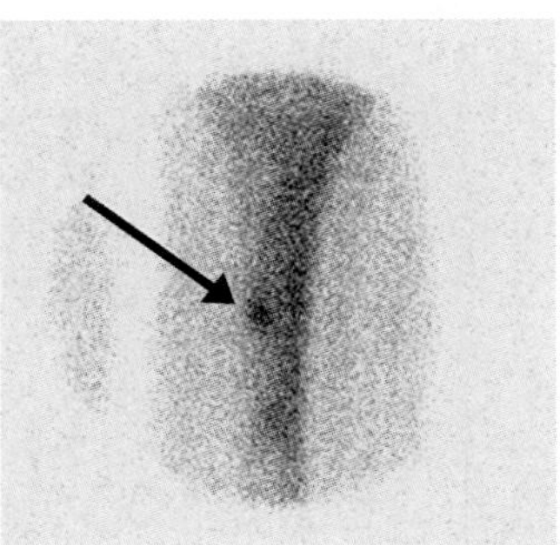

Anterior, posterior, and pinhole views from a bone scan demonstrate a small, cortically based focus of mildly to moderately increased radiotracer accumulation at the proximal left tibia medially (*arrow*).

Differential Diagnosis

- ***Stress fracture:*** The focal, cortically based uptake in a lower extremity makes this the most likely diagnosis, given the history. The fairly mild uptake suggests this may represent an early stress fracture/reaction.
- *Shin splints:* These will also show increased cortically based uptake in the lower extremities but are always located in the mid tibia, and the activity is segmental, running parallel to the bone.
- *Bone metastasis:* This will usually not be found distal to the middle femoral level and much more commonly involves the medullary, not cortical, bone (follows red marrow distribution; see Case 62).

Essential Facts

- Repetitive activity, typically in the lower extremity and with athletes, can lead to a spectrum of skeletal stress responses ranging from early stress reaction to a completed fracture.
- Patients will present with pain at or near the site of involvement and give a history of repetitive and/or recent change in activity.
- Stress fractures on bone scan will appear as *focal* or *fusiform* cortically based lesions and also usually appear hot on blood flow and blood pool images if acquired.
- Bone scan can help distinguish stress fractures involving the tibiae from shin splints, which are also caused by exercise and will produce pain in the posteromedial mid tibial level.
- Shin splints are thought to be caused by repetitive tugging of Sharpey fibers—tendinous insertions—of the soleus muscle on the bone.
- Bone scan of shin splints shows very linear, nonfocal cortical/periosteal uptake in the posteromedial mid tibiae; involvement is often bilateral but may be asymmetric or symmetric, as in this other patient (*arrows*) shown bottom left.

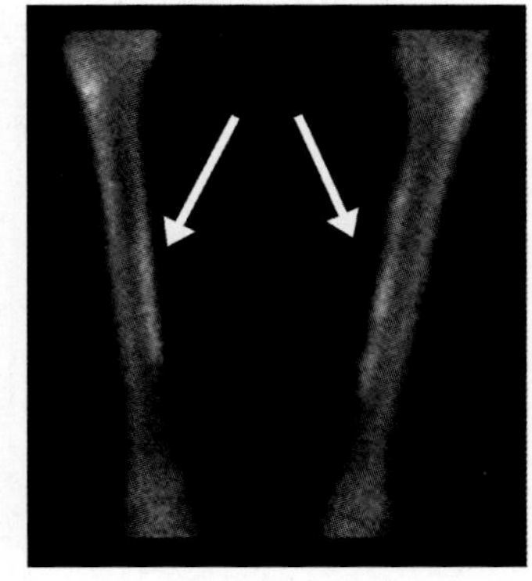

- Management is less aggressive for shin splints than for stress fractures, for which prolonged rest is required to avoid more significant injury (i.e., completed fracture).

Other Imaging Findings

- Plain radiographs are much less sensitive than scintigraphy for stress fractures but can demonstrate focal cortical thickening, sometimes with a lucent linear "Looser zone" perpendicular to the cortex; CT can demonstrate similar findings.
- MRI can sensitively demonstrate marrow edema (high T2 signal) and a linear low T1 signal for stress fractures.

✓ Pearls & ✗ Pitfalls

✓ Stress fractures, like completed fractures, tend to be hot on all three phases of a bone scan. Shin splints are hot only on delayed phase.

✗ In the small tubular bones of the feet, stress fractures may appear to involve the entire width of a bone, as in this different patient:

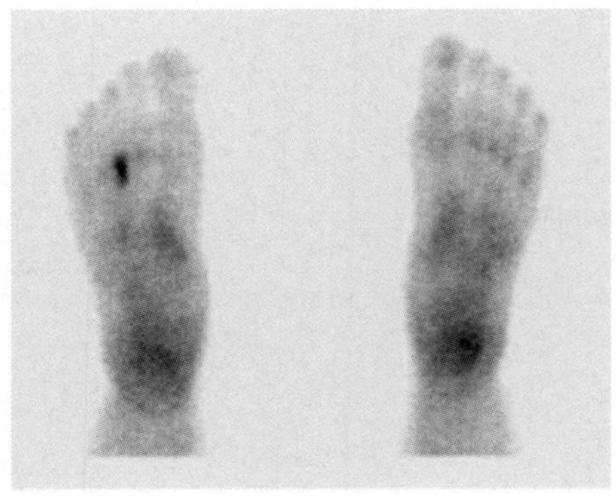

Case 23

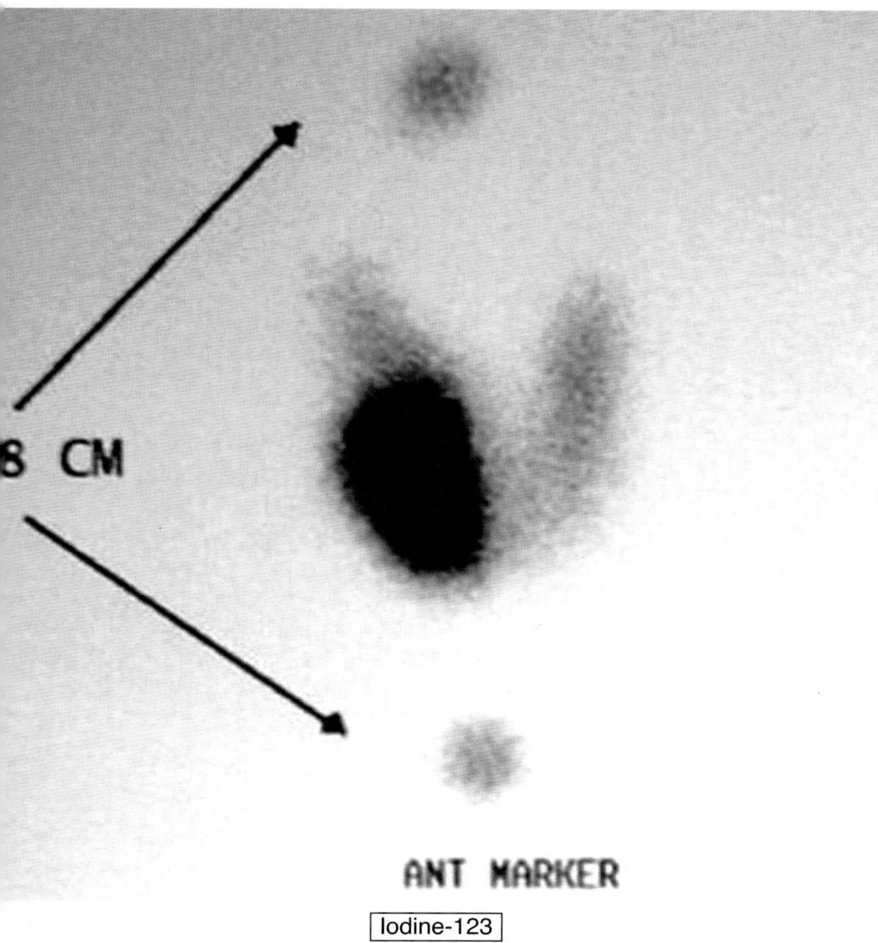

Iodine-123

Clinical Presentation

30-year-old man presents with a palpable nodule in the right neck and clinical hyperthyroidism.

Imaging Findings

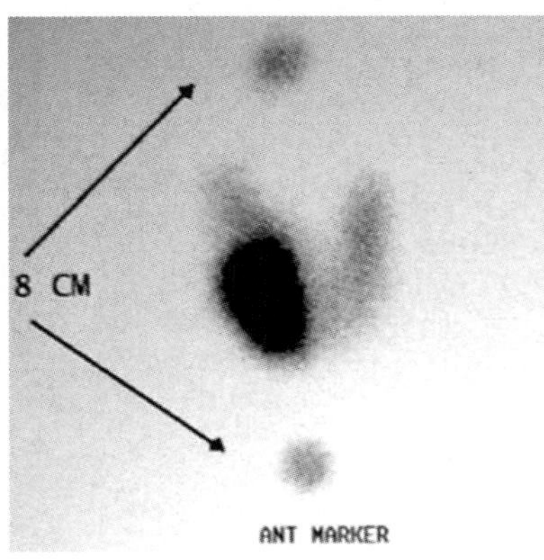

Iodine 123 thyroid scan image demonstrates a focus of increased activity at the right lower pole, with some suppression of the remainder of the gland.

Differential Diagnosis

- ***Toxic hyperfunctioning adenoma ("hot nodule"):*** Significant radioiodine accumulation by the nodule and some suppression of uptake in the remainder of the gland make this the correct diagnosis.
- *Functioning adenoma ("warm nodule"):* This will also have significant iodine accumulation but will not cause significant suppression of the remainder of the gland and is not typically toxic (does not cause hyperthyroidism).
- *Thyroid cancer:* Warm or hot nodules on a radioiodine scan (I123 or I131) are benign. Warm or hot nodules on a Tc99m pertechnetate thyroid scan *may* also be benign but require follow-up with a radioiodine scan to rule out a discordant nodule, which carries a 15 to 20% risk for malignancy (see Case 73).

Essential Facts

- Toxic hyperfunctioning adenomas are hot nodules with variable suppression of the remainder of the gland
- They account for 5% of solitary palpable nodules and are essentially always benign.
- A hot nodule is more likely to cause overt hyperthyroidism when it reaches 2.5 cm in size.
- Can be single or multiple, such as in this different patient with three hyperfunctioning nodules:

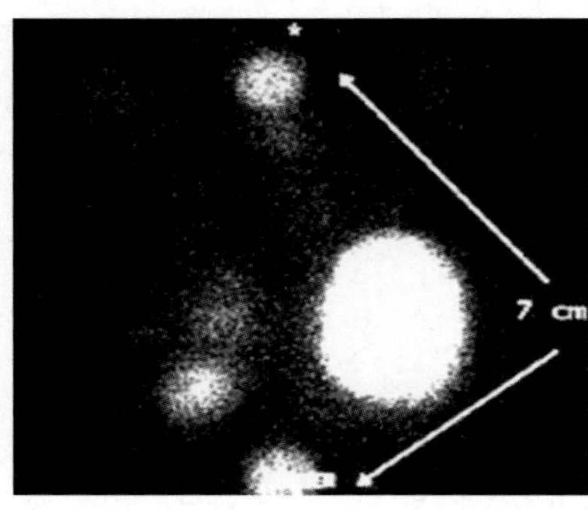

- Thyroid uptake values for a single hot nodule are typically normal (10–30%). Uptake values for multiple hot nodules may be mildly to moderately elevated, with clinical hyperthyroidism more common than for a single nodule.
- I131 ablation is the standard treatment for most hot nodule(s), although surgery is also an option. Toxic nodules are more resistant to radiotherapy than is Graves disease, so higher doses are typically used (often up to 33 mCi).

Other Imaging Findings

- US, CT, or MRI can demonstrate solid nodule(s). However, these are entirely nonspecific without the functional radioiodine thyroid scan.

✓ Pearls & ✗ Pitfalls

- ✓ Hot nodule(s) account for only 10% of patients with thyrotoxicosis. Graves disease is most common (70% of cases), followed by thyroiditis (20%).
- ✓ Both "warm" (functioning) and "hot" (hyperfunctioning) nodules are benign, but warm nodules are not associated with thyrotoxicosis and so typically are not treated.
- ✗ Nodules that are hot on radioiodine (organification) scan are benign; those that are hot on pertechnetate (trapping) are usually benign but should be followed with a radioiodine scan to rule out discordancy (cold on iodine). Discordant nodules remain indeterminate for malignancy.
- ✗ A known thyroid nodule (e.g., by palpation or ultrasound) that is not visible (as hot or cold) on a thyroid scan should be called warm (benign) only if one is certain that the appearance does not actually reflect a cold (indeterminate) nodule overlying normal thyroid tissue. For this reason, some authors insist that regarding a nodule, "if it's not hot, it's cold."

Case 24

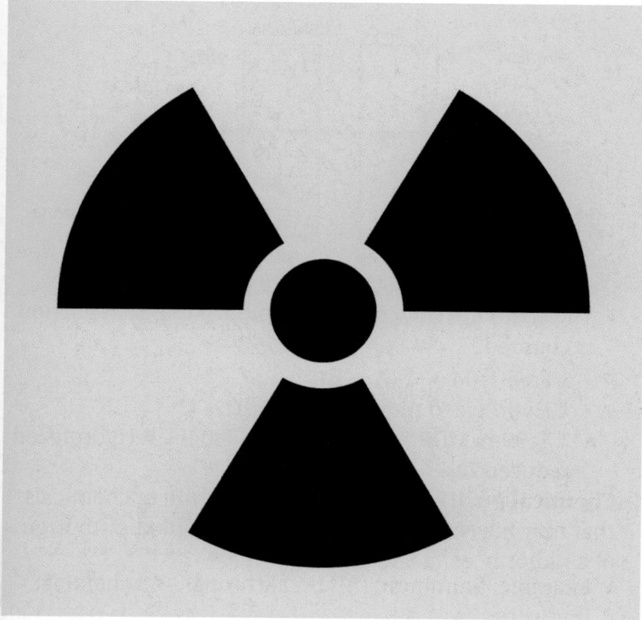

Clinical Presentation

The technologist is called in at 6:00 amto perform a Tc99m-MDP bone scan. Because unit doses are not available, the radiopharmaceutical must be made from a kit, and quality control needs to be performed.

Essential Facts

- **Radionuclidic purity** must be checked after elution of the generator. This is the fraction of the total radioactivity present in a radiopharmaceutical that contains the desired radionuclide.
  - Example: molybdenum 99 is a radionuclidic impurity found in Tc99m pertechnetate.
  - Testing method: dose calibrator
  - Allowable limits: < 0.15 µCi of Mo99 per mCi of Tc99m *at the time of administration.* Because of the longer half-life of Mo99, this ratio changes with time.
  - Adverse effects: increased radiation dose to the patient

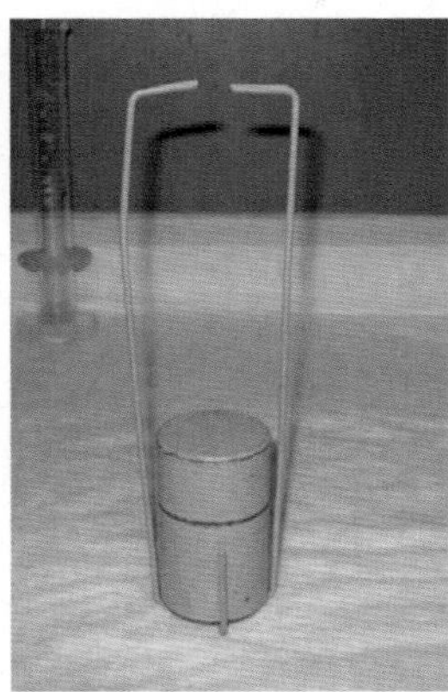

  - Procedure: A calibrated lead pig designed to work with the dose calibrator is used to measure the activity of the elution. This lead pig shields the 140-keV photons of the Tc99m and allows penetration of the higher-energy Mo99 (739 and 778 keV). This gives the activity (µCi) of Mo99. The elution is then measured in the dose calibrator directly, which gives the activity (mCi) of Tc99m. A ratio of Mo99 to Tc99m is then recorded.
- **Radiochemical purity** must also be checked. This is the fraction of the total radioactivity in a radiopharmaceutical that is present in the desired chemical from.
  - Example: free pertechnetate is a radiochemical impurity found in Tc99m-MDP.
  - Testing method: thin-layer chromatography
  - Allowable limits: the U.S. Pharmacopeia, not the Nuclear Regulatory Commission (NRC), sets limits for purity.
    - Tc99m pertechnetate (Tc04) ≥ 95%
    - Tc99m-SCOL ≥ 92%
    - Other Tc99m agents ≥ 90%.
  - Adverse affects: Altered biodistribution. Free pertechnetate can be seen as gastric and thyroid/salivary uptake.
  - Procedure: Silica gel and paper strips are used to separate radiochemicals. A drop of the radiopharmaceutical is placed near the bottom of each strip. The bottom of each strip is then placed in a solvent. Saline is used for the silica gel strip and acetone is used for the paper strip. Radiochemicals then separate to the top and bottom of each strip as follows:

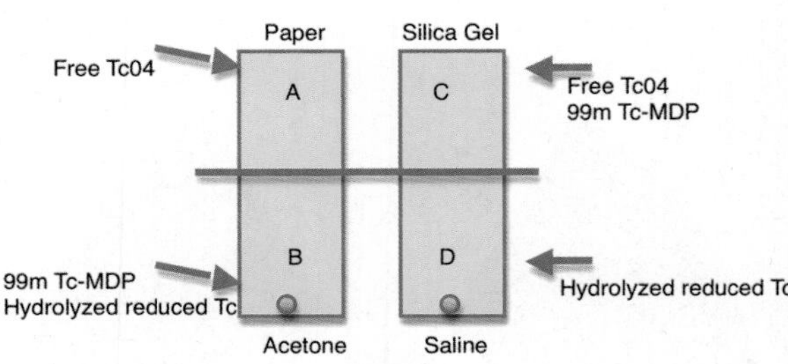

  - The strips are then cut in the middle and each portion is counted.
    - % Free Tc04 = A/(A + B)
    - % Hydrolyzed reduced Tc = D/(D + C)
    - % Tc99m-MDP = 100 − (% Free Tc04 + % Hydrolyzed reduced Tc)
- **Chemical purity:** this is the concentration of chemicals that may adversely affect labeling or the biodistribution of a radiotracer.
  - Example: aluminum (Al) breakthrough is a chemical impurity.
  - Testing method: colorimetry
  - Allowable limits: aluminum must be < 10 ppm.
  - Adverse affects: Altered biodistribution. Al+ in Tc99m MDP causes liver uptake (due to colloid formation) and Al+ in Tc99m-SCOL causes lung uptake.
  - Procedure: A standard 10-ppm solution of aluminum is used and compared with the elution. A drop of each is placed on a test strip, and visual comparison of the color is made. Intensity of the elution should be less than that of the aluminum standard.

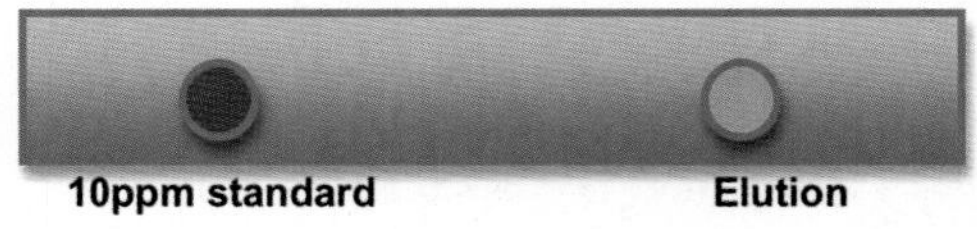

✓ Pearls & × Pitfalls

✓ With Tc99m-MAA and Tc99m-SCOL, only free pertechnetate is tested for when radiochemical purity is checked.

✓ Chemical purity testing is no longer mandatory in NRC states.

× The Mo99:Tc99m ratio must be known at the time of *injection*, not elution.

× When molybdenum breakthrough is tested for, the Mo99 must be assayed before the Tc99m to prevent error due to residual charge in the calibrator.

Case 25

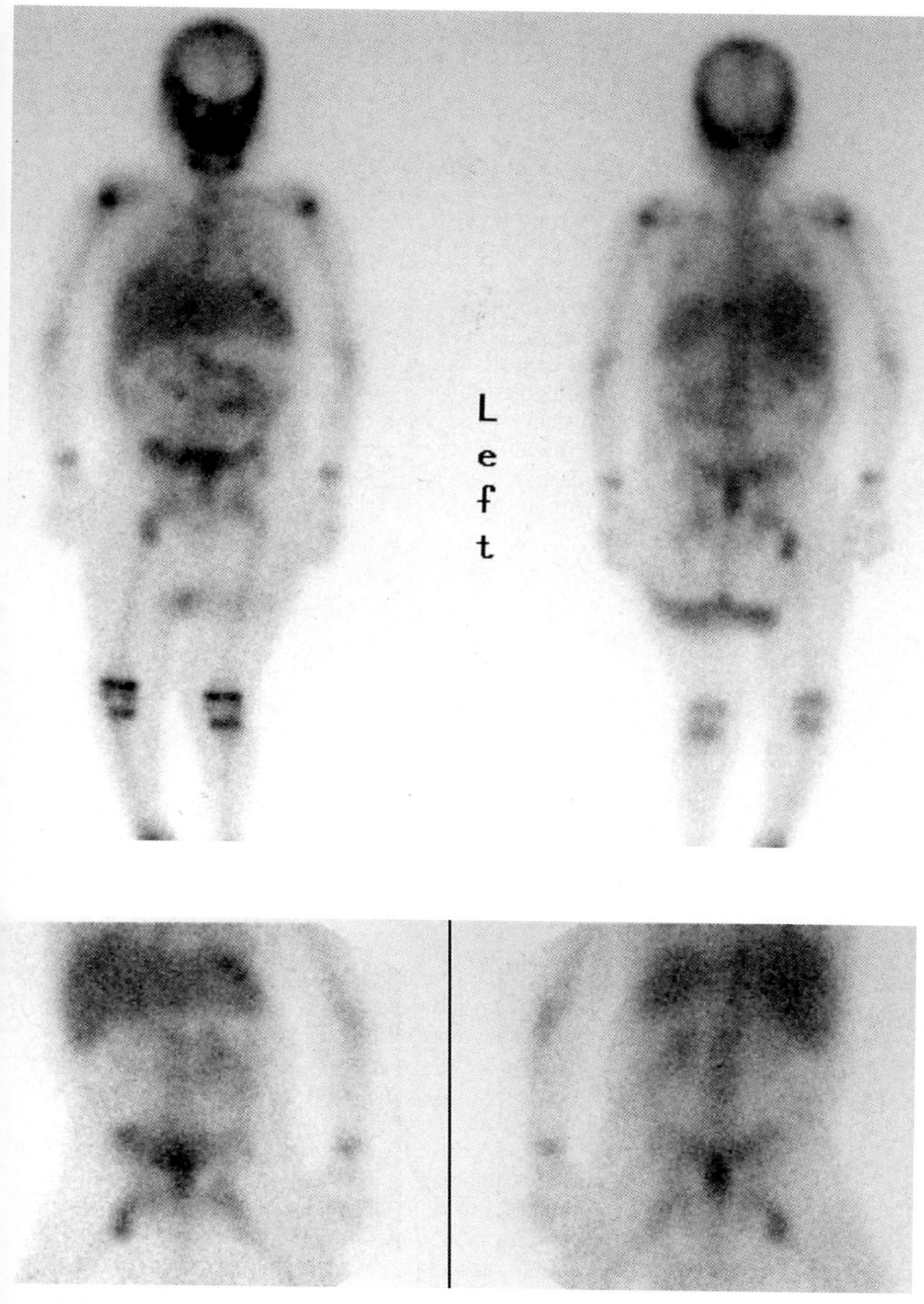

Clinical Presentation

6-year-old boy with a fever of unknown origin.

Imaging Findings

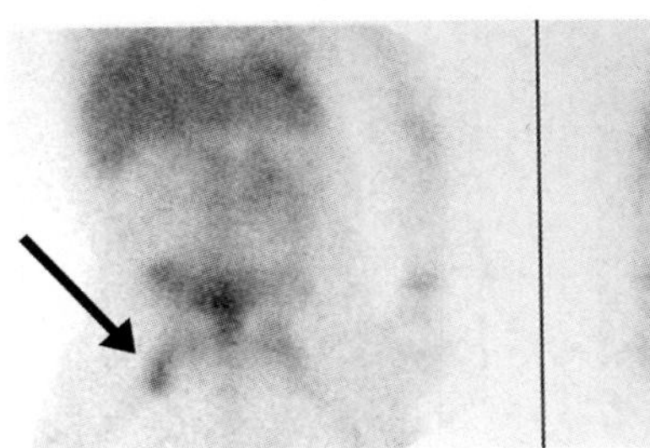
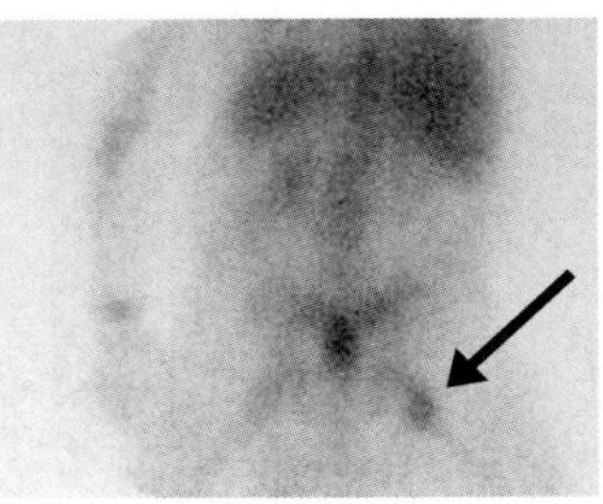

Anterior and posterior whole-body and spot pelvic views demonstrate focally increased activity in the right proximal femur (*arrows*). Physiologic salivary, hepatic, splenic, osseous, and bowel activity is seen.

Differential Diagnosis

- ***Gallium scan showing osteomyelitis:*** Focally increased osseous activity makes this the most likely diagnosis, given the history.
- *Gallium scan showing a bone metastasis:* This could have a similar appearance, but without additional foci or a history of malignancy, it is less likely.
- *Gallium scan showing a hip fracture:* This could have a similar appearance but is less likely, given the history.

Essential Facts

- Ga67, an iron analogue with uptake mediated by transferrin receptors, is a nonspecific neoplasm and infection/inflammation imaging agent.
- In addition to imaging tumors like lymphoma, gallium is used to assess for sarcoid, pulmonary infections including *Pneumocystis carinii/jiroveci* pneumonia (PCP), fever of unknown origin (FUO), and diskitis/spinal osteomyelitis.
- Given the significant physiologic bowel excretion, Ga67 sensitivity for abdominal infection is decreased, and indium 111 WBCs may be superior if the CT result is negative.
- Osteomyelitis is typically due to bacteria such as *Staphylococcus aureus*, can be multifocal, and is most common in children and immunocompromised adults.

Other Imaging Findings

- Three-phase bone scintigraphy is a good test for osteomyelitis, assuming the underlying bone is otherwise normal. However, for this FUO work-up, gallium is more appropriate to survey both bone and soft tissue for infection or tumor.
- To assess for infected joint prostheses, dual In111 WBC/Tc99m SCOL imaging looking for *discordant* WBC accumulation is most specific.
- For diabetic feet, dual bone scan/WBC scan imaging looking for *concordant* uptake in osteomyelitis is most specific to avoid false-positives from neuropathic joints (on bone scan) or cellulitis (with WBC alone).
- Plain radiographs can demonstrate bone destruction and periostitis in advanced osteomyelitis but are insensitive for early infection.
- MRI is sensitive for osteomyelitis but can be nonspecific (e.g., with neuropathic joint or bone marrow edema without infection) and cannot easily assess the entire skeleton. Here is the fat-suppressed MRI for this same patient showing the lesion (*circle*):

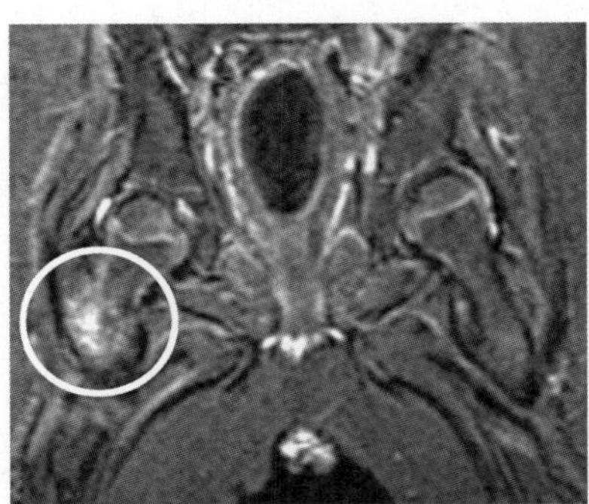

✓ Pearls & × Pitfalls

- ✓ Whole-body gallium and whole-body WBC scans as an unknown can look similar with normal liver, spleen, and bone marrow. However, WBC has spleen > liver and no bowel (with In111 label), and gallium has liver ≥ spleen with lacrimal uptake (see "Interpreting Whole-Body Scans").
- ✓ Although there is considerable overlap between gallium and WBC imaging for infection, gallium tends to be superior to WBC for spinal osteomyelitis/diskitis, more chronic infections, and some pulmonary infectious/inflammatory processes, including PCP and sarcoid.
- ✓ Rotational artifact can produce asymmetric uptake, especially at the hips, on any type of nuclear scan. However, uptake that is increased on both anterior and posterior projections must be real.
- × Normal gallium biodistribution includes bone *cortex* in addition to bone *marrow* (Ga67 is also a "poor man's bone scan"). Hence, anything that can be hot on a (cortical) bone scan, including degenerative joint disease, simple fractures, and normal growth plates in children, will be hot on gallium.

Case 26

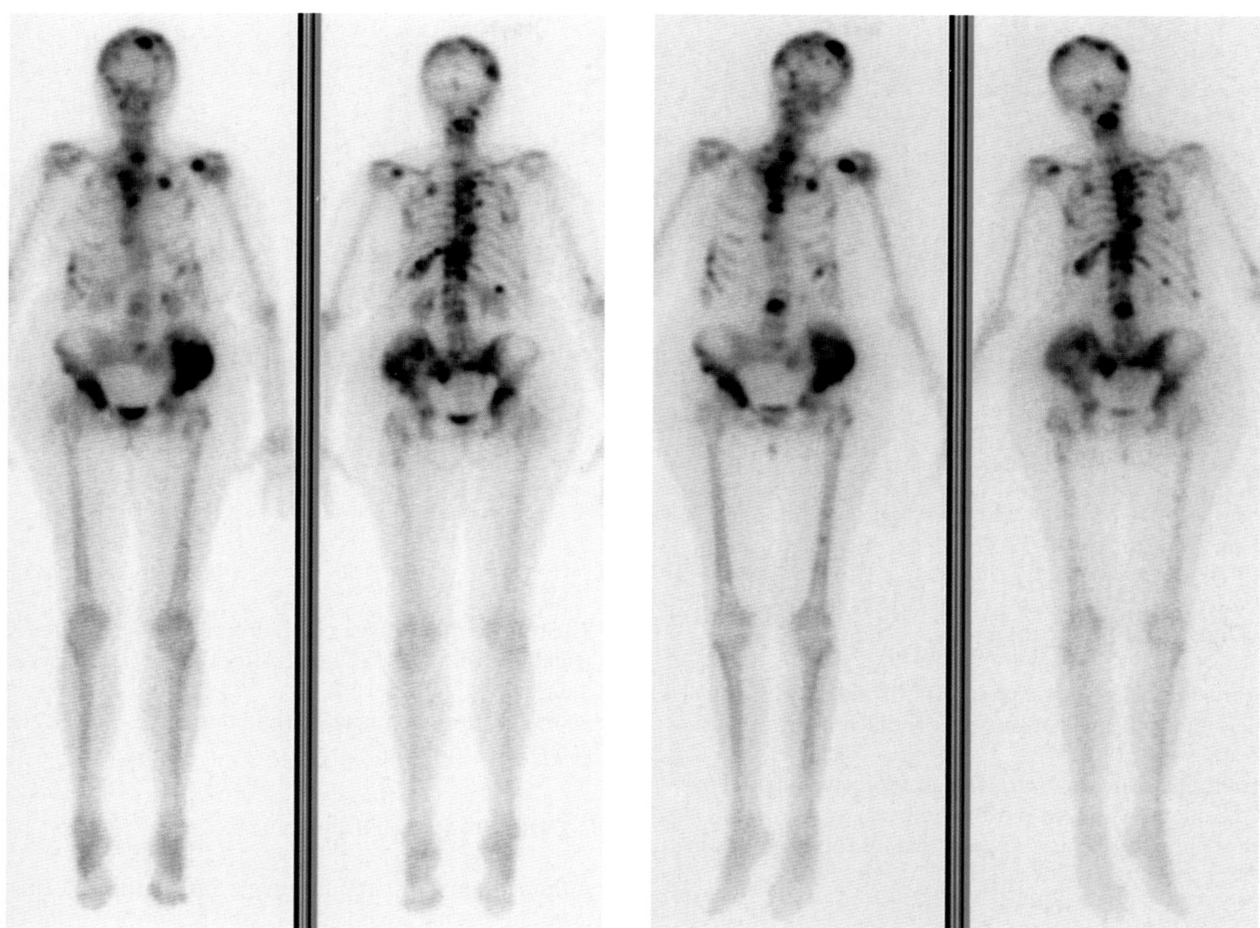

Clinical Presentation

. 67-year-old woman with breast cancer and severe bone pain from multiple bony metastases. Figure A demonstrates ne patient's standard bone scan. The patient then received a palliative radionuclide therapy, and the scan in Figure B was btained. What therapy did the patient receive?

Imaging Findings

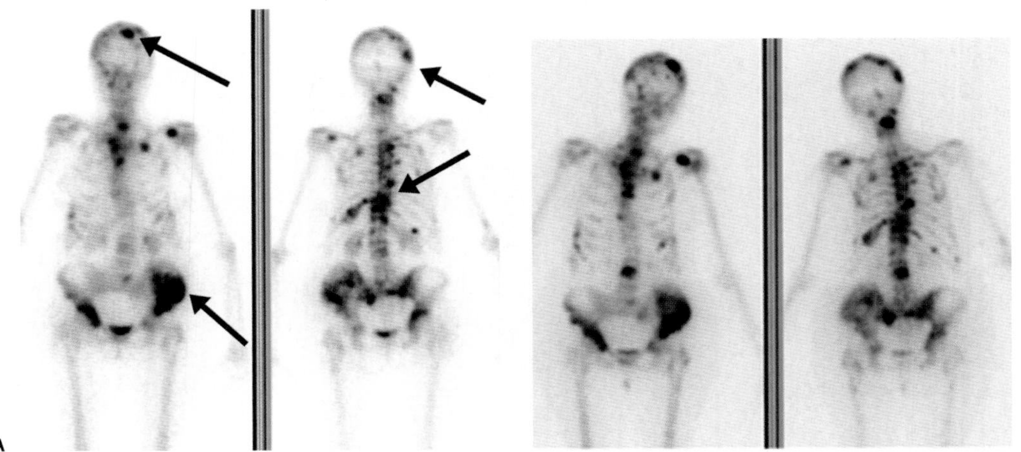

(A) Three-hour delayed anterior and posterior whole-body bone scan images demonstrate innumerable osteoblastic metastases to the axial skeleton (*arrows*). **(B)** Anterior and posterior whole-body post-therapy images demonstrate uptake patterns similar to those in the whole-body bone scan, again revealing innumerable axial osteoblastic bony metastases.

Differential Diagnosis

- ***Samarium 153 (Quadramet):*** This is the only osseous therapeutic agent that can be adequately imaged (both β- and γ-emitter).
- *Strontium 89 (Metastron):* This is approved for therapy but cannot be imaged (pure β-emitter).
- *Phosphate 32:* This is also approved for therapy but cannot be imaged (pure β-emitter).

Essential Facts

- Patients with significant pain from widespread osteoblastic metastases are candidates for palliative treatment of symptoms with bone-seeking, β-emitting radiopharmaceuticals.
- All three radiopharmaceuticals above are approved by the U.S. Food and Drug Administration and can be used for this type of therapy. (Patients with local bone pain from limited lesions can undergo external-beam radiation.)
- These tracers bind to increased osteoblastic sites surrounding tumor and undergo β-emission; osseous prostate and breast cancer metastases are most commonly treated.
- Pain reduction is likely achieved through cytoreduction, decreased intramedullary pressure, and radiation-induced apoptosis of lymphocytes secreting pain-modulating cytokines.
- Eighty percent of patients may have a partial or complete symptomatic response.
- Myelotoxicity is the primary adverse event, causing thrombocytopenia and leukopenia. A transient increase in pain can also occur early, before eventual pain reduction.
- The transient increase in pain occurs in 10% of patients, usually within 48 to 72 hours after therapy, and lasts 2 to 3 days.
- Pain relief does not usually begin until after 1 week and can last up to a year.

Other Imaging Findings

- Although some institutions image Sm153 therapy, this is not necessary. No imaging can be performed using the other agents (because they are not γ-emitters).

✓ Pearls & × Pitfalls

- ✓ A *plastic* syringe shield should be used. With a lead shield, the lead–β-particle interaction would increase the radiation dose to the injecting individual.
- ✓ This therapy improves quality of life, not survival.
- ✓ If a patient has a positive response but pain has returned, additional doses may be given at ~3- to 6-month intervals.
- ✓ Radiation safety: Most undergo outpatient treatment with only verbal instruction of radiation safety precautions. Documented written instructions are usually not required unless higher-than-normal doses of Sm153 are given.
- × If the metastatic bone lesions are not osteoblastic or the cause of the pain is not skeletal, these therapies will not be effective. Documentation of blastic lesions on bone scan before therapy is preferable.
- × Therapy is contraindicated in patients with low platelet or WBC counts.
- × Myelosuppression can occur in any patient. The nadir for platelets is at ~4 weeks. The nadir for WBCs is at 2 to 4 weeks, with levels normalizing by 7 weeks.

Case 27

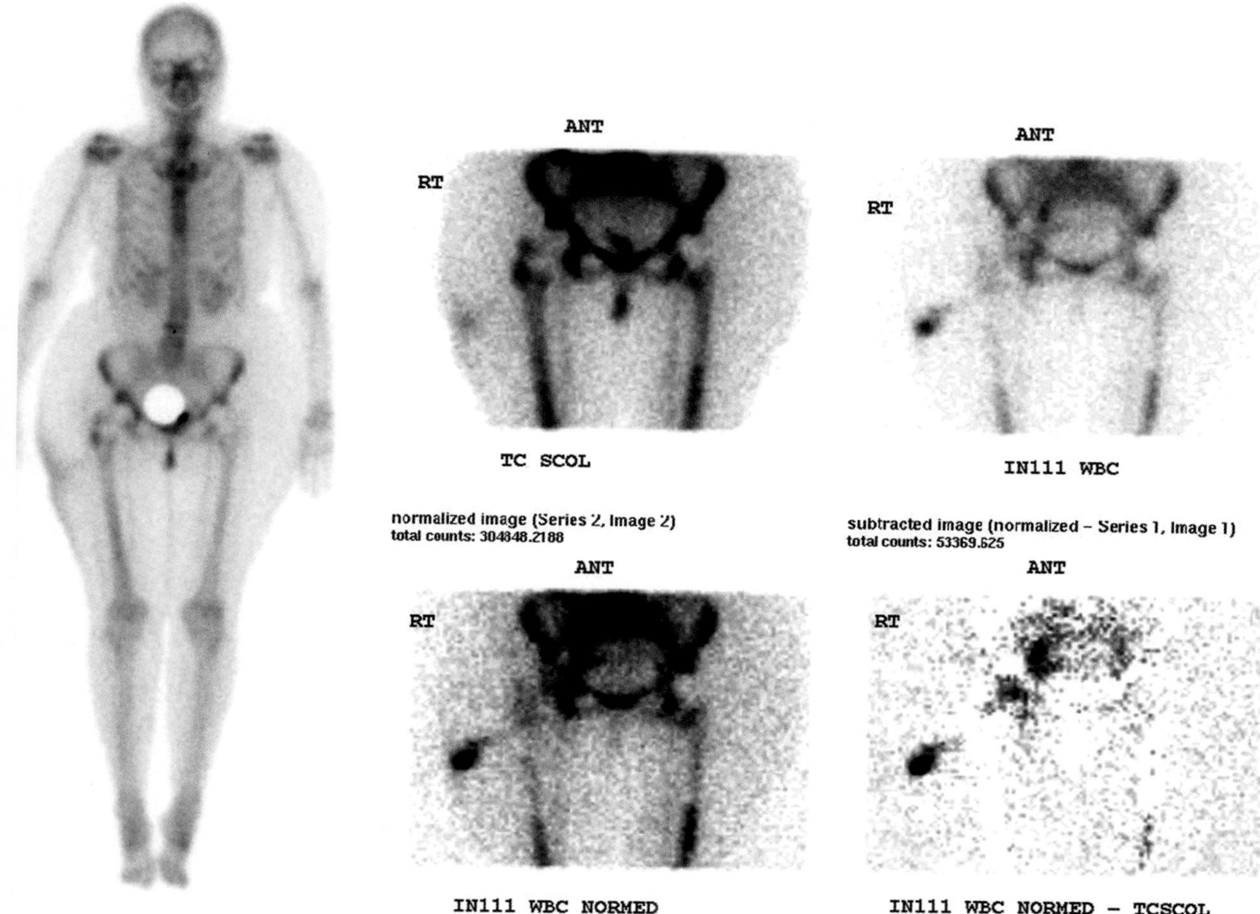

A

B

Clinical Presentation

A 65-year-old woman with right hip pain.

Imaging Findings

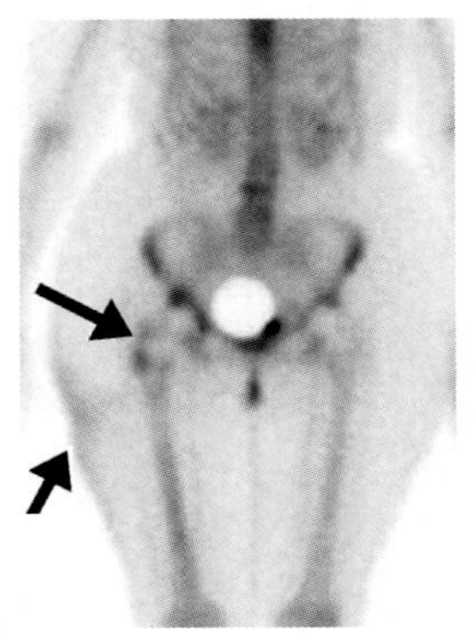

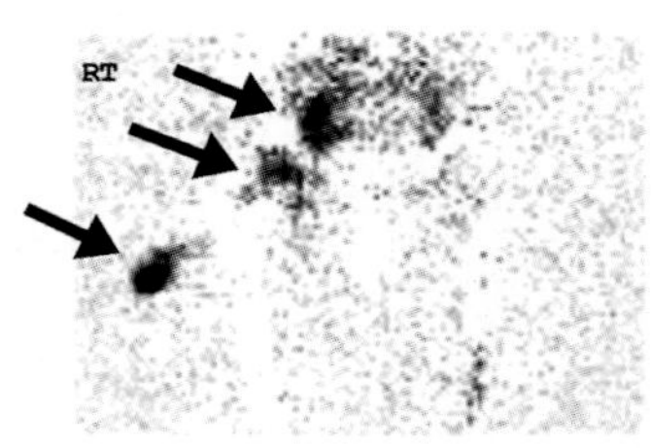

(A) Anterior image from a Tc99m whole-body bone scan reveals increased uptake in the region of the greater trochanter as well as in the region of the femoral neck on the right (*long arrow*). Photopenic hip hardware is noted bilaterally. Soft-tissue uptake is noted on the lateral aspect of the right upper thigh (*short arrow*). Mildly increased activity at the right acetabulum is likely degenerative. **(B)** Simultaneously obtained Tc99m-SCOL and indium 111–tagged WBC scans with different energy windows. Once the two images were obtained, the In111-tagged WBC image was normalized to the Tc99m SCOL study by counts, and the latter image was subtracted from the former on a pixel-by-pixel basis. The subtracted image reveals discordantly increased In111-tagged WBCs in the lateral thigh soft tissues, right hip joint, and pelvis adjacent to the right hip (*arrows*).

Differential Diagnosis

- ***Infected prosthesis (with right thigh cellulitis and pelvic abscess):*** WBC accumulation out of proportion to SCOL accumulation indicates an infected joint, which is also usually increased on bone scan. Abnormal WBCs in the right thigh as well as pelvic soft tissues indicate additional sites of infection.
- *Prosthetic loosening:* This would also have increased uptake on bone scan but would not have increased WBC accumulation.
- *Normal marrow packing:* This would have regions of increased and decreased activity on SCOL but would not have increased discordant WBC uptake and would not be increased on bone scan (after completion of postoperative healing).

Essential Facts

- A painful prosthesis may indicate infection or loosening.
- A negative bone scan argues against both, but a positive bone scan may indicate either.
- WBC scan alone is inaccurate because of the marrow replacement ("packing") or proliferation/activation that follows prosthetic placement.
- SCOL scan will map only the patient's normal marrow. WBC scan goes to normal marrow as well as infected bone and soft tissue.
- An infected prosthesis can be in an early or late stage. The early-stage infection occurs within 3 to 8 weeks. Treatment consists of washing out the joint and treating with intravenous (I.V.) antibiotics.
- The late-stage infection can occur months to years later. During this stage, the hardware is removed and I.V. antibiotics are instituted until the infection is cured, at which time the prosthesis can be replaced.
- The total hip replacement infection rate is ~1 to 2%.

Other Imaging Findings

- Plain films can show bony resorption with loosening and destruction/periostitis with infection but are insensitive.
- Typically, MRI and CT are also limited because of metallic artifacts.
- Increased gallium 67 uptake (out of proportion to bone scan) can also suggest infection.
- FDG-PET has also shown promise in detecting active infection involving hardware and other sites.

✓ Pearls & ✗ Pitfalls

✓ When looking at bone scans, ensure that the soft tissue are evaluated for pathology (e.g., cellulitis, deep vein thrombosis), as demonstrated by this case.

✓ Concordant uptake of WBC and SCOL is consistent with marrow packing/activation, *not* infection.

✗ Following uncomplicated prosthesis placement, the bone scan is typically hot for 1 to 2 years, but this can persist for much longer in some cases.

✗ Following antibiotic therapy, a positive bone scan does not necessarily indicate persistent infection, as this can also be seen with bone healing.

Case 28

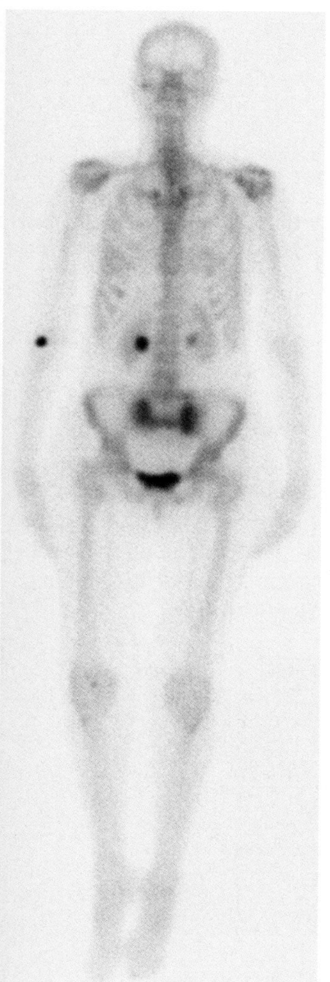

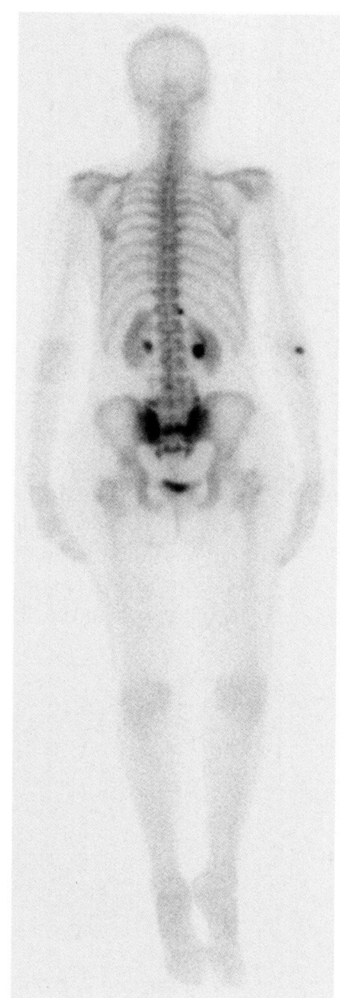

Clinical Presentation

A 66-year-old woman with a history of breast carcinoma and new low back pain.

Imaging Findings

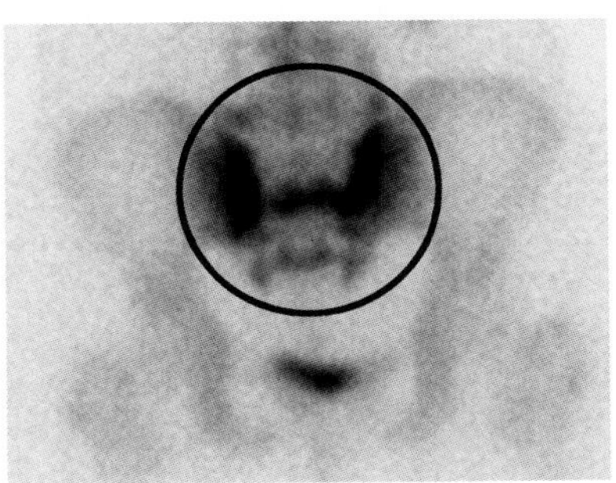

Tc99m-MDP bone scintigraphy demonstrates symmetric, linear, vertically oriented increased uptake through the sacral alae and a horizontal lesion through the sacral body (*circle*). A punctate focus at right T12 is likely degenerative.

Differential Diagnosis

- ***Sacral insufficiency fracture:*** Linear vertical uptake involving both sacral alae with horizontal uptake through the sacral body ("Honda" sign) is virtually pathognomonic for this entity.
- *Sacroiliitis:* This can look similar if bilateral but is centered at the sacroiliac joints themselves (slightly more laterally) and lacks the horizontal component.
- *Metastatic disease:* This commonly involves the pelvic bones but is not as linear or symmetric as seen here.

Essential Facts

- Sacral insufficiency fractures are seen most commonly in elderly women with osteoporosis, but can result from any cause of osteomalacia, such as steroid use or pelvic radiation.
- Presents with sudden and severe low back, groin, and/or hip pain following minor or unrecalled trauma
- May be associated with additional fractures in the pelvic ring as well as in other locations, such as a vertebra or rib
- Conservative management is usually sufficient, with healing often taking 6 to 9 months.

Other Imaging Findings

- Plain radiographs are insensitive for sacral insufficiency fractures but may demonstrate subtle lucent lines or sclerosis.
- CT may also demonstrate subtle fracture lines or sclerosis but is also fairly insensitive.
- MRI is sensitive, showing nonspecific edema and/or enhancement; linear fracture lines can also be seen.

✓ Pearls & ✗ Pitfalls

✓ Sacral insufficiency fractures can also be unilateral, demonstrating only one or two of the three "Honda" lines. Any linear, vertically oriented lesion involving a sacral ala, although not as specific as a bilateral fracture appearance, should have this entity included in the differential. Here is another patient's bone scan showing two-thirds of the "Honda" sign (*arrows*):

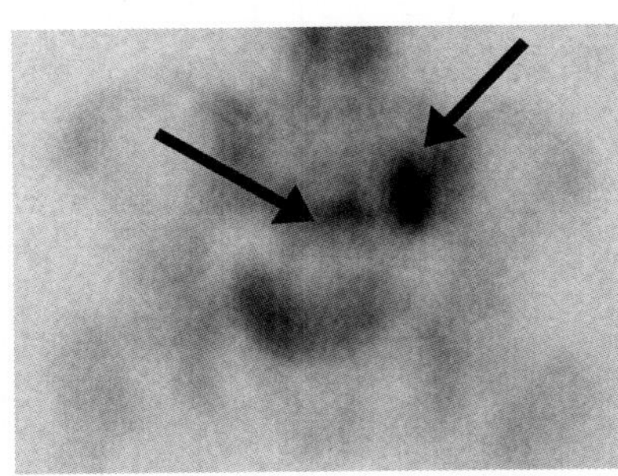

✗ The normal sacroiliac joints appear slightly more intense than the adjacent bones and should not be confused with pathology.

✗ Paget disease can also demonstrate curvilinear abnormal uptake in the pelvis. However, the location and symmetry seen in this patient would be unusual.

Case 29

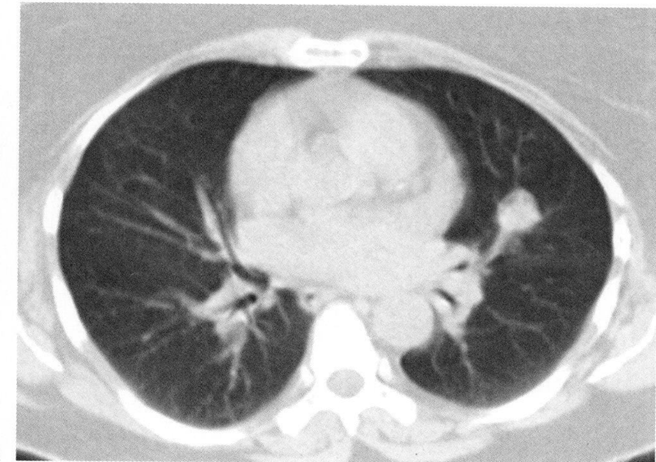

A

Clinical Presentation

A 53-year-old woman presents with a newly diagnosed solitary pulmonary nodule.

Further Work-up

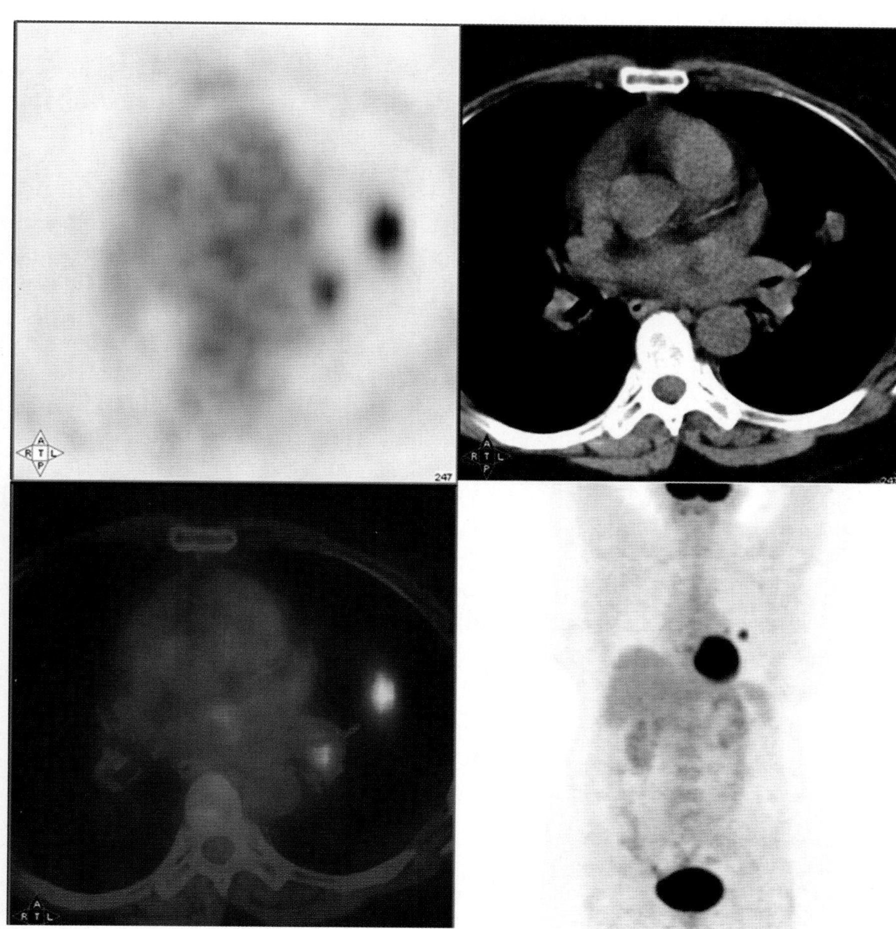

B

Imaging Findings

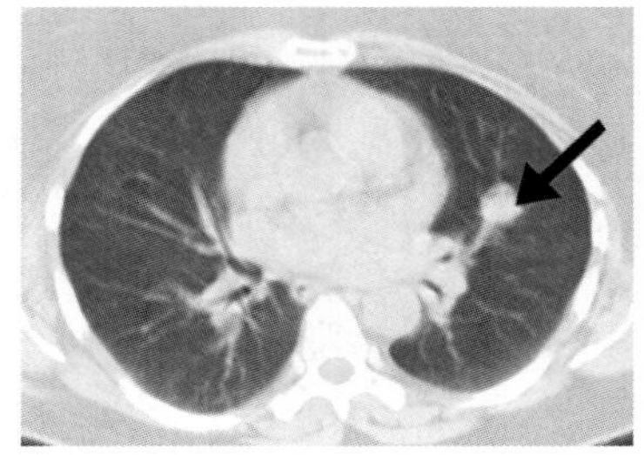
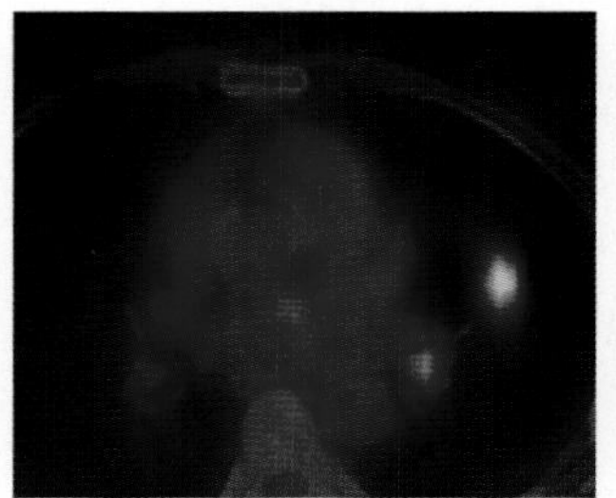
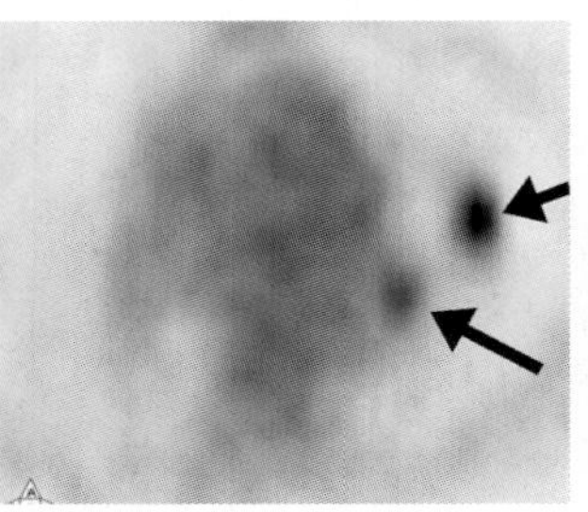

(A) Chest CT demonstrates a 1.5-cm noncalcified nodule in the left upper lobe (*arrow*). **(B)** FDG-PET/CT and PET demonstrate markedly increased activity to both the left lung nodule and a left hilar lymph node (*arrows*).

Differential Diagnosis

- ***Lung cancer with ipsilateral hilar metastasis*:** A hypermetabolic solitary pulmonary nodule (SPN) is lung cancer until proven otherwise; ipsilateral hypermetabolic mediastinal lymph nodes usually indicate regional metastases.
- *Tuberculosis (TB):* Active TB can be markedly hypermetabolic in the parenchyma and hila. However, the parenchymal lesion is often more infiltrative or cavitary; inactive TB may be calcified on CT and have lower FDG uptake.
- *Sarcoid:* This can demonstrate hypermetabolic pulmonary parenchymal and mediastinal soft tissue; however, the mediastinal activity is typically more symmetric with bilateral hilar and paratracheal uptake.

Essential Facts

- SPNs can be benign or malignant. Common calcification patterns (e.g., central, diffuse, "popcorn," laminated) on chest x-ray (CXR) or CT favor benign lesions such as granulomas or hamartomas; spicules favor lung cancer.
- SPNs indeterminate on CT can be further assessed by FDG-PET, which has a high positive predictive value and negative predictive value for malignancy and can also stage the whole body.
- Malignant SPNs have increased FDG uptake above the mediastinal blood pool and can represent small-cell or non–small-cell bronchogenic cancers and less commonly pulmonary carcinoid, lymphoma, or solitary pulmonary metastases.
- Benign SPNs have uptake ≤ blood pool with etiologies that include healed granuloma, hamartoma, avascular necrosis, and rheumatoid nodule.
- A history of tobacco or asbestos exposure and hemoptysis are often associated with lung cancer.

Other Imaging Findings

- CXR can detect and characterize an SPN (e.g., calcification, borders), but not as sensitively as CT.
- Chest CT can sensitively detect and characterize an SPN as well as guide percutaneous biopsy.
- Dynamic-contrast CT can assess for malignancy by identifying significant enhancement of the SPN; this is less expensive and may be more available than FDG-PET at some centers but is not as accurate.

✓ Pearls & ✗ Pitfalls

✓ SPNs as small as 7 to 10 mm can be accurately assessed on FDG-PET, depending on the type of scanner and location of the nodule (more breathing motion "artifact" at the lung bases).

✓ An SUV ≥ 2.5 is the most common indicator of suspicion for malignancy on PET, although some centers use SUV > 2.0, uptake > mediastinal blood pool, or significant uptake on the non-attenuation corrected images as suspicious.

✓ Besides malignancy, active infectious or inflammatory processes, including pneumonia and granulomatous diseases, can have markedly increased SUVs.

✗ Low-grade malignancies such as bronchoalveolar cancers can be falsely negative on PET; SPNs that are PET-negative have a low, but not zero, risk for malignancy and therefore should be followed on CT and biopsied if there is continued growth.

✗ SUV measurements can be variable and imprecise, fluctuating with a number of factors including patient body surface area and serum glucose.

Case 30

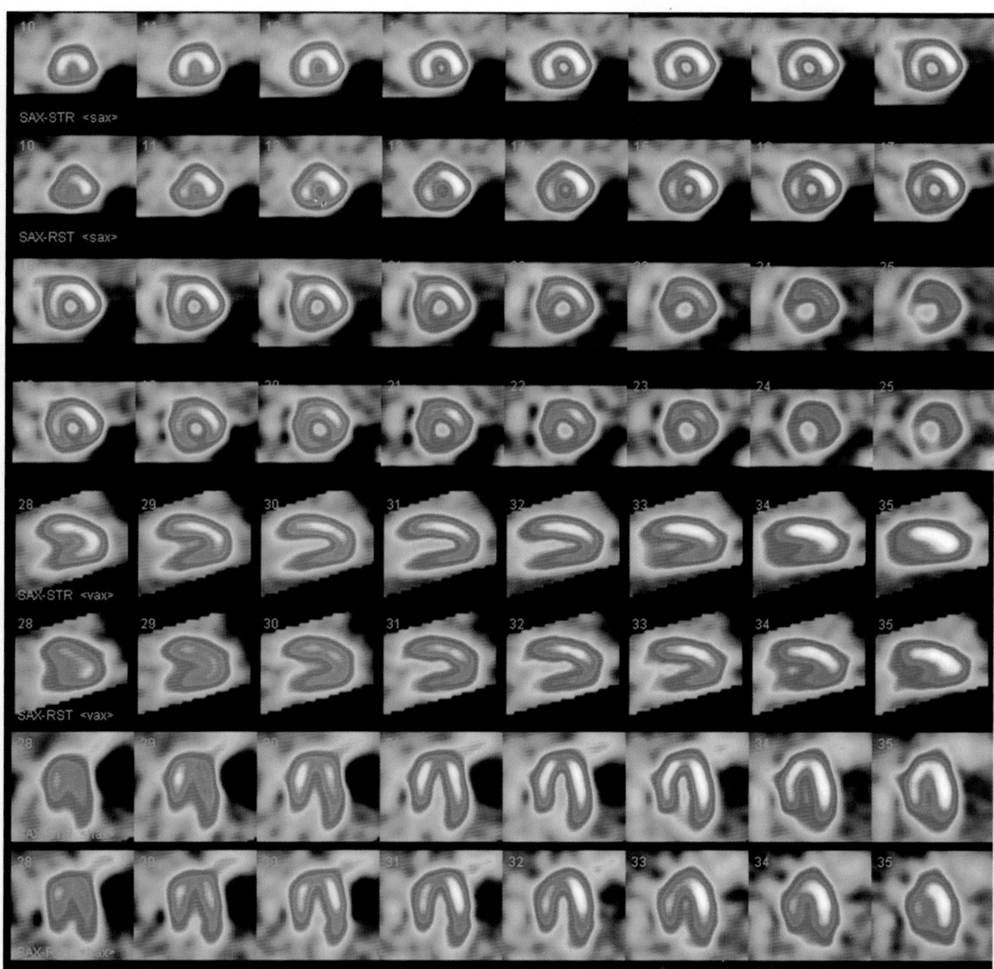

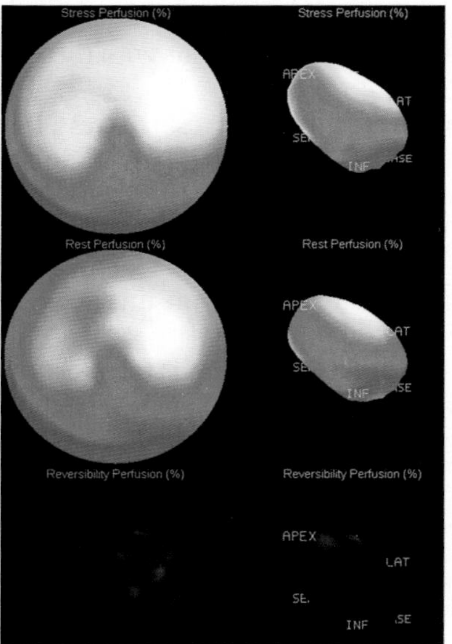

Clinical Presentation

55-year-old man with intermittent chest pain. Gated images were normal, and the left ventricular ejection fraction was 58%.

Imaging Findings

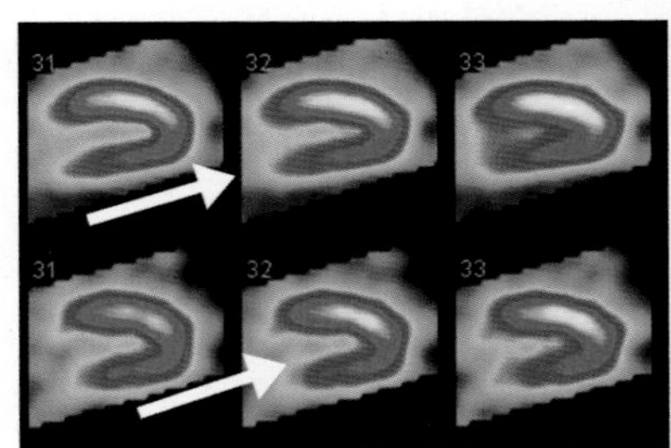

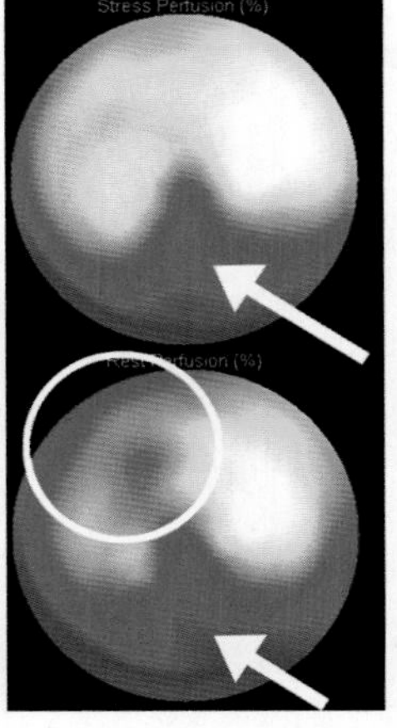

A B **(A)** Rest and stress myocardial perfusion scintigraphy demonstrate a large, moderately severe defect of the inferior left ventricula wall that appears identical on both resting and post-stress image (*arrows*). **(B)** Rest and stress polar maps and surface renderings dis play the same nonreversible abnormality (*arrows*). A mild anterio wall decrease at rest is not present at stress, consistent with mil chest wall attenuation (*circle*).

Differential Diagnosis

- ***Diaphragm attenuation artifact:*** Fixed inferior wall defects with normal wall motion are most commonly due to this artifact.
- *Inferior myocardial infarction:* This would look identical on these images (a nonreversible defect). However, an infarct this large should have an associated wall motion abnormality.
- *Hibernating inferior myocardium:* This would have an identical appearance on these images but would also be expected to have a regional wall motion abnormality (also known as resting ischemia).

Essential Facts

- Stress–rest myocardial perfusion scintigraphy is an accurate method for identifying coronary artery disease, both ischemia (generally reversible defects) and infarction (fixed).
- Although very sensitive, this technique can be limited by several types of artifacts, many related to patient soft-tissue attenuation, which decreases the number of photons reaching the gamma camera.
- Diaphragm attenuation is seen inferiorly ("right coronary artery territory"), whereas breast (or chest wall) attenuation involves the anteroseptal apex ("left anterior descending territory"). Both appear as fixed defects, similar to infarct and hibernating tissue.
- However, on gated imaging, defects from attenuation artifact should have normal wall motion. Infarct and hibernating tissue will both have regional wall motion abnormalities (on *both* resting and post-stress gated SPECT images).
- Diaphragmatic attenuation is encountered more commonly in larger patients, in men, and in patients who are imaged while supine.

Other Imaging Findings

- Resting echocardiography can also be used to evaluate regional wall motion. A normal echo would support the absence of an infarct or hibernation.
- Cardiac PET is less prone to attenuation artifacts, given the higher-energy photons used as well as the standard availability of attenuation correction in PET.
- Recently, there has been more widespread use of attenuation correction with both SPECT (gamma-based correction) and SPECT/CT.

✓ Pearls & ✗ Pitfalls

✓ Given its lower photon energies, attenuation artifacts are more commonly encountered when thallium 201, as opposed to Tc99m-labeled MIBI/TETRO, is used, although attenuation artifacts still occur with these tracers.

✓ If a defect improves somewhat from rest to stress, it is more likely attenuation artifact, particularly if a dual tracer protocol has been used (Tl201 rest, Tc99m-MIBI/TETRO stress).

✓ If diaphragmatic attenuation is suspected following supine imaging, immediate repeat prone imaging can demonstrate "defect" resolution.

✗ Although normal regional wall motion is the most reliable indicator of attenuation artifact, a true infarct may not show a regional wall motion abnormality on cardia SPECT or PET if it is small.

✗ Attenuation correction, although useful, can *introduce* artifactual defects due to misregistration. Carefully ensure that the attenuation map is properly aligned. If a defect is seen only after attenuation correction, it is likely an introduced artifact.

Case 31

A

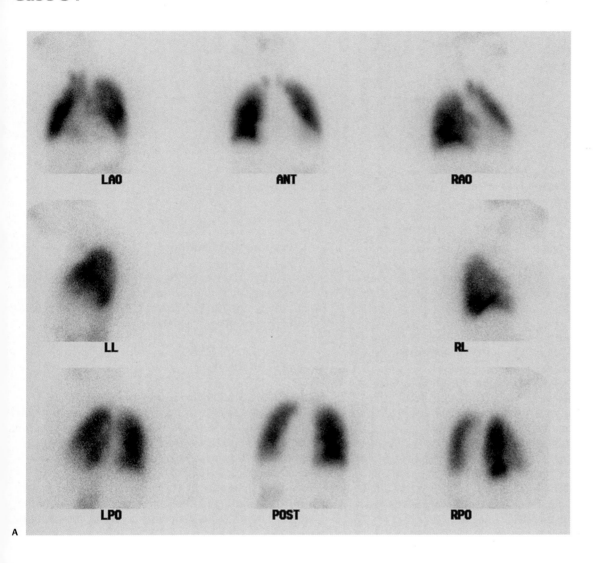

Clinical Presentation

A 62-year-old woman with acute shortness of breath.

Further Work-up

Given the extrapulmonary activity, an additional spot image of the head was obtained to assess for intracranial activity.

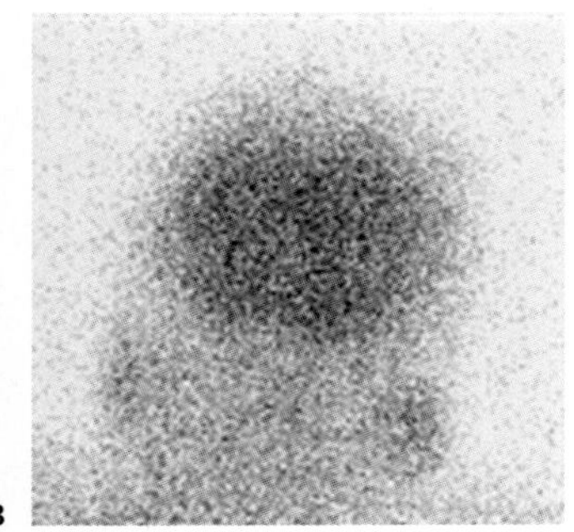

B

Imaging Findings

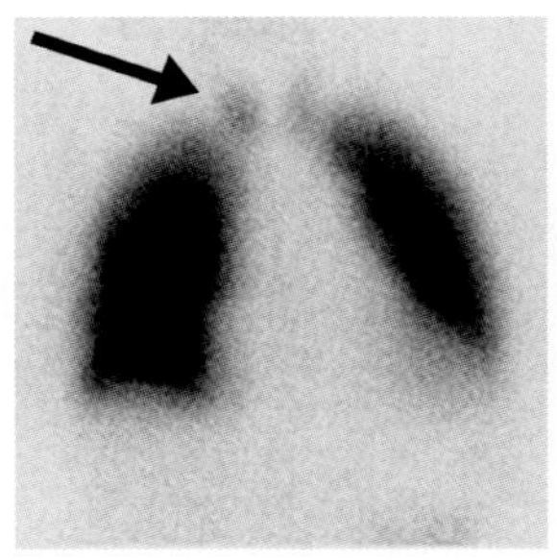
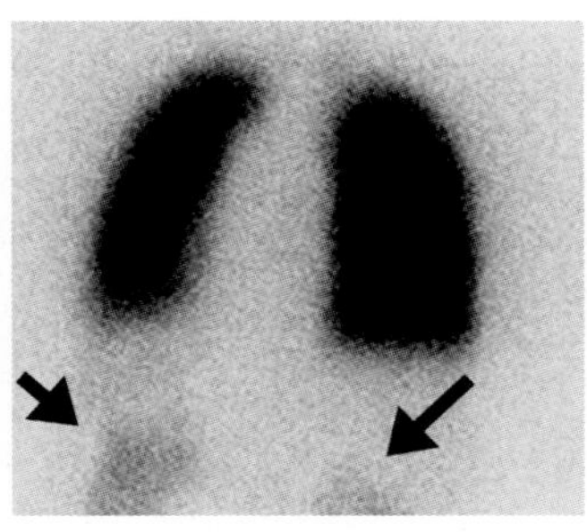
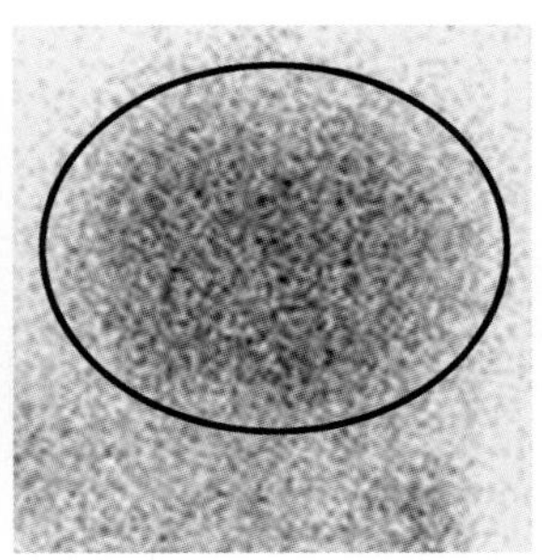

(A) Multiple Tc99m-MAA perfusion images demonstrate no moderate or large perfusion defects but show abnormal extrapulmonary activity in the thyroid and kidneys (*arrows*). **(B)** Spot image of the head demonstrates MAA accumulation in the cerebral cortex (*circle*).

Differential Diagnosis

All three demonstrate extrapulmonary activity in the kidneys and thyroid. However, only a shunt will demonstrate uptake in the brain.

- ***Right-to-left shunt:*** Extrapulmonary uptake including kidneys, thyroid, and most importantly brain indicates a right-to-left shunt.
- *Free pertechnetate:* Poor MAA radiolabeling can result in free pertechnetate, which will accumulate most notably in the kidneys and/or thyroid in a typical chest field of view. However, a spot image of the head will reveal no significant intracranial uptake.
- *Recent prior nuclear study:* Concurrently present Tc99m-labeled radiotracer (e.g., a Tc99m-RBC MUGA scan the prior afternoon) can yield extrapulmonary uptake similar to free pertechnetate. However, a spot image of the head should again reveal no intracranial uptake.

Essential Facts

- Shunts can be pre-, post-, or intracardiac.
- Common etiologies include patent ductus arteriosus (PDA), atrial septal defect (ASD) or other congenital heart diseases (CHDs), pulmonary arteriovenous malformations, and cirrhosis resulting in tiny intrapulmonary shunts.
- In addition to the abnormal anatomic communication, right-to-left shunt flow typically requires the development of elevated right pressures (Eisenmenger physiology).
- Pulmonary capillaries are 7 to 8 µm and MAA particles are 10 to 100 µm and thus lodge in the first capillary bed they encounter (i.e., the pulmonary capillaries, normally).
- With a right-to-left shunt, MAA enters the systemic circulation and lodges in systemic capillaries in proportion to perfusion.
- Percentage shunt fraction can be accurately quantified by obtaining whole-body MAA perfusion scans and comparing background-corrected lung and whole-body regions of interest.

Other Imaging Findings

- Chest radiographs can be suggestive of certain CHDs and can demonstrate shunt perfusion.
- Echocardiography and cardiac MRI can demonstrate and quantify shunts from ASDs and other CHDs.

✓ Pearls & × Pitfalls

✓ In patients with known right-to-left shunt, some authors suggest decreasing the number of injected MAA *particles* (with a fresher MAA labeling kit or by lowering the injected radioactive dose). However, no iatrogenic neurologic deficits have ever been convincingly documented in these patients.

✓ Free pertechnetate will not localize intracranially and can be differentiated from shunt by a spot image of the head, as in this patient showing no intracranial activity:

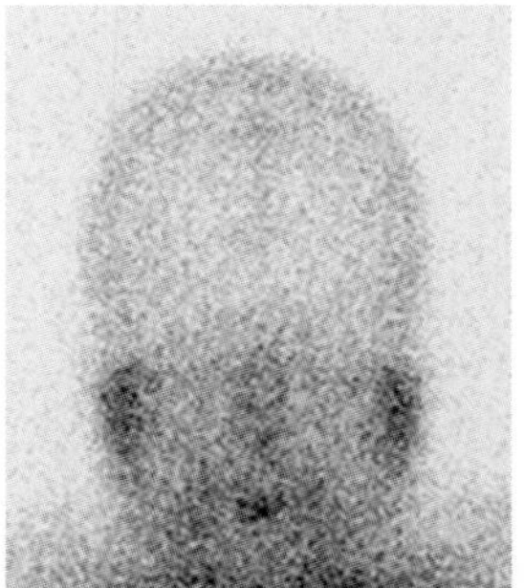

✓ In addition to causing extrapulmonary uptake on lung ventilation–perfusion scanning, free pertechnetate should always be a consideration for unusual uptake on any Tc99m-labeled examination, such as gastric uptake on a bone or RBC scan. In such cases, uptake in the thyroid or salivary glands can distinguish free pertechnetate from true pathology.

Case 32

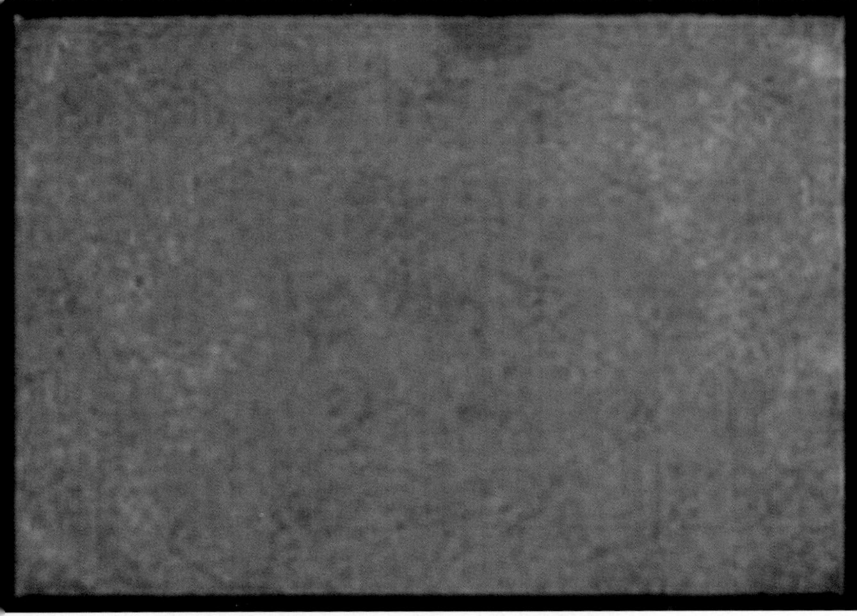

Clinical Presentation

A technologist performing weekly gamma camera quality control obtained an intrinsic flood image.

Imaging Findings

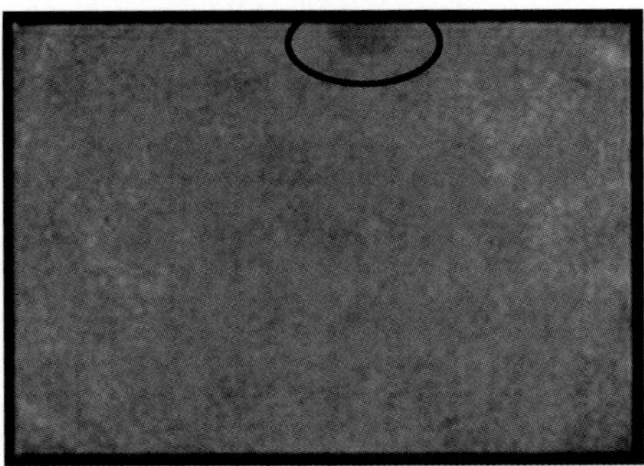

A flood image performed without the collimator (intrinsic) reveals a subtle semicircular region of nonuniform decreased activity along the upper edge of the camera head (*circle*).

Differential Diagnosis

Areas of nonuniformity on a flood image can be due to an abnormality in the collimator, crystal, or electronics of the camera.

- ***Faulty photomultiplier tube:*** In this case, the area of nonuniformity has a half-hexagonal configuration and thus follows the pattern of photomultiplier tubes, which are hexagonal in cross-section.
- *Damaged collimator:* Although this may cause a similar appearance, this is an intrinsic flood, which is performed with the collimator off.
- *Cracked crystal:* The pattern will not have a smooth edge or follow the photomultiplier tube. It is typically linear in appearance.

Essential Facts

- Intrinsic flood images are acquired with the collimator off and measure the performance of the crystal and electronics. They also allow electronic compensations to different areas of the crystals to create more uniformity.
- Extrinsic flood images are acquired with the collimator on and measure performance of the entire system. This should be done daily before clinical use.
- Factors that can affect uniformity include the following:
  - A count rate that is too high and beyond the capabilities of the camera
  - An incorrectly set energy window for the isotope being imaged
  - An artifact from a nearby source, such as an injected patient in a nearby room
  - Multiple-energy isotopes such as gallium and thallium are more prone to uniformity errors.
  - Photomultiplier tube voltage drift

Other Imaging Findings

- This is a flood field image acquired with the same camera head with correction applied. This compensates for the photomultiplier tube abnormality. However, it does not correct the underlying problem:

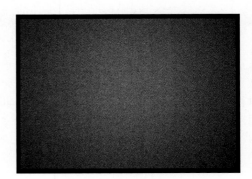

✓Pearls & ✗ Pitfalls

✓ Improvements in intrinsic camera resolution are unlikely to make a significant clinical image improvement as overall system resolution (R, expressed as full width half maximum, or FWHM) is also limited by the collimator and scatter.

- $R\ system = \sqrt{(R\ intrinsic^2 + R\ collimator^2 + R\ scatter^2)}$

✓ Using an energy window shifted to the high side of the photopeak can decrease the effect of scatter. The trade-off is a lower count rate, however, which will require a longer imaging time.

✗ Intrinsic flood images must be acquired with the source at a distance of least five times the useful field of view of the camera head. This ensures a uniform distribution of energy across the head.

✗ Poor flood uniformity leads to a higher false-positive rate when lesions are evaluated.

Case 33

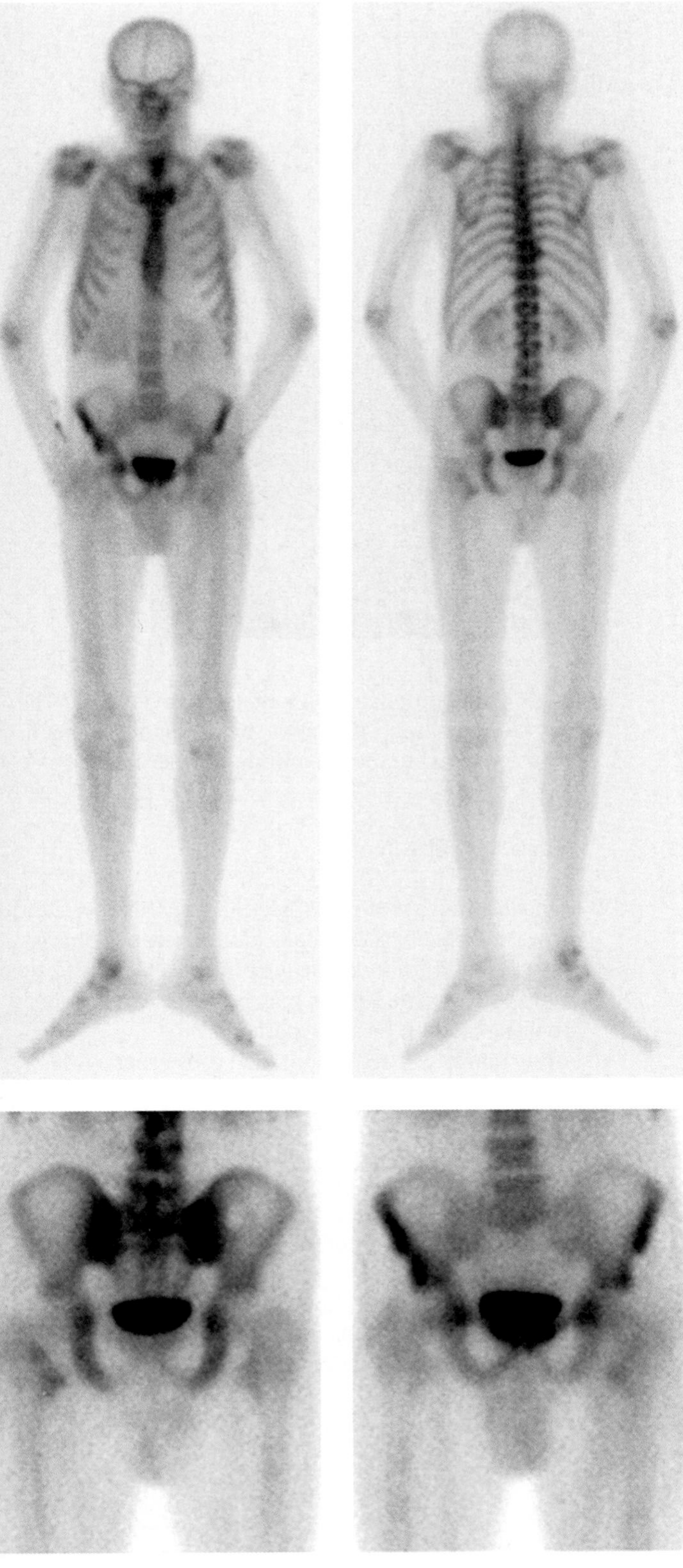

Clinical Presentation

A 54-year-old man with a history of renal cell carcinoma, now with right gluteal region pain.

Imaging Findings

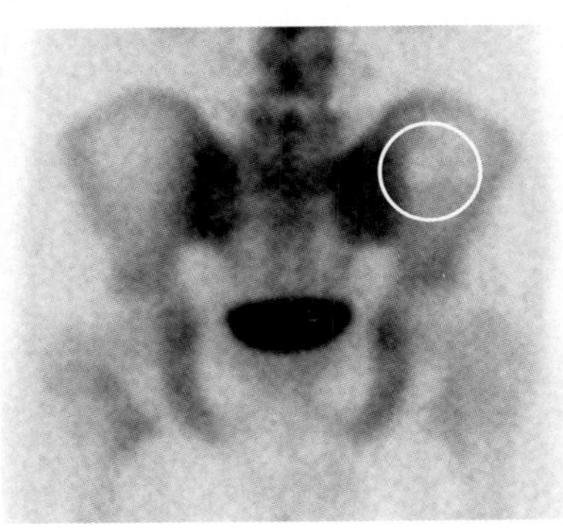

Anterior and posterior whole-body and spot pelvic images from a bone scan demonstrate a subtle round cold defect in the right iliac wing (*circle*).

Differential Diagnosis

- ***Lytic metastasis:*** Renal cell metastases are commonly lytic and therefore cold on bone scan, making this the most likely diagnosis, given the history.
- *Myeloma:* Solitary plasmacytoma or multiple myeloma is also commonly lytic (cold) but less likely, given the history.
- *Acute bone infarct:* Bone infarcts are usually cold if acute but are not generally seen in this location. Femoral heads and diaphyses are more typically involved.

Essential Facts

- Most bone lesions, including metastases, have a significant osteoblastic component and are therefore increased on bone scan.
- However, a minority of lesions, including predominantly lytic and/or highly aggressive ones, can be isointense or cold on bone scan given that they do not result in increased osteoblastic activity.
- Common examples include renal cell and thyroid cancer metastases and plasmacytoma/multiple myeloma.
- Acute bone infarcts can also have decreased uptake due to decreased radiotracer delivery (blood flow). (Subacute to chronic infarcts will generally have some mildly *increased* uptake as they heal.)

Other Imaging Findings

- Plain radiographs, CT, and MRI can demonstrate the lytic lesion(s). Here is the CT scan of this patient showing the larger right iliac lesion seen on bone scan (*circle*) and a second smaller one more posteriorly that was occult on bone scan (*arrows*):

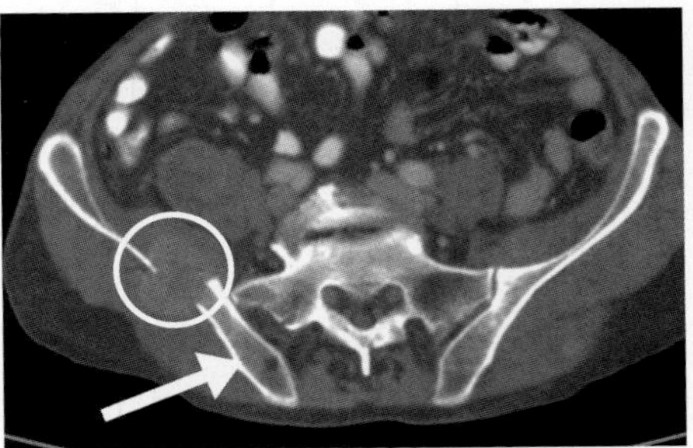

- FDG-PET can demonstrate a lytic lesion even when the bone scan does not (PET shows the lesion metabolism itself as opposed to the surrounding skeletal reaction).

✓ Pearls & × Pitfalls

✓ Some lesions that are mostly lytic may still have subtly increased osteoblastic uptake along their periphery.

✓ Accordingly, with multiple lytic lesions, like those seen in myeloma, some lesions may be occult while others are visualized in the same patient.

✓ Purely marrow space lesions, like those seen with lymphoma, may not be lytic or sclerotic and be occult on bone scan and CT. These, however, may be seen on MRI or PET.

× External-beam radiation, often to the spine, can also cause regional decreased activity on bone scan. A defect configured to a radiation port will be seen, with the appropriate history (see Case 100).

× Metallic artifact, including items worn or in pockets, can simulate a cold defect on bone scan. Reviewing multiple image projections and/or assessing the patient can distinguish.

Case 34

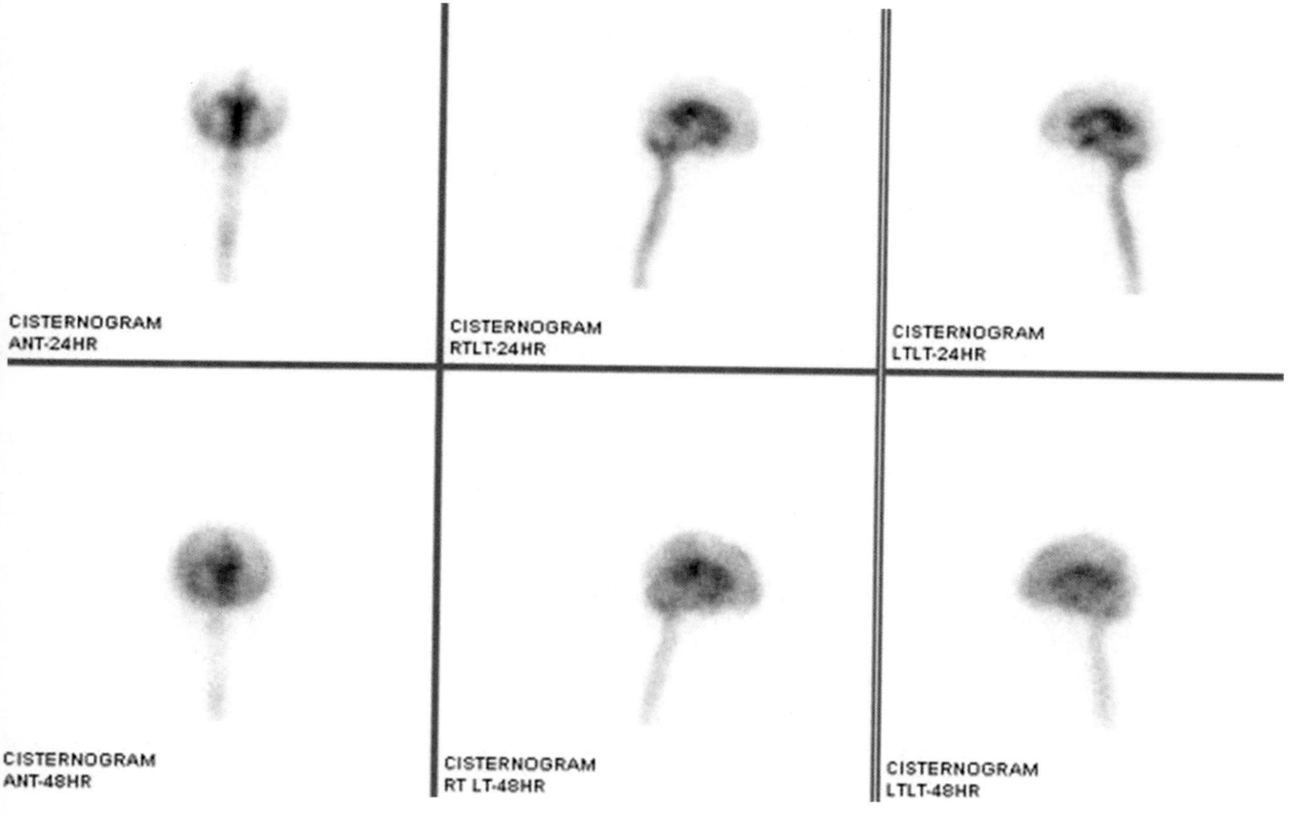

Clinical Presentation

A 65-year-old woman with cognitive decline, incontinence, and difficulty walking.

Imaging Findings

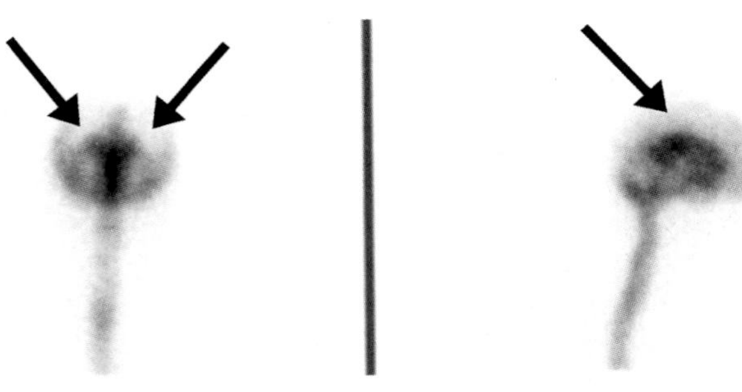

Anterior and lateral images from a radionuclide cisternogram obtained with indium 111 DTPA reveal incomplete migration of radiotracer over the convexities by 24 hours. Lateral ventricular reflux is also noted (*arrows*). By 48 hours, further but incomplete migration is noted, and persistent reflux is seen in the lateral ventricles.

Differential Diagnosis

- ***Obstructive communicating hydrocephalus:*** Delayed flow over the convexities with reflux into the ventricles is indicative of this diagnosis. Normal-pressure hydrocephalus (NPH) is a subtype of obstructive communicating hydrocephalus.
- *Cerebrospinal fluid (CSF) leak:* Although this is another common indication for radionuclide cisternography, there is no evidence of extracranial passage of radiotracer.
- *Normal variant:* Persistent reflux of radiotracer into the ventricles is never normal.

Essential Facts

- NPH is a type of obstructive communicating hydrocephalus without increased CSF pressure. On cisternography, this is characterized by delayed migration of radiotracer over the convexities and persistent reflux of ventricular activity. This pattern may benefit from shunting.
- NPH is a disease of extraventricular obstruction: impaired CSF resorption by the arachnoid granulations. This may be due to prior subarachnoid hemorrhage or meningitis.
- Classic clinical triad: dementia, gait disturbance, and incontinence
- Prediction of response to shunting is the goal of diagnostic testing; however, cisternography has limited value for this. (It is no better than clinical examination plus CT.)
- There are four cisternographic appearances:
  - Type 1: normal; migration seen over the convexities (by 24 hours, no later than 48 hours) and no ventricular reflux
  - Type 2: delayed migration and no reflux
  - Type 3: transient reflux and delayed clearance
    - 3A: clearance over the convexities but may be delayed
    - 3B: clearance by an alternate pathway (transependymal)
  - Type 4: poor clearance and persistent ventricular activity; benefits from shunting

Other Imaging Findings

- CT and MRI can show dilated ventricles and subarachnoid spaces, but this may be difficult to distinguish from generalized atrophy.
- MRI may help in defining patients who will respond to shunting. Characteristic features are a CSF flow void in the cerebral aqueduct and third ventricles, and ventricular dilatation out of proportion to sulcal atrophy.

✓ Pearls & × Pitfalls

✓ Activity should never be seen in the ventricles normally.

✓ Activity should normally surround the brain by 24 hours. However, it may take up to 48 hours in older patients. Here is a normal for comparison showing tracer extending over the convexities and no ventricular activity at 24 hours:

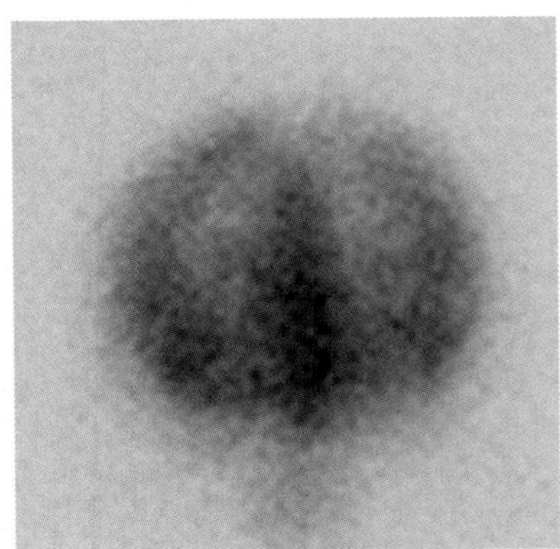

× DTPA does enter the cerebral cortex, and images after 24 hours begin to reflect cerebral uptake rather than CSF.

× Cisternography cannot differentiate obstructive communicating hydrocephalus with normal pressure (i.e., NPH) from that with elevated pressure. Spinal tap pressure measurements can be used to distinguish.

× Delayed clearance over the convexities without refluxed ventricular activity is *not* compatible with a diagnosis of NPH and may indicate a noncommunicating hydrocephalus.

Case 35

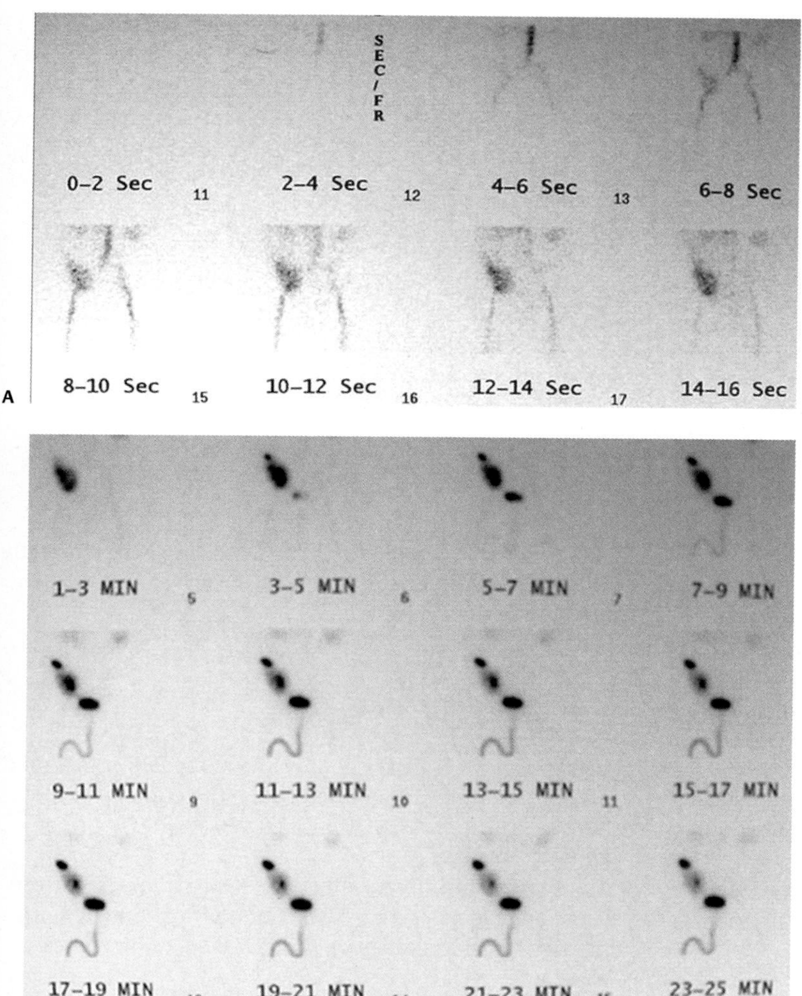

A

B

Clinical Presentation

A rising creatinine despite good urine output status post renal transplant.

Further Work-up

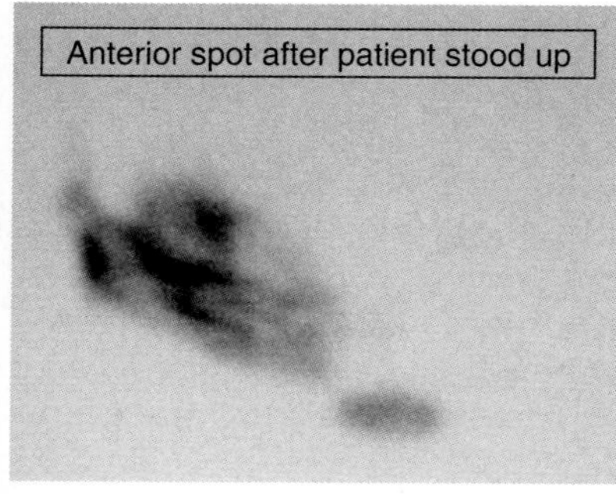

C

Imaging Findings

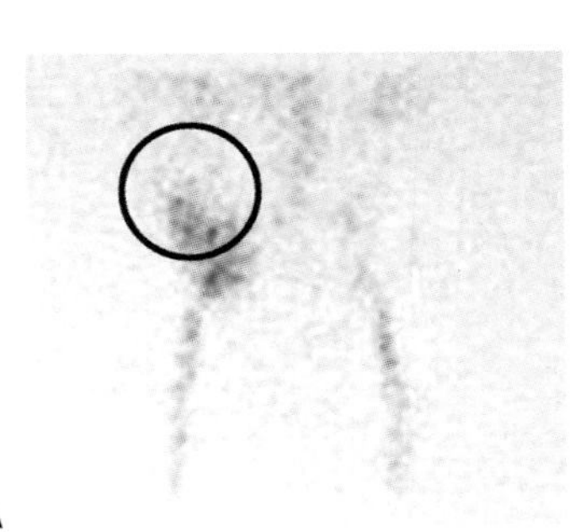
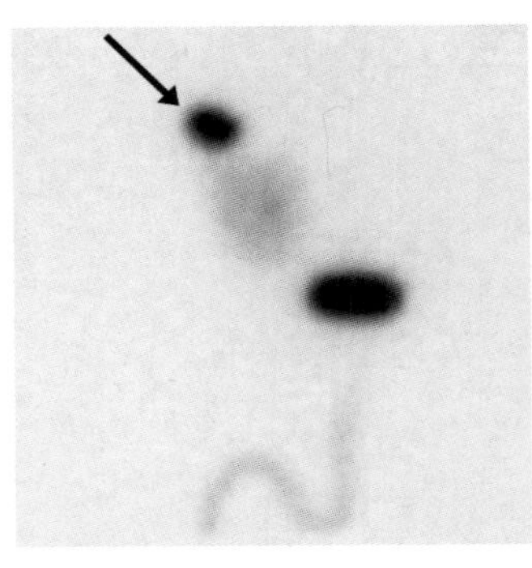
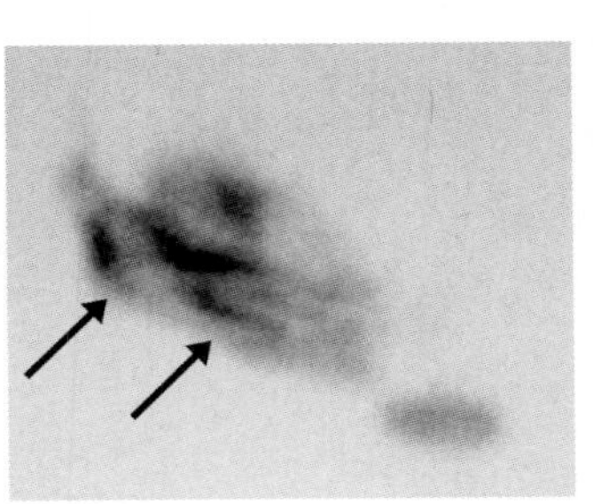

(A) Anterior pelvic angiographic phase images from a Tc99m MAG3 scan demonstrate prompt perfusion (within 2 seconds of iliac perfusion) to a renal transplant in the right iliac fossa. However, there is a lack of demonstrable flow to the upper pole. As a result, the superior portion ends with an unusual concave appearance (*circle*). **(B)** Function-phase images demonstrate normal uptake and excretion by the middle and inferior renal portions. However, there is progressive focal accumulation of radiolabeled urine at the superior portion (*arrow*). **(C)** Following patient repositioning, there is free spillage of the collection within the pelvic peritoneal cavity (*arrows*).

Differential Diagnosis

- ***Upper pole infarct and partially contained urinary leak:*** Lack of blood flow or parenchymal function indicates upper pole infarct. The eventual free spillage of urinary tracer indicates leakage of urine formed by the functioning lower renal parenchyma.
- *Compound kidney with upper pole hydronephrosis:* This may look similar on the functional phase but would have better flow and parenchymal function, and urine would not spill freely.
- *Large upper pole cyst:* This could look similar only if the cyst communicated with the urinary collecting system. But again, fluid would not spill freely.

Essential Facts

- Scintigraphy is commonly employed to evaluate renal transplants with evidence of decreasing function.
- Dysfunction can be categorized as medical or surgical.
- Medical diseases include acute tubular necrosis (ATN; early after transplant) and immunosuppressive drug toxicities and rejection (later after transplant).
- Surgical diseases include vascular compromise (arterial or venous), urinary obstruction, leak, hematoma, and lymphocele.
- Medical diseases typically appear as homogeneous flow and uptake but with delayed or diminished urinary excretion, depending on the tracer used (DTPA vs. MAG3) and on the precise medical disease.
- Infarcts demonstrate no blood flow or function to all or a portion of the transplanted kidney. Diminished transplant perfusion may appear as flow delayed beyond 4 seconds of iliac perfusion.
- A urinary leak can be contained or free-flowing and can be further evaluated by altering patient position, as in this case above.
- A hematoma or lymphocele may not be visualized directly scintigraphically, but either can distort the appearance or function of the adjacent kidney.

Other Imaging Findings

- US can also assess arterial flow and detect abnormal fluid collections, but it cannot determine the etiology of the fluid (e.g., urinoma). US is also used to guide biopsy of a failing transplant.
- More typically, infarcts affect the entire transplant. Here is the angiographic phase from another patient showing no blood flow to the entire transplanted kidney (*circle*):

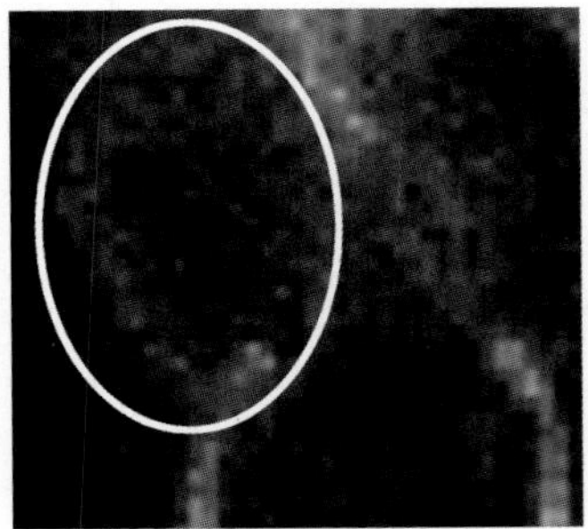

✓ Pearls & ✗ Pitfalls

✓ As with any renal scan, Tc99m-labeled DTPA or MAG3 may be used for transplant evaluation. MAG3 often has superior uptake and excretion but is more expensive and may not be as readily available.

✗ On the flow phase, significant renal perfusion should be seen within 2 to 4 seconds of adjacent iliac artery perfusion. However, a tight injection bolus is crucial for interpretation of this phase. The renogram curves are useful to assess bolus adequacy.

Case 36

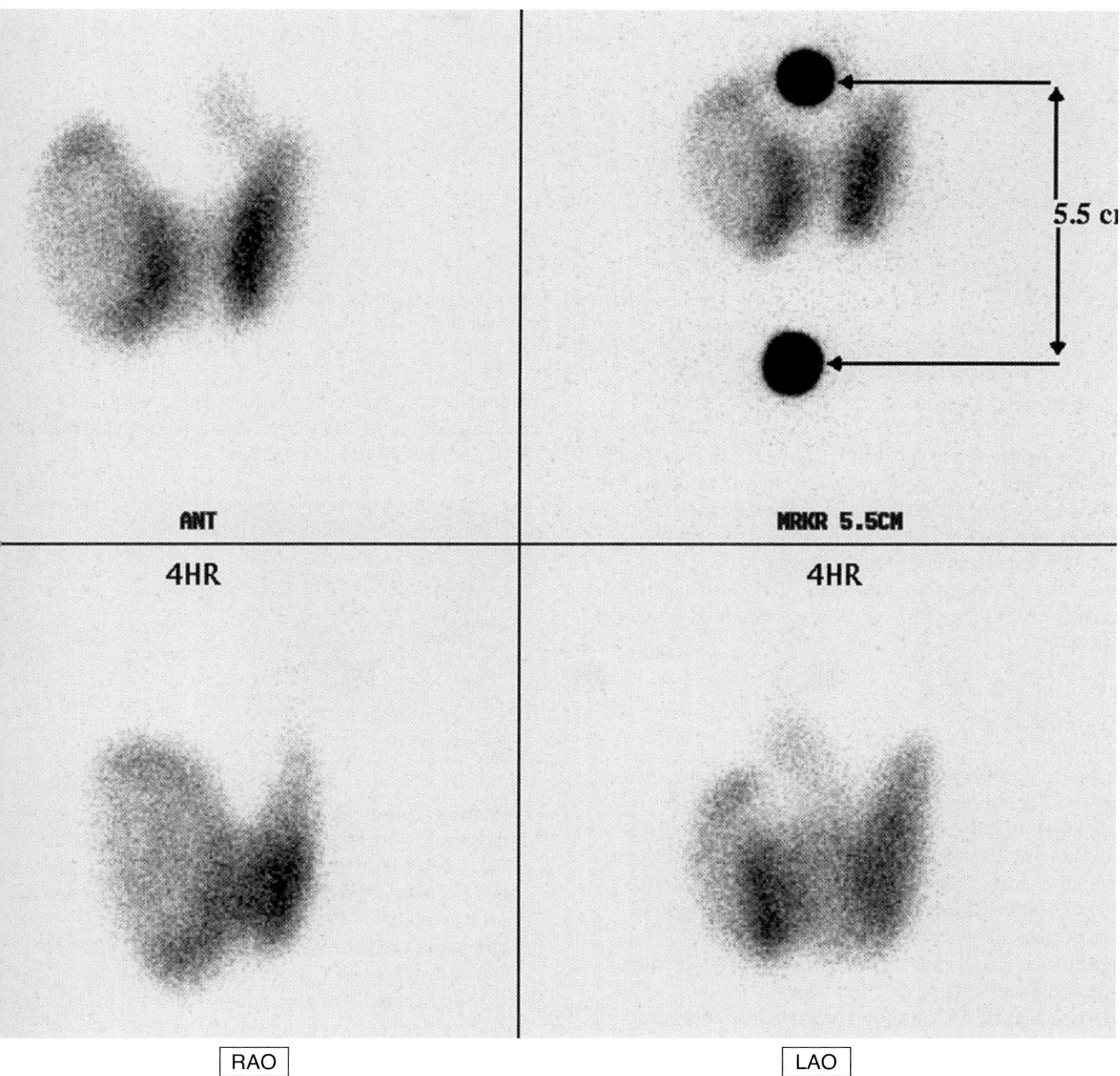

Clinical Presentation

A 38-year-old woman presents with a palpable nodule in her right neck.

Imaging Findings

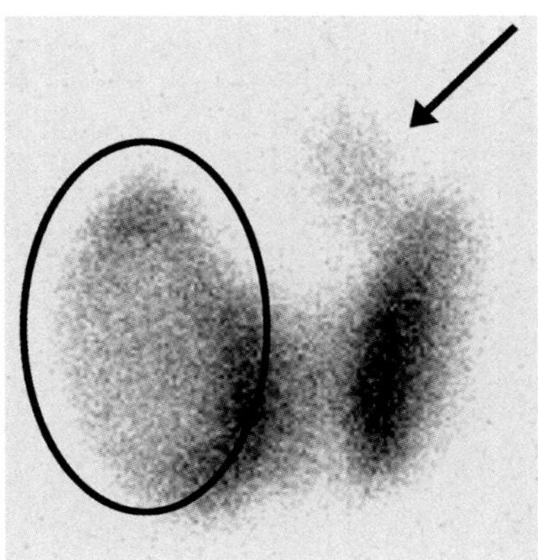

Iodine 123 thyroid scan demonstrates a large "cold" nodule within the right thyroid lobe (*circle*). A sma[ll] pyramidal lobe is incidentally noted superiorly (*arrow*).

Differential Diagnosis

- ***Thyroid carcinoma:*** This is the diagnosis of exclusion for any dominant hypofunctioning cold thyroid nodule(s).
- *Colloid cyst:* This is a very common etiology for a cold thyroid nodule, but unless it is entirely cystic on US, tissue confirmation is generally needed.
- *Hypofunctioning thyroid adenoma:* This is also a common etiology of cold nodules, but biopsy is needed to exclude cancer.

Essential Facts

- Fifteen to twenty percent of cold nodules (on pertechnetate or radioiodine scans) are thyroid cancer.
- Papillary and follicular cancers are most common, followed by medullary, Hürthle cell, and anaplastic cancers.
- Papillary cancers tend to metastasize regionally (lymphatics), whereas follicular cancers are more likely to metastasize distantly (hematogenous).
- Medullary thyroid cancers arise from C (parafollicular) cells and have elevated calcitonin levels.
- Increased cancer likelihood: young, male, nodule growing, prior neck radiation
- Most cold nodules are ultimately benign (colloid nodule, simple cyst, hypofunctioning thyroid adenoma) but should be considered cancer until proven otherwise.
- Other less common etiologies for cold nodules include focal thyroiditis, hematoma, abscess, metastasis to the thyroid, lymphoma, and large parathyroid lesions.

Other Imaging Findings

- US: Cold nodules that are completely cystic on US are benign; however, those that are partially or completed solid need to be biopsied to exclude malignancy.
- Consider scintigraphically "marking" the location of a palpable nodule on a thyroid scan. Here is a thyroid scan in another patient demonstrating a second occult but visually dominant and therefore suspicious cold nodule. Both nodules should be biopsied:

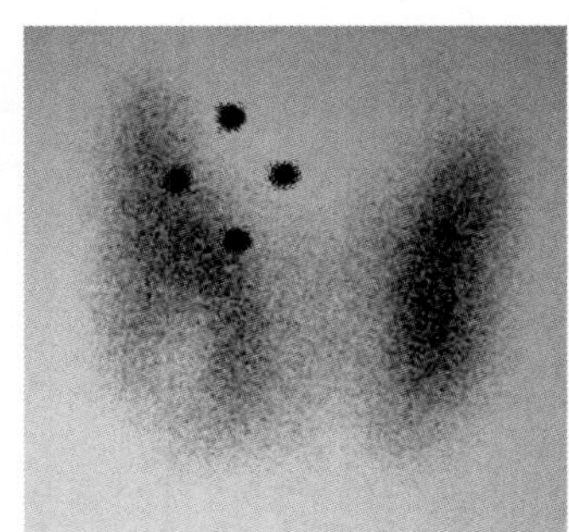

- Medullary thyroid cancers are neuroendocrine in origin and can occasionally have focally increased uptake on MIBG or octreotide imaging (but are cold on thyroid scans). They can be associated with multiple endocrine neoplasia types IIa and IIb.
- Primary and metastatic thyroid cancers can often be visualized on FDG-PET, particularly higher-grade papillary and anaplastic tumors. Lower-grade thyroid cancers (primary or metastatic) will be cold on FDG-PET.

✓ Pearls & × Pitfalls

✓ Nodules that are warm (significant iodine uptake) or hot (significant uptake with suppression of the rest of the gland) are considered benign.

✓ Although multiple similar cold nodules in a gland are most likely benign, any "dominant" cold nodule(s) by imaging or physical examination should be considered suspicious.

× A known nodule (by US or palpation) that is *not visualized* on thyroid scan (see previous figure, upper nodule) is considered "indeterminate" and treated as cold: 15 to 20% risk for cancer ("if it's not hot, it's cold").

Case 37

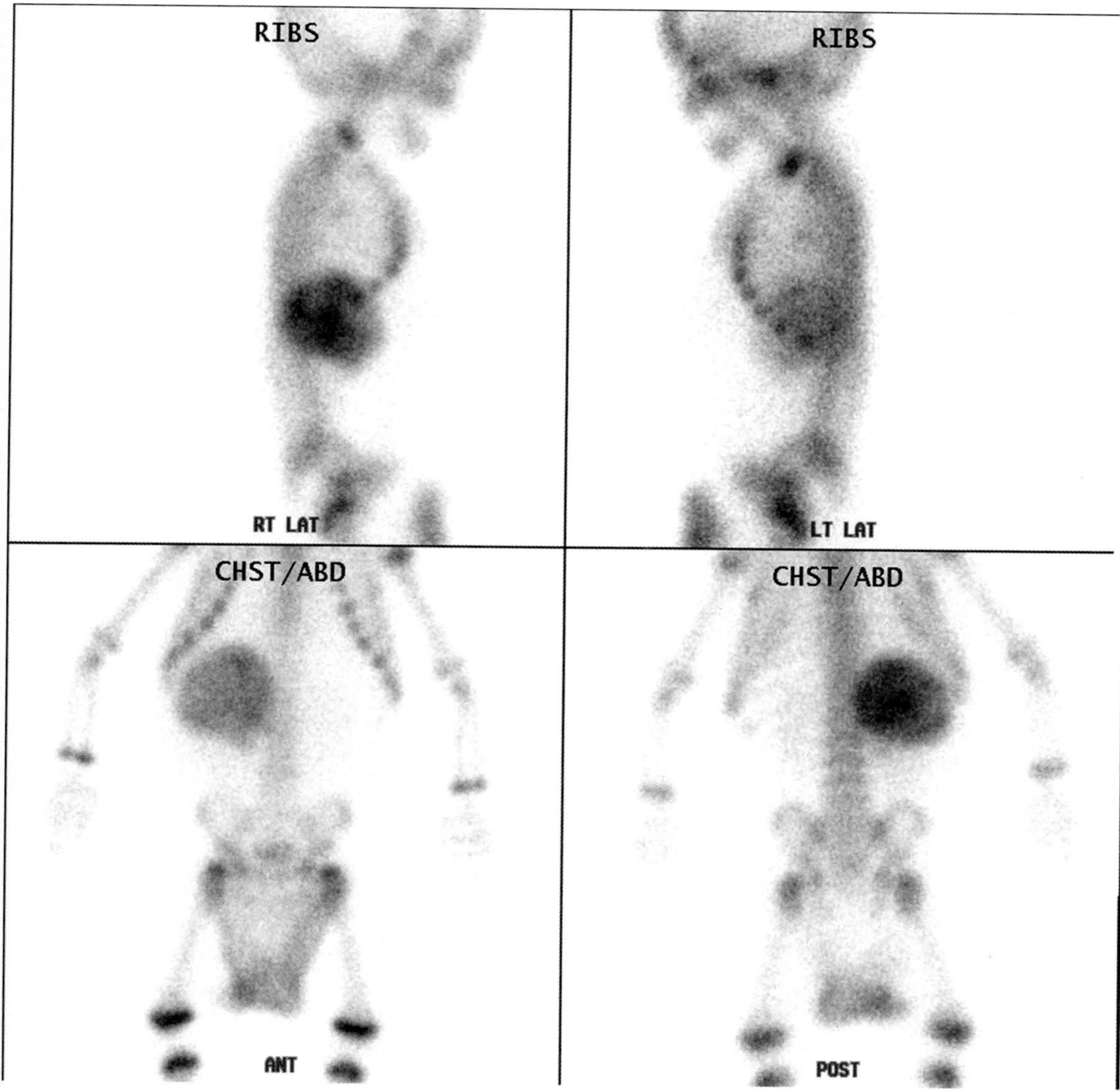

Clinical Presentation

History withheld.

Imaging Findings

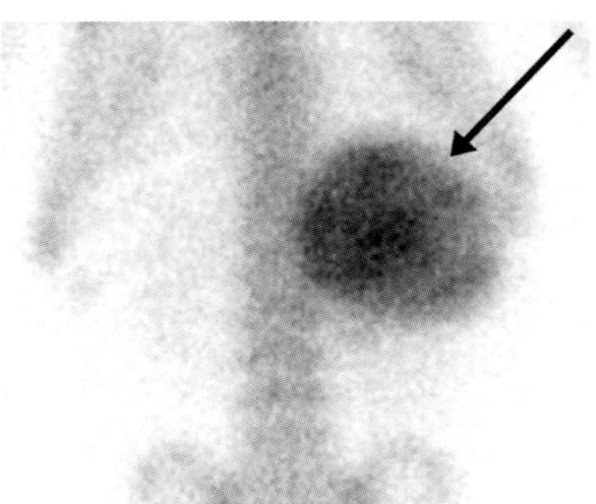

Tc99m HDP bone scintigraphy demonstrates intense growth plate activity and a large head-to-body size ratio, indicating that this is a young child. A large, markedly increased focus is seen in the right upper abdominal soft tissues. It is more intense on the posterior view, indicating that it is more posteriorly located (*arrow*). No abnormal bone foci are seen.

Differential Diagnosis

- ***Primary neuroblastoma (NB):*** Soft-tissue uptake on bone scan in a posterior abdominal mass in a young child makes this the most likely diagnosis.
- *Liver metastasis:* Some liver metastases can be seen *focally* on bone scan, such as with mucinous or calcifying lesions. However, this lesion is much more intense posteriorly, suggesting a retroperitoneal location. Furthermore, such liver metastatic primary tumors are less commonly childhood cancers (e.g., colon cancer).
- *Colloid formation artifact:* Excess reducing agent (usually tin) in the radiopharmaceutical preparation can lead to colloid formation, which can be seen as *diffuse* liver uptake. Again, the uptake here appears more likely behind the liver (and more focal).

Essential Facts

- Several soft-tissue pathologic processes can accumulate radiotracer on bone scan, including benign lesions (e.g., meningiomas), primary and metastatic malignancies, soft-tissue necrosis (e.g., strokes and myocardial infarctions), inflammation, myositis, amyloid deposition, and hypercalcemia.
- In a young child, abdominal/retroperitoneal soft-tissue uptake will often represent NB.
- Of neural crest origin, NB is a common tumor in young children, typically presenting with a retroperitoneal mass that is often calcified.
- A significant proportion of primary NB lesions will be evident on bone scan and can be visualized while a known tumor is staged or can be detected incidentally.
- NB most commonly metastasizes to bone. Bone metastases can be seen on bone scan but are even better assessed on MIBG scan.

Other Imaging Findings

- Soft-tissue uptake on bone scan can often be further defined on CT or MRI. For example, uptake in hepatic metastases, meningiomas, and cerebral infarcts can be confirmed on anatomic imaging.
- NB is also staged/restaged with MIBG for both soft-tissue and osseous disease.
- Here are the CT and MIBG scans in this same patient showing the calcified retroperitoneal NB mass, which is MIBG-avid (*arrows*). Note the myocardial uptake that is normally seen on MIBG (*arrowhead*).

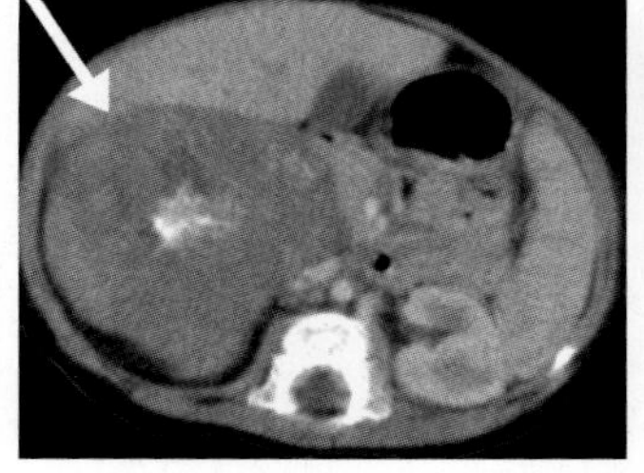

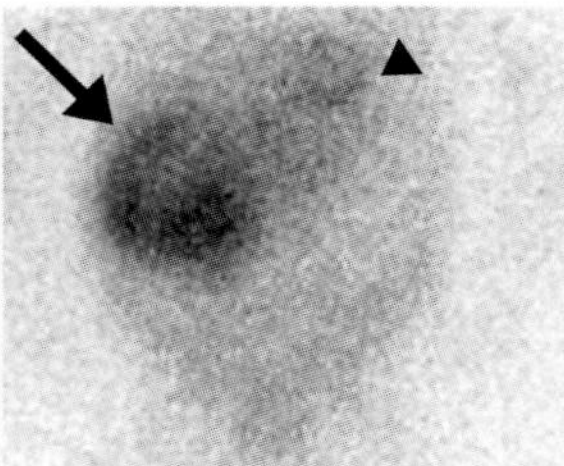

✓ Pearls & ✗ Pitfalls

✓ Calcified/mucinous tumors and other calcifying pathologic processes are commonly avid for bone scan tracers. However, lesions with microscopic calcifications that cannot be visualized by CT and even noncalcifying lesions can also have increased uptake.

✓ MIBG is more sensitive and specific for detecting bone metastases than bone scan. However, the combination of the two may be even more accurate in some patients.

✗ Other common artifactual causes of soft-tissue uptake on bone scan include urine contamination on the skin and lymphatic axillary nodal uptake due to an infiltrated dose injection.

Case 38

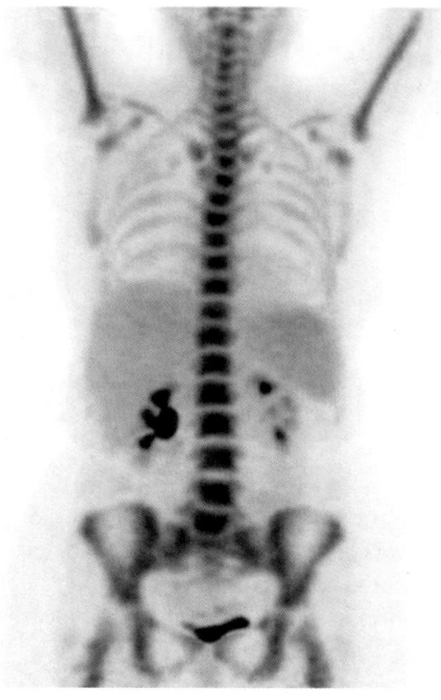

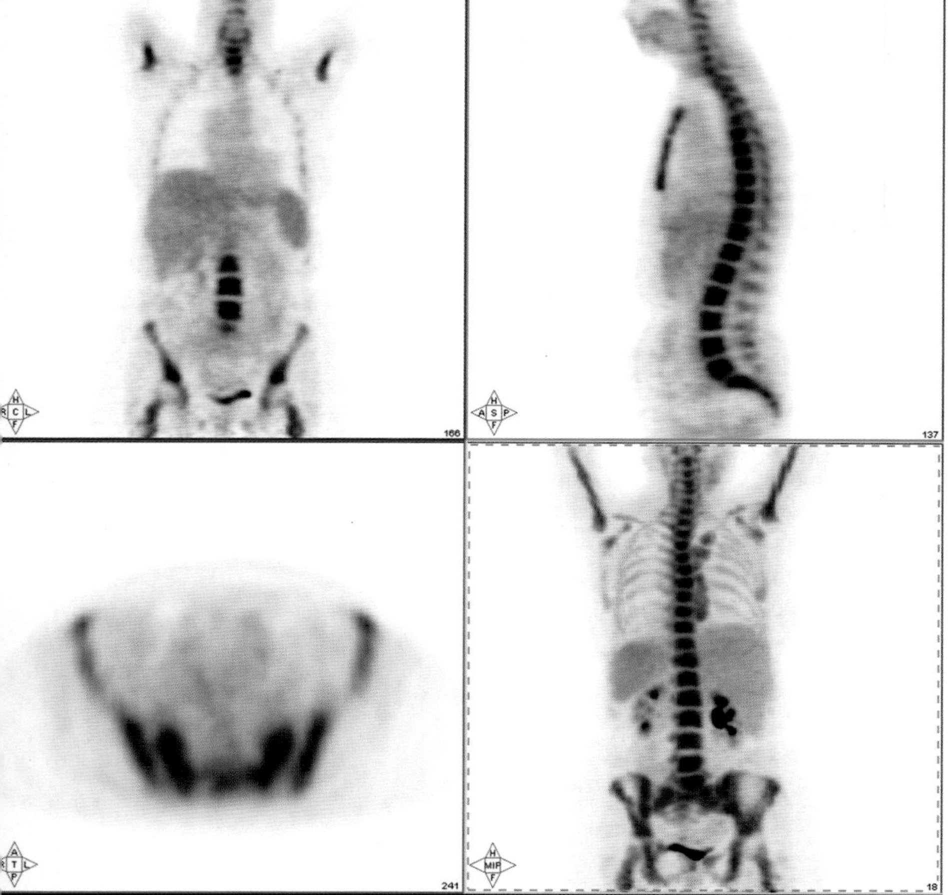

Clinical Presentation

26-year-old man with a history of lymphoma presents for restaging.

Imaging Findings

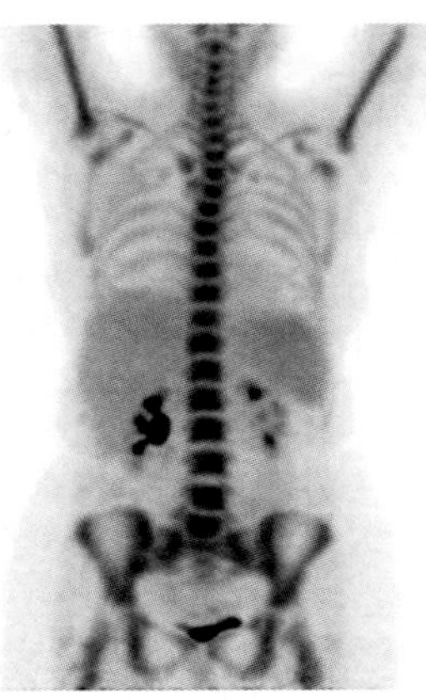

Coronal, sagittal, axial, and MIP images from FDG-PET demonstrate diffusely increased uptake in the entire visualized marrow distribution.

Differential Diagnosis

- ***Benign marrow stimulation:*** Homogeneous, intensely increased uptake in the axial and proximal appendicular skeleton (red marrow) diffusely makes this the most likely diagnosis.
- *Widespread osseous tumor:* This can look similar if severe, but uptake will usually be more heterogeneous.
- *Altered biodistribution:* Elevated patient insulin or glucose levels during the examination can cause diffuse alterations in FDG uptake but usually result in increased peripheral muscle (not skeletal) uptake (see Case 6).

Essential Facts

- Oncology patients are often anemic from chemotherapy regimens or as a result of the tumor itself and can be given a granulocyte colony–stimulating factor (G–CSF) such as filgrastim (Neupogen; Amgen, Thousand Oaks, CA) to boost marrow function.
- The increase in marrow metabolism and cellularity associated with G–CSFs (or that may be an endogenous response to anemia itself) can cause diffusely increased FDG uptake throughout the red marrow, which in adults is confined to the axial and proximal appendicular skeleton (red marrow extends more distally in children).

Other Imaging Findings

- Bone scintigraphy will be essentially negative in patients with pharmacologic marrow stimulation (although in chronic severe anemias like sickle cell anemia it can show increased uptake around the major peripheral joints and skull because of marrow expansion).
- Bone scintigraphy may be positive for diffuse osseous tumor or negative if the tumor involves the marrow exclusively (e.g., lymphoma).
- CT and MRI can be used to distinguish benign uptake from diffuse tumor; MRI is more sensitive than CT for osseous tumor, and plain radiographs are relatively insensitive. Marrow biopsy may be required, however.

✓ Pearls & × Pitfalls

✓ Diffuse marrow stimulation on FDG-PET can obscure true superimposed skeletal metastases. When possible, the patient should be off short-acting marrow-stimulating agents like filgrastim for approximately 1 week before the PET examination (and longer for longer-acting agents).

× Diffusely increased splenic uptake greater than liver can also be seen with marrow stimulation (spleen is a red marrow equivalent).

× However, focal splenic uptake or diffuse splenic uptake *without* increased marrow likely indicates splenic tumor involvement, particularly in lymphoma.

× Very widespread osseous tumor can approximate benign marrow stimulation on PET but will appear slightly more heterogeneous; additionally, the tumor is often (but not always) evident on the CT portion, as in this different patient:

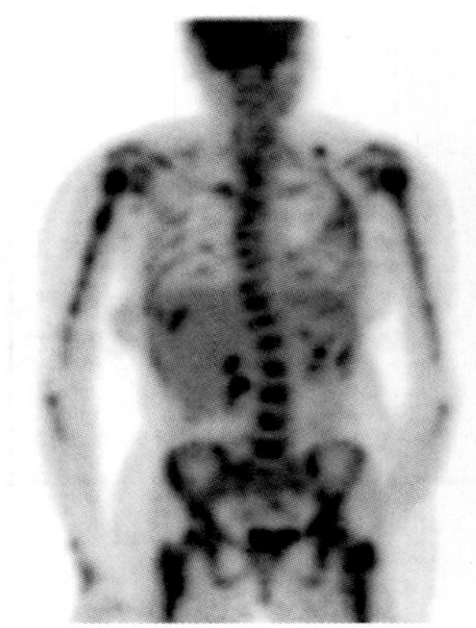

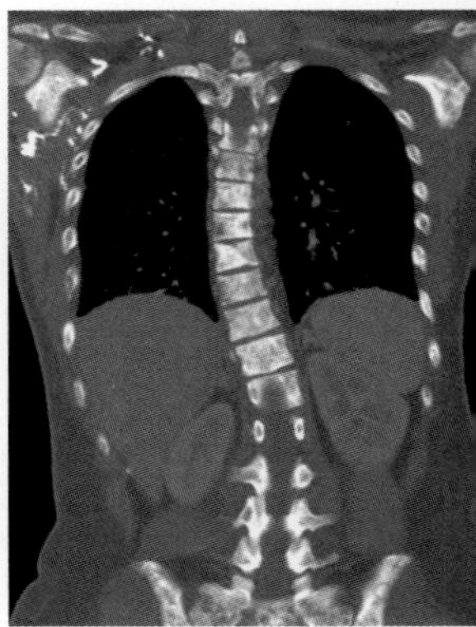

Case 39

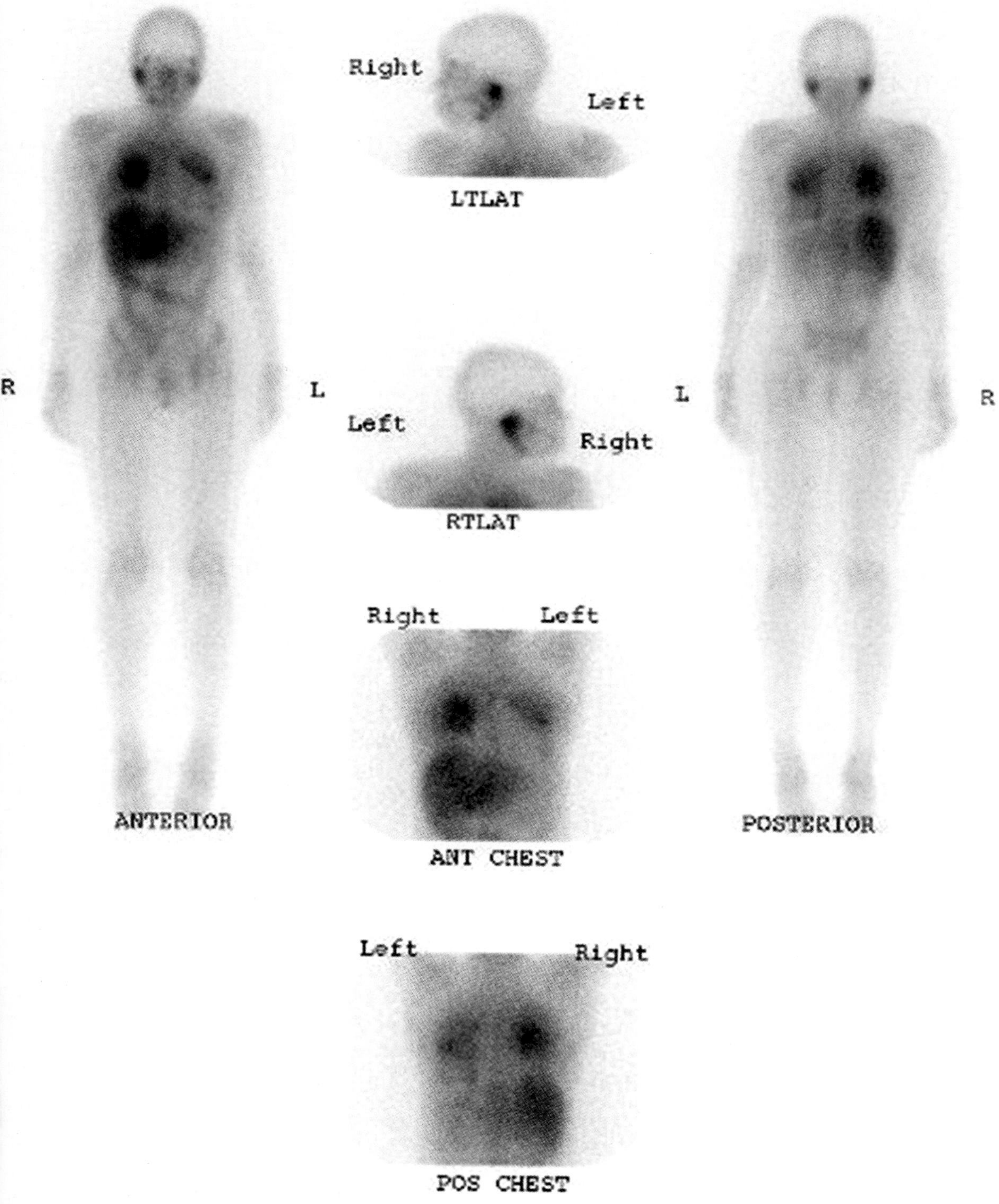

Clinical Presentation

42-year-old woman with human immunodeficiency virus and shortness of breath. A chest radiograph was normal. nages were acquired at 48 hours after injection of radiotracer.

Imaging Findings

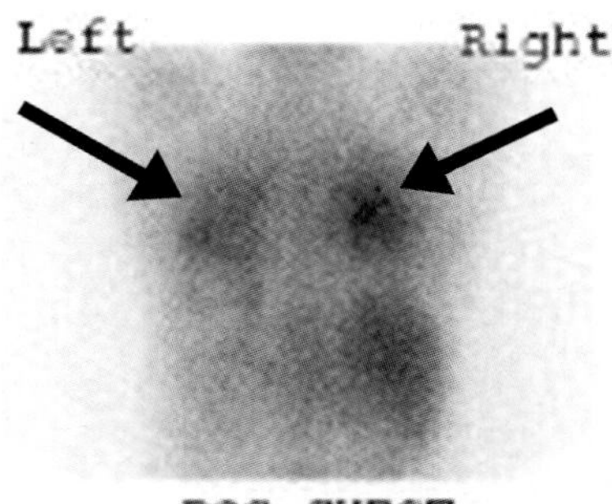

Forty-eight–hour delayed whole-body planar images as well as spot views of the chest demonstrate physiologic uptake in the liver, bowel, and lacrimal and salivary glands. Diffuse, intense uptake (greater than liver) is seen throughout both lungs, most notably in the upper lobes (*arrows*).

Differential Diagnosis

- ***Gallium scan demonstrating* Pneumocystis carinii/ jiroveci *pneumonia (PCP):*** The physiologic distribution makes Ga67 the correct radiopharmaceutical. Diffuse, intense pulmonary parenchymal uptake is most likely PCP (or other atypical infection), given the history.
- *Sarcoid:* This is typically associated with paratracheal and bilateral hilar lymph node uptake on Ga67, often with increased salivary and lacrimal involvement ("panda" sign). It can also, however, present with diffuse pulmonary parenchymal uptake alone.
- *Tumor:* Several malignancies, including lung cancer, lymphoma, melanoma, and sarcoma (except Kaposi), are Ga67-avid. These are typically more focal, however.

Essential Facts

- Ga67 is a nonspecific radiotracer avid for many infectious, inflammatory, and neoplastic processes. A number of infections, including PCP, can be imaged, as well as tumors, sarcoidosis, and lung inflammation, such as from drug toxicities.
- Increased Ga67 uptake is due to increased vascular permeability, increased tissue permeability, neutrophil activation, and binding to transferrin and lactoferrin.
- The degree of gallium uptake corresponds to the degree of inflammation seen on histology but not necessarily the degree of symptoms or radiographic findings. With PCP, intense, diffuse uptake can be present with a normal chest radiograph.
- A grading system of gallium lung uptake can be used:
  - Grade 0: no uptake after 48 hours
  - Grade 1: uptake less than liver
  - Grade 2: uptake equal to liver
  - Grade 3: uptake greater than liver

Other Imaging Findings

- In patients with PCP, chest radiography and CT typically have nonspecific findings and are normal in 10 to 15% of patients. The most common finding on chest CT is a bilateral reticular interstitial pattern.
- FDG-PET can image the majority of diseases historically imaged with Ga67, including pulmonary infection/ inflammation, with an overall greater sensitivity. However, insurance reimbursement for infection/inflammation can be problematic with PET, so it is uncommonly performed for this indication.

✓ Pearls & × Pitfalls

- ✓ Kidneys may be seen normally on 24-hour gallium images; however, significant activity seen after 48 hours is abnormal.
- ✓ Gallium uptake will indicate active pulmonary disease, even with a normal chest radiograph.
- ✓ Gallium can be used to monitor response to therapy. A classic gallium scan appearance following PCP therapy with aerosolized pentamidine shows persistent bilateral apical activity and resolution elsewhere—the apices have less ventilation and thus less therapy is delivered.
- ✓ A negative gallium scan makes the diagnosis of PCP unlikely.
- × Sarcoid can alternatively present with diffuse lung uptake and no lymph node activity.
- × Physiologic breast activity in women may mimic lung uptake. Posterior images will help differentiate the two.
- × Gallium imaging performed within 24 hours after tracer injection will commonly show normal physiologic diffuse lung uptake. Lung uptake on more delayed images is abnormal, however.
- × *Pneumocystic jiroveci* is now known to be the causative agent in humans, although the term PCP is still commonly used.

Images courtesy of Dr. Lionel Zuckier, Department of Radiology, University of Medicine and Dentistry of New Jersey, Newark, NJ.

Case 40

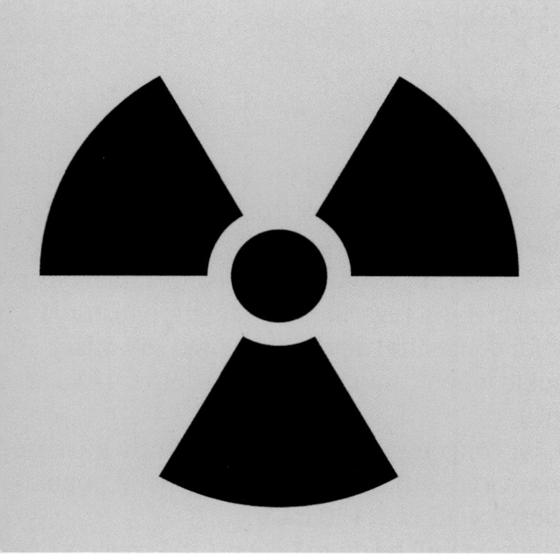

Clinical Presentation

A nuclear medicine technologist informs you that she is pregnant.

Further Work-up

She estimates that conception was 6 weeks ago. Her current cumulative dose since that time is 0.47 rem.

What Needs to Be Done?

Carefully monitor her exposure for the rest of the year.
Nothing. Return to work as before.
She can no longer work handling radiation doses anymore this year.

Differential Diagnosis: Discussion

What Needs to Be Done?

- ***Carefully monitor her exposure for the rest of the year.*** Correct, the technologist will require continued monitoring and may receive no more than 0.03 rem during the remainder of the pregnancy. See below for discussion.
- *Return to work as before.* Incorrect.
- *She can no longer work handling radiation doses for this year.* Incorrect.

Essential Facts

- The dose equivalent to the embryo/fetus during the entire pregnancy must not exceed 0.5 rem (5 mSv).
- The dose equivalent to the embryo/fetus is the sum of the deep dose equivalent to the pregnant woman and the dose equivalent to the embryo/fetus resulting from radionuclides in the embryo/fetus and radionuclides in the pregnant woman.
- A fetal badge should be provided to the declared pregnant worker. Exposure should be uniform throughout the pregnancy.
- Because this worker already has an exposure of 0.47 rem (4.7 mSv), she is not allowed > 0.03 rem (0.3 mSv) for the remainder of this pregnancy.
- Pregnant women with exposures already > 0.5 rem (5 mSv) at the time they declare pregnancy are allowed an additional embryo/fetal dose equivalent of up to 0.05 rem (0.5 mSv).

✓ Pearls & × Pitfalls

✓ Based on the National Council on Radiation Protection:
- The risk for congenital defect from doses < 10 rad (100 mGy) at any stage of pregnancy is very small compared with the normal risk for congenital defects (estimated at 4–6% regardless of radiation history).
- The risk for congenital defect at ≤ 5 rad (50 mGy) is negligible when compared with the other risks of pregnancy.
- The risk for congenital defect is significantly increased when compared with the that of the general population at doses > 15 rad (150 mGy).

✓ The fetal thyroid will begin to take up and concentrate iodine only after the 10th week.

× The 3- to 5-week period of pregnancy is the time when the fetus is most sensitive to death from radiation.

Case 41

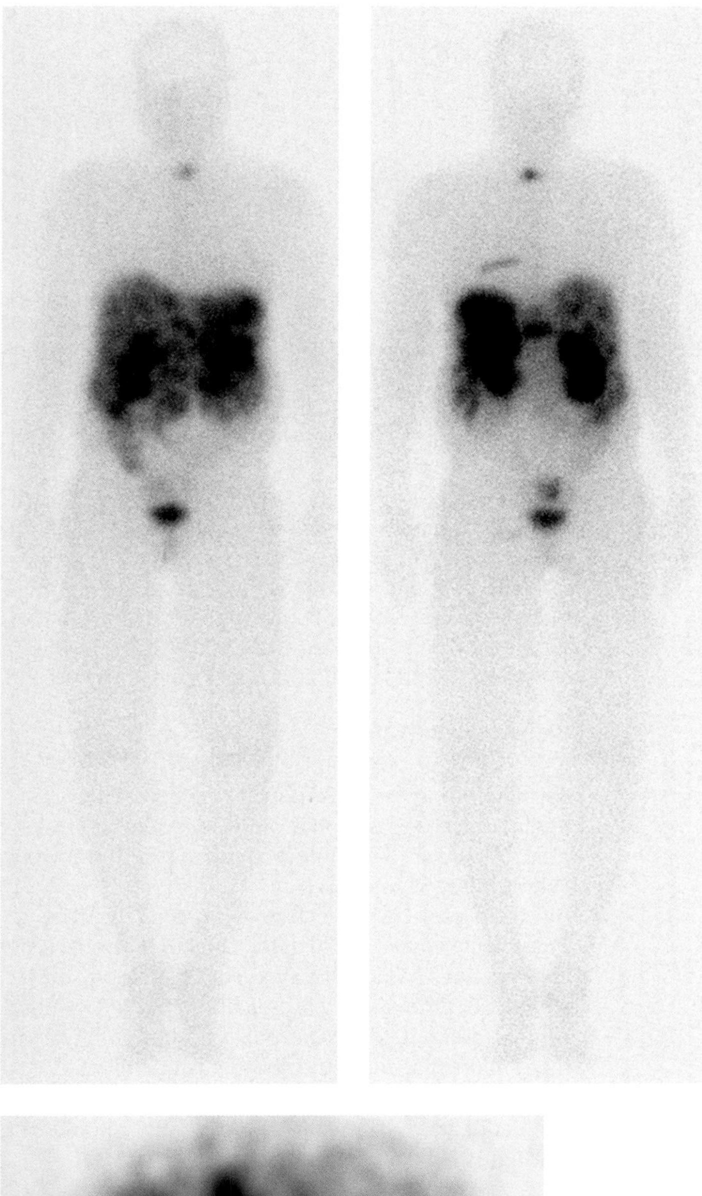

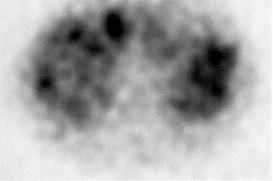

Clinical Presentation

43-year-old man with a history of malignancy presents for restaging.

Imaging Findings

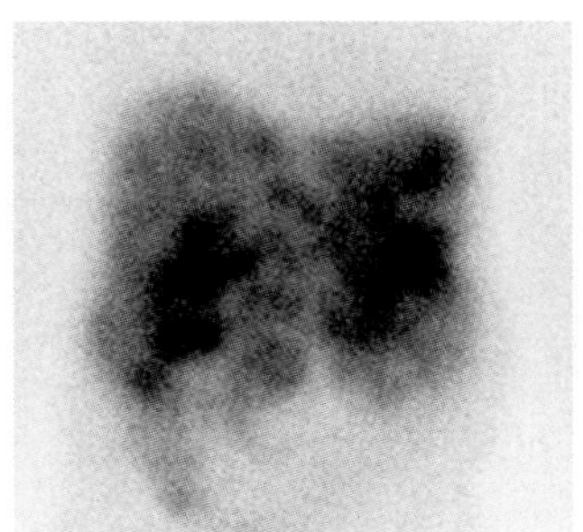
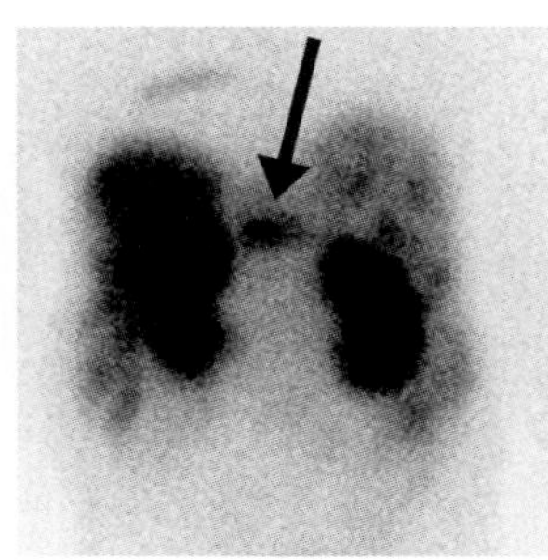
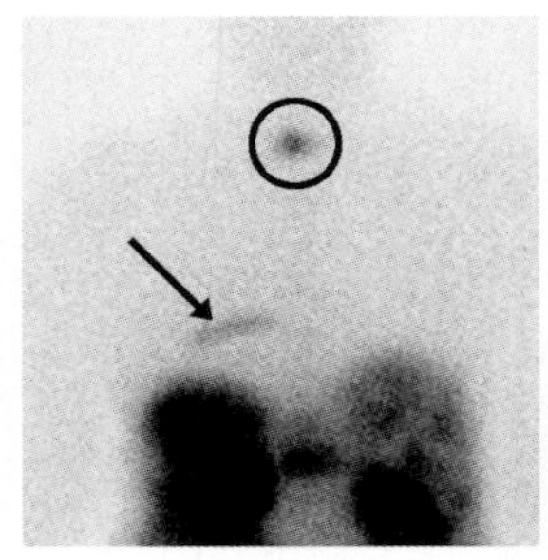
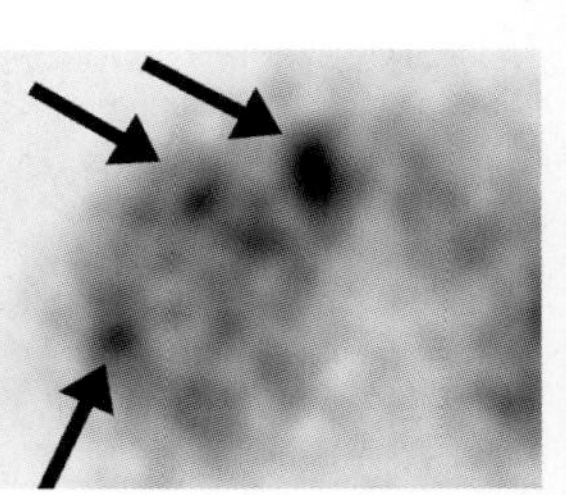

(A) Anterior and posterior whole-body views demonstrate multiple abnormal skeletal (rib and spine; *arrows*), abdominal, soft-tissue, and hepatic lesions. A focus seen over the neck on the anterior view is most likely a shine-through artifact from an upper spine lesion, best seen on the posterior view (*circle*). Intense physiologic renal cortical and splenic activity is seen diffusely. **(B)** An axial SPECT image better demonstrates the multiple hepatic lesions (*arrows*).

Differential Diagnosis

- ***OctreoScan showing metastatic islet cell carcinoma:*** The intense splenic and renal cortical activity and lack of normal skeletal uptake make OctreoScan imaging of a metastatic neuroendocrine tumor (NET) the most likely diagnosis.
- *MIBG scan showing metastatic neuroblastoma:* This can also be used for NET imaging and also does not have normal marrow uptake. However, intense physiologic splenic and renal cortical uptake should not be seen.
- *Gallium scan showing metastatic melanoma:* Ga67 will also show physiologic liver, spleen, and bowel activity. However, spleen is not greater than liver and will also show normal bone and lacrimal uptake.

Essential Facts

- Pentetreotide (OctreoScan) is a somatostatin analogue (eight–amino acid fragment) labeled with indium 111.
- Most NETs, such as most islet cell tumors (gastrinoma, carcinoid, VIPoma, glucagonoma), pituitary adenomas, and pheochromocytomas, are OctreoScan-avid.
- Other potentially avid tumors include small-cell lung carcinomas, meningiomas, astrocytomas, and certain lymphomas and breast cancers.
- Two NETs—insulinomas and medullary thyroid cancers—have a significantly lower OctreoScan avidity.
- Islet cell tumors often originate in the pancreas, bowel, or elsewhere in the abdomen, but the primary lesion may not been seen.
- Metastases include those to the skeleton and liver, where they may become particularly symptomatic, causing, for example, flushing and diarrhea with carcinoid syndrome.

Other Imaging Findings

- Bone scintigraphy can be used in conjunction with octreotide to assess for skeletal metastases.
- CT or MRI can demonstrate the primary lesion or hepatic or peritoneal metastases; the hepatic lesions are typically hypervascular and best seen on arterially weighted imaging (they may not be apparent on standard portal venous–phase imaging).
- MIBG scanning can be used to detect many NETs, with significant overlap with OctreoScan in tumor avidity (see Case 12).
- FDG-PET can also be attempted for imaging these tumors. As a very general rule, more differentiated (lower-grade) subtypes will be better seen with OctreoScan (or MIBG) and less well-differentiated tumors better seen with FDG-PET.

✓ Pearls & ✗ Pitfalls

✓ For whole-body scans, if normal skeletal activity is *absent*, the study is probably an OctreoScan, MIBG scan, or iodine 131 whole-body scan (see "Interpreting Whole-Body Scans").

✓ Although most NETs are OctreoScan-avid, the intense physiologic renal cortical uptake makes perirenal lesions (e.g., adrenal) hard to visualize. For this reason, MIBG should be contemplated for renal/adrenal NET evaluation.

✗ Any skeletal uptake on OctreoScan, MIBG, or I131 imaging is abnormal and indicates metastatic disease.

✗ Physiologic biliary excretion of pentetreotide into the gallbladder, as in this case below (*arrow*), should be distinguished from a true liver metastasis:

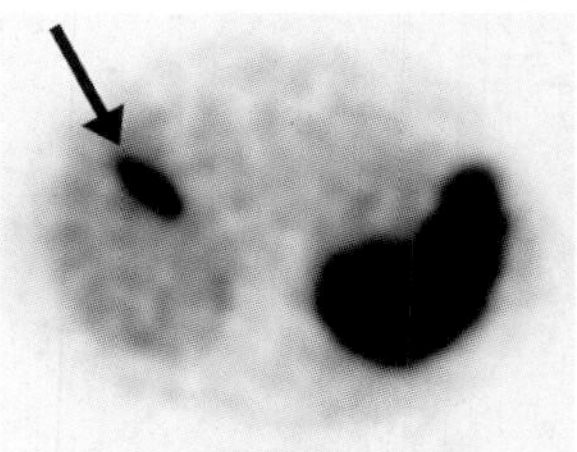

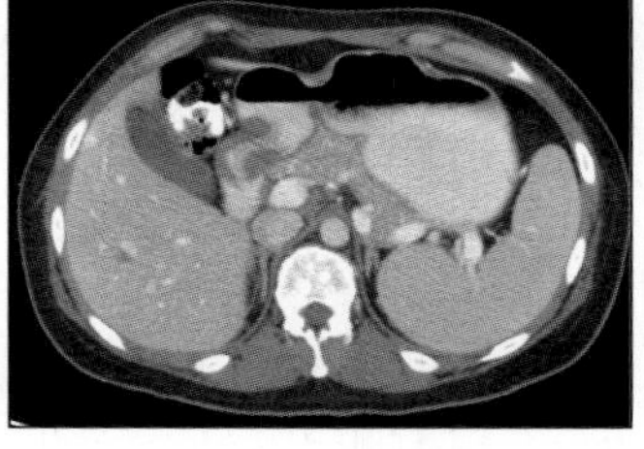

Case 42

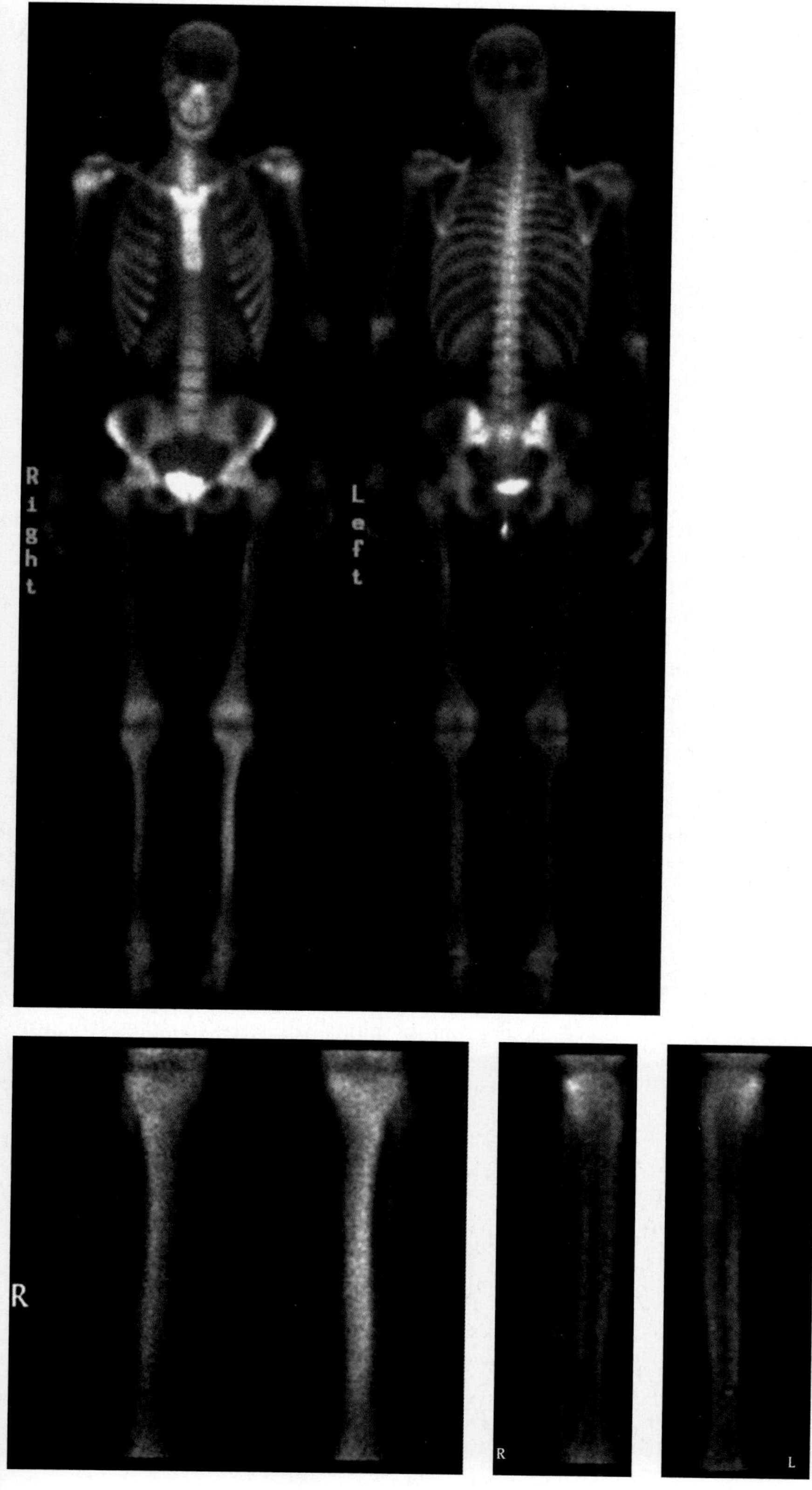

Clinical Presentation

19-year-old woman with recent left leg pain.

Imaging Findings

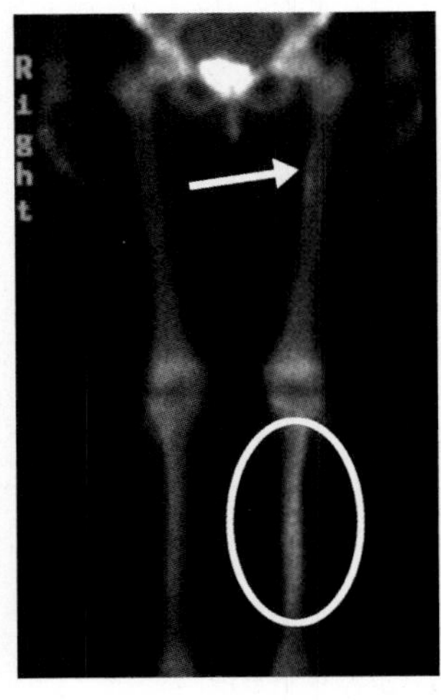

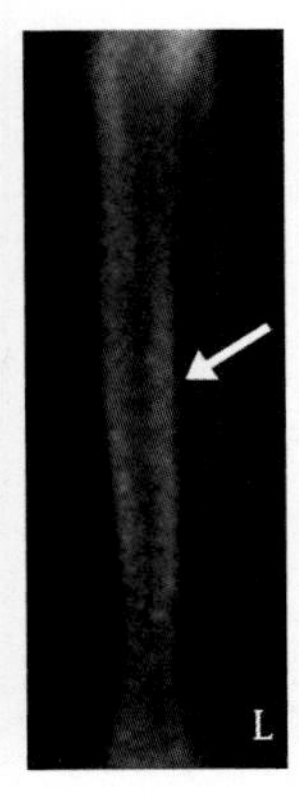

A B

(A) Anterior and posterior whole-body bone scan images demonstrate linear increased uptake along the medial cortical surface of the left proximal femur (*arrow*). Additionally there is less-well-defined increased uptake at the mid tibiae, the left greater than the right (*circle*). **(B)** Anterior and lateral spot views of the tibiae/fibulae demonstrate that the increased uptake is most pronounced along the posterior cortical surfaces of the tibiae the left greater than the right, in a linear distribution (*arrow*).

Differential Diagnosis

- ***Shin and hip "splints":*** Linear uptake along the posterior periosteal surface of the mid tibia is essentially pathognomonic for shin splints. A similar appearance can be seen along the medial surface of the proximal femur.
- *Hypertrophic osteoarthropathy:* This is also characterized by uptake along the periosteum of the extremities. However, it is usually much more extensive, typically involving bilaterally the femora, tibiae, fibulae, and often the upper extremities, with more diffuse involvement of each bone (see Case 13).
- *Venous stasis/thrombosis:* This will also have uptake along the periosteum of a lower extremity. However, uptake tends to be more irregular and is not confined to the mid posterior tibia.

Essential Facts

- Shin splints (also known as medial tibial stress syndrome) are an overuse injury at the site of the soleus muscle tendinous insertion along the tibial periosteum ("Sharpey fibers").
- Result in regional periostitis along the posteromedial surface of the mid to distal third of the tibia
- Patients experience diffuse soreness in this region that is exacerbated by exercise.
- Can be unilateral or bilateral
- Management involves rest (several weeks) and anti-inflammatories and need not be as aggressive as with stress fractures, which require longer rest and immobilization.
- The less common but analogous "hip (or quad) splint" can be seen along the tendinous insertions of the hip adductors along the medial periosteal surface of the proximal femur, as in this patient.

Other Imaging Findings

- No plain radiographic or CT findings are typically visualized
- MRI can demonstrate abnormal signal or enhancement along the tibial periosteum in more advanced cases.

✓ Pearls & × Pitfalls

✓ Shin splints are not hyperemic and thus typically not hot on blood flow or blood pool phases, unlike fractures (stress or completed), which tend to be hot on all three phases.

✓ Despite the name, the symptoms and imaging findings of shin splints are along the medial *posterior* tibial surface.

✓ On bone scan, lateral views are often necessary (as in this patient) to demonstrate that the abnormal uptake is along the cortical/periosteal surface of the bone, as opposed to the more central medulla (which carries a very different differential diagnosis, including infection and tumor).

× Do not confuse splints with stress fractures, which are also an overuse injury of the lower extremities with abnormal uptake at the bone periphery. Stress fractures appear as much more focal lesions and may occur anywhere in the lower extremities, as in this other patient below (*arrow*):

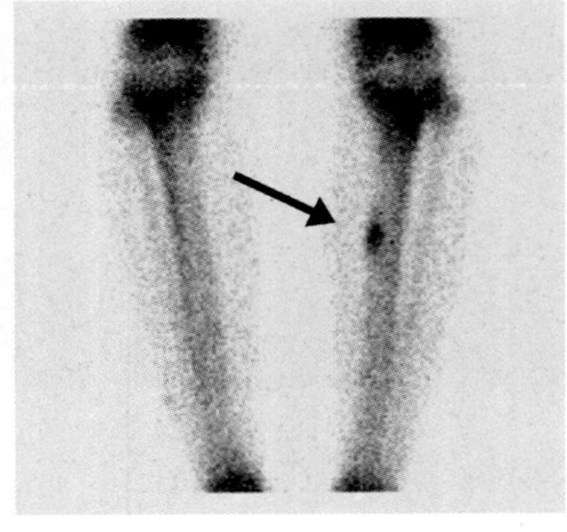

Case 43

Clinical Presentation

A 65-year-old man has undergone near complete thyroidectomy for stage III papillary thyroid cancer. You are requested to administer 150 mCi of iodine 131, and radiation precautions must be considered.

Considerations

- He could most likely be treated as an outpatient.
- He must be treated as an inpatient.
- He cannot be treated with this amount of radiation.

Differential Diagnosis: Discussion

- ***He could most likely be treated as an outpatient:*** Correct.
- *He must be treated as an inpatient:* Incorrect.
- *He cannot be treated with this amount of radiation:* Incorrect.

Essential Facts

- Because the patient is being dosed with > 30 µCi of iodine 131, a written directive (signed prescription) is required from an authorized user.
  - A written directive is also required for administration of any therapeutic dose of unsealed by-product material or any therapeutic dose of radiation from by-product material.
  - Diagnostic studies performed with other forms of I131, such as I131-MIBG, do not require a written directive, even if the dose is > 30 µCi.
- The Nuclear Regulatory Commission no longer requires hospitalization for patients treated with high-dose I131, and a patient may be released from the department based on several criteria (covered under 10 CFR 35.75):
  - A given dose is < 33 mCi or a patient external measurement of < 7 mR/h at 1 m.
  - Alternatively, patient-specific dose calculations can be made. These are based on the dose given and estimated occupancy factor for that patient (E). The total annual projected dose to an individual member of the public from a released patient *cannot exceed 0.5 rem* (500 mrem or 5 mSv), and if exposure to others is likely to exceed 0.1 rem (1 mSv), verbal and written instructions must be given on minimizing this exposure—as low as reasonably achievable (ALARA)—to ensure that it does not exceed the 0.5-rem annual limit.
- E = 0.75 when a physical half-life, an effective half-life, or a specific time period under consideration (e.g., bladder holding time) is ≤ 1 day.
- E = 0.25 when an effective half-life is > 1 day or if the patient has been given instructions, such as:
  - Maintain a prudent distance from others for at least the first 2 days.
  - Sleep alone in a room for at least the first night.
  - Do not travel by airplane or mass transportation for at least the first day.
  - Do not travel on a prolonged automobile trip with others for at least the first 2 days.
  - Have sole use of a bathroom for at least the first 2 days.
  - Drink plenty of fluids for at least the first 2 days.
- E = 0.125 when an effective half-life is > 1 day or if the patient has been given instructions, such as:
  - Follow the instructions for E = 0.25.
  - Live alone for at least the first 2 days.
  - Have few visits by family or friends for at least the first 2 days.
- Based on the patient described above and an occupancy factor of 0.25, he may be indeed be released after dosing with the requested 150 mCi based on the following calculation: $D(\infty) = 0.007612 \times 150\text{ mCi} \times 0.299 = 0.341\text{ rem}$.
- If the patient is admitted for his treatment (will not or cannot follow radiation precautions):
  - Radiation precaution signs must be posted outside his room.
  - Instructions must be given to nursing.
  - Room surveys must be recorded.
- On discharge: if it is likely that individuals may be exposed to > 0.1 rem (1 mSv), written instructions must be provided to patients on how to maintain doses to others ALARA.
- The technologist administering the dose of I131 does not necessarily require bioassay. Only adults likely to receive an intake in excess of 10% of the annual limit require bioassay. For I131, this value is 3 µCi, which is unlikely if capsules are used rather than liquid.
- Maintain records containing the following information for 3 years:
  - Radiopharmaceutical
  - Patient name
  - Dose
  - Date/time of administration
  - Name of person administering the dose

✓ Pearls & ✗ Pitfalls

- ✓ Calculation of the prescribed dose of I131 for thyroid cancer treatment is usually based on the extent of disease.
  - Thyroid bed remnant: 30 to 100 mCi
  - Local lymph node metastases: 150 mCi
  - Lung metastases: 175 mCi
  - Bone metastases: 200 mCi
- ✓ To avoid radiation toxicity:
  - Dose to the blood should not exceed 200 rad.
  - Whole-body retention at 48 hours should be < 120 mCi (< 80 mCi if extensive pulmonary metastases are present to avoid pulmonary fibrosis).
- ✓ Assessment of cancer risk due to exposure to I131 is difficult; however, several studies have shown that this is significant only at high doses (> 500 mCi).
- ✗ Remember that radioiodine is administered orally.
- ✗ Ensure elevated thyroid stimulating hormone (TSH) levels before any radioiodine administration (diagnostic or therapeutic). This may be accomplished by thyroid hormone withdrawal (making the patient hypothyroid, resulting in serum TSH > 30 mIU/L) or intramuscular Thyrogen injections 1 and 2 days before iodine dosing. This regimen also improves FDG PET detection of metastatic thyroid cancer.
- ✗ Ensure that a pregnancy test is performed in all women of childbearing potential before dosing.
- ✗ Patients who are incontinent or require round-the-clock nursing care may not be eligible for high-dose outpatient therapy and may need to be admitted.

Case 44

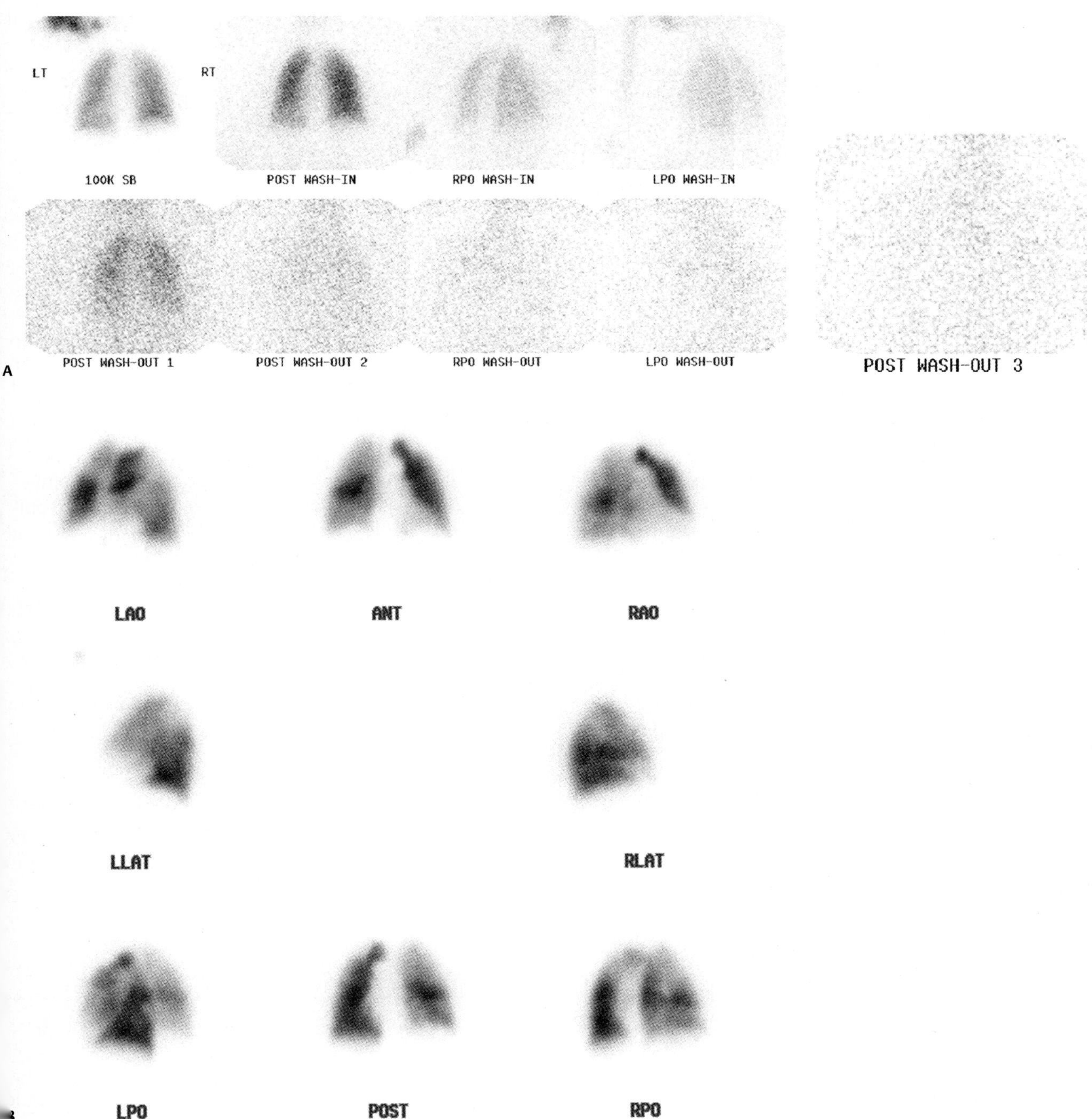

A

B

Clinical Presentation

A 25-year-old pregnant woman with acute shortness of breath. Chest radiograph was normal.

Imaging Findings

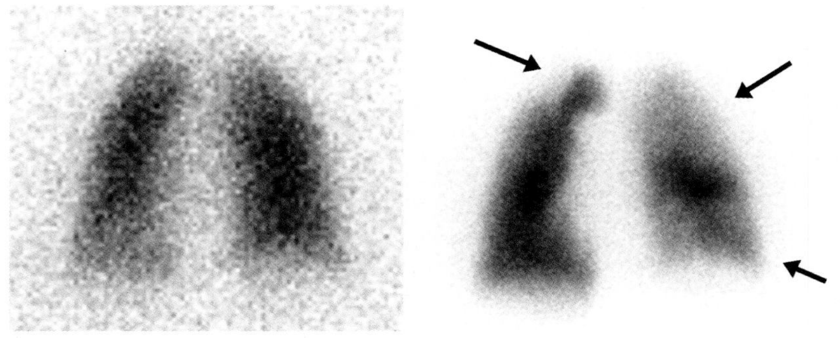

(A) Sequential posterior and posterior oblique xenon 133 ventilation images are normal. There are no defects on single-breath or early wash-in imaging, and there is no abnormal retention on washout. **(B)** Tc99m-MAA images demonstrate multiple medium and large subsegmental and segmental perfusion defects (*arrows*)—some are decreased and others are completely absent.

Differential Diagnosis

- ***High probability of pulmonary embolism (PE):*** At least two large (or the equivalent) mismatched perfusion defects meet the criteria for high probability.
- *Pulmonary vasculitis:* This is also in the differential for multiple mismatches but is rare and less likely given the history.
- *Mediastinal adenopathy compressing pulmonary vessels:* This is also in the differential for mismatches but usually does not result in this many widespread defects; furthermore, it is unlikely, given the normal chest x-ray (CXR).

Essential Facts

- Most perfusion defects seen-in lung ventilation–perfusion (VQ) scans are not due to PE but are secondary to reflex vasoconstriction from a primary matched airway abnormality (e.g., asthma, mucous plug, chronic obstructive pulmonary disease).
- However, the greater the number and/or size of *mismatched* perfusion defects, the more likely they are due to PE as classified by PIOPED.
- PIOPED I, II, and III have been completed. PIOPED II (which added CTA/CT venography [CTV] data) is typically used for the assessment of VQ scans. (PIOPED III includes MRA/magnetic resonance venography [MRV]).
- Highlights of PIOPED II classification:
  - Normal: no perfusion (Q) defects
  - Very low probability: one to three small Q defects (matched or not)
  - Low probability: more than three all small Q defects
  - Intermediate probability: mismatched one moderate (25–75% segment) to one large plus one moderate or equivalent Q defects (one large = two moderate)
  - High probability: mismatched two or more large or equivalent Q defects
- Clinicians should then combine the scan result with their clinical suspicion to determine overall probability.

Other Imaging Findings

- CXRs are nonspecific and insensitive for PE and may be normal. Associated findings include a small pleural effusion, atelectasis, enlarged and sharply defined central pulmonary artery, regional oligemia ("Westermark" sign), and focal peripheral density from infarct ("Hampton hump").
- CTA will demonstrate intraluminal filling defect(s) and has emerged as the modality of choice for most patients who can tolerate intravenous contrast. CTV can also evaluate the extremities for deep vein thrombosis at the same time.
- Catheter angiography is the historic gold standard but uncommonly used today unless intervention is considered.
- MRA/MRV is also being used at some centers.
- On VQ, a "triple match" of V, Q, and CXR abnormalities in the lower lungs is intermediate probability (but is very low probability in middle and upper lungs).
- A "stripe sign" on VQ (preserved peripheral perfusion with a more central defect) is very low probability.

✓ Pearls & × Pitfalls

✓ On perfusion scans, a true defect may have absent or merely decreased uptake (down = out, as seen in this case). Also, the lungs should normally get hotter as you go lower, as there is more lung volume and thus there are more pulmonary capillaries inferiorly (if not, then a likely defect).

× Remember to obtain CXR shortly before or after VQ.

× When Xe133 is used for ventilation, a perfusion match can be made to early defects (wash-in), late retention (washout), or both. For example, normal wash-in but abnormal retention on washout qualifies as a *matched* defect.

Case 45

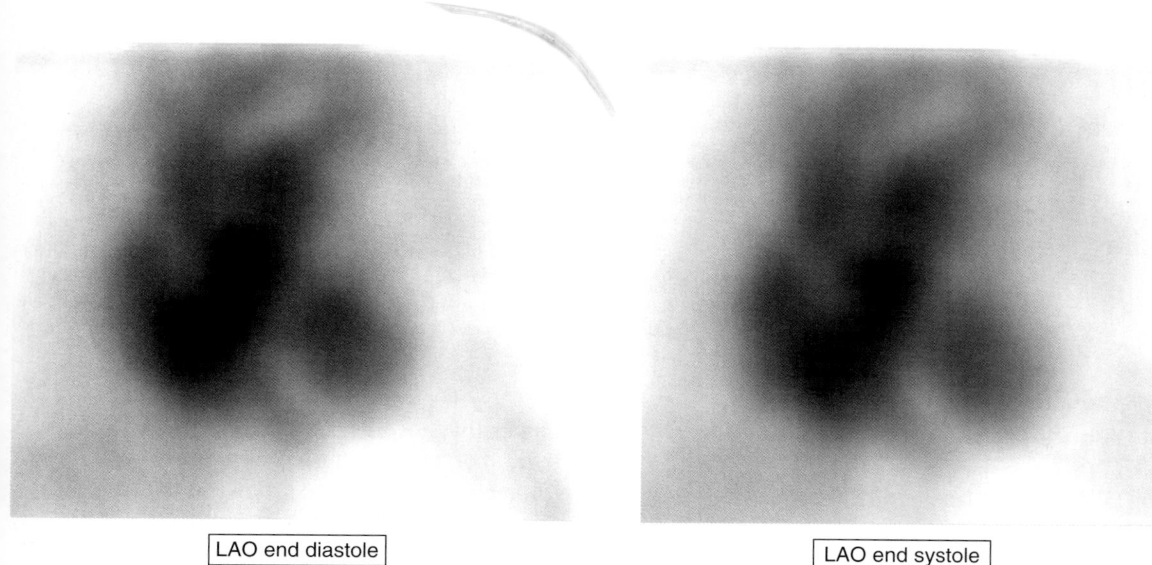

LAO end diastole

LAO end systole

Clinical Presentation

A 64-year-old man with progressive shortness of breath.

Imaging Findings

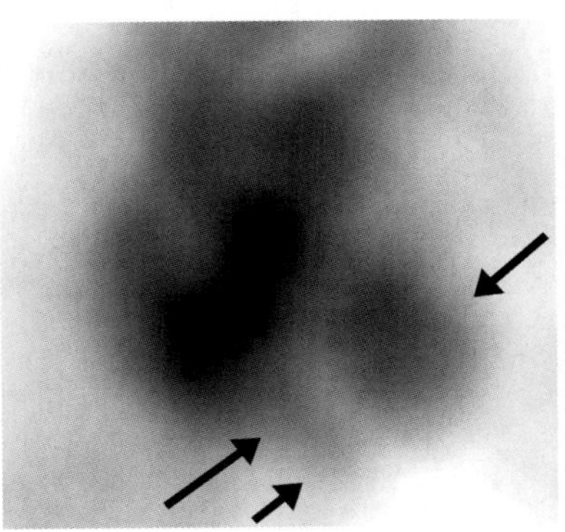

Two left anterior oblique (LAO) frames at end diastole (ED) and end systole (ES) from a Tc99m RBC MUGA scan demonstrate a significantly dilated left ventricle (LV; *single arrow*) compared with the normal right ventricle (RV; *double arrows*). Only a slight decrease in LV size is seen on end systole compared with end diastole (left ventricular ejection fraction [LVEF] calculated to be 32%). The visualized portions of the RV demonstrate normal size and wall motion.

Differential Diagnosis

Decreased resting LVEF and ventricular dilatation are nonspecific and can be seen with ischemic disease, valvular disease, and cardiac toxicity.

- ***Ischemic cardiomyopathy:*** A regional wall motion abnormality is most specific for ischemic disease, although global wall motion abnormalities can also be seen, as in this case. The RV is typically spared, as also in this case.
- *Chemotherapy:* Certain regimens, such as doxorubicin, are potentially cardiotoxic. Effects are dose-dependent and usually transient. RV and LV dilatation may be seen. Alcohol is another toxin that can cause this same dilated cardiomyopathic appearance.
- *Aortic regurgitation:* LV dilatation is a common finding; however, early in the disease, LVEF is normal. As the disease progresses, LVEF drops. This pattern can also be seen with mitral regurgitation and prolonged aortic stenosis.

Essential Facts

- Radionuclide ventriculogram (also known as RVG, RNV, or MUGA) can be used to assess LV function in several conditions, including ischemic or valvular heart disease and cardiomyopathies, and to assess ventricular function during chemotherapy. RV function can also be evaluated.
- RVG can be performed via two methods: first pass or equilibrium. First pass is rapid bolus imaging of Tc99m-pertechnetate or Tc99m-DTPA as tracer passes through the cardiac chambers over several beats. Equilibrium requires Tc99m-RBC imaging over many more cycles, gated to the electrocardiogram (ECG).
- Both methods provide images of the cardiac chambers, from which wall thickness and motion can be inferred and ejection fractions calculated. Diastolic filling rates can also be determined to assess for diastolic dysfunction.
- Currently, the examination is most commonly performed for chemotherapy, which may result in a global wall motion abnormality. Ischemic disease more commonly shows regional wall motion abnormalities.
- Cardiomyopathy due to *pressure* overload, such as in hypertension or aortic stenosis, will show concentric LV hypertrophy (small cavity and septal thickening seen as photopenia between the chambers) with a normal-to-hypernormal LVEF initially. Only later in the disease will the LVEF drop and the ventricle dilate.
- Cardiomyopathy due to *volume* overload causes earlier chamber dilation and more eccentric muscle hypertrophy (which is less severe than hypertrophy from pressure overload).

Other Imaging Findings

- Resting myocardial perfusion gated SPECT (e.g., with thallium 201 or MIBI) images the cardiac *wall* motion directly (as opposed to the *chambers*). The examination is longer, more expensive, and not quite as reproducible for following chemotherapy effects, however.
- Echocardiography can measure LV size and LVEF without ionizing radiation. However, it uses several geometric assumptions that are not as accurate for EF calculation and can be even less accurate for heavy patients.
- Cardiac MRI is an accurate means of assessing LVEF and also provides good anatomic evaluation without radiation. This modality is more costly and technically difficult, however.

✓ Pearls & × Pitfalls

✓ The RV should normally have a slightly larger volume than the LV.

✓ Equilibrium images are acquired in the LAO ("best septal view"), anterior, and left lateral projections.

✓ First pass (typically performed in right anterior oblique) is more accurate for RV evaluation (no chamber overlap as with equilibrium).

✓ In patients taking cardiotoxic chemotherapy (e.g., doxorubicin), a relative drop in LVEF of $>$ 10% from previous *plus* an absolute LVEF of $<$ 50% is an indication to stop treatment.

✓ MUGA can also be performed during stress. Developing a wall motion abnormality or not increasing LVEF during stress is consistent with coronary disease/ischemia.

Case 46

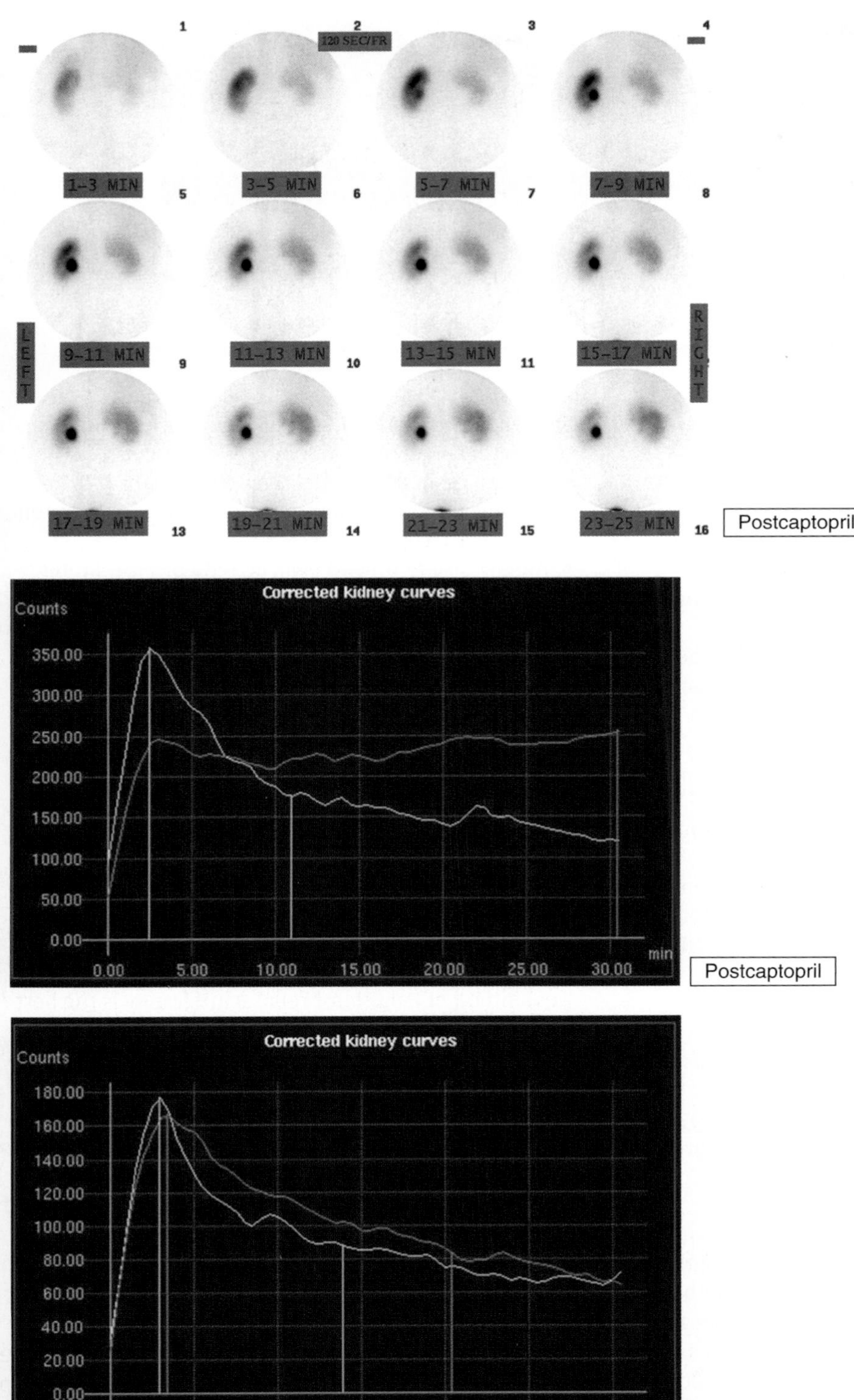

Clinical Presentation

A 42-year-old man with uncontrolled hypertension. Examination was performed post captopril (images and curves shown in Figs. A and B). Baseline examination was normal symmetric (baseline curve shown in Fig. C; right is red, left green; baseline images not shown).

Imaging Findings

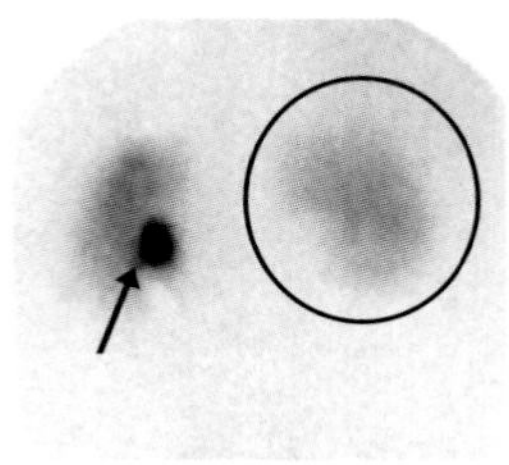

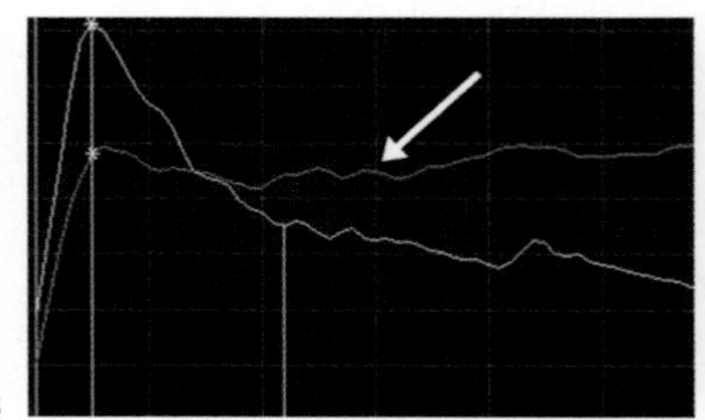

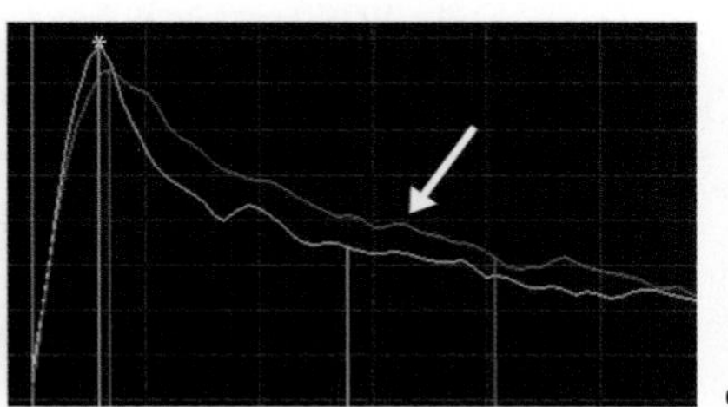

(A,B) Posterior images and renogram curves from a Tc99m-MAG3 captopril renal scan demonstrate normal uptake and excretion by the left kidney into an extrarenal pelvis (A, *arrow*), which progressively clears over time, arguing against obstruction. On the right, there is progressive radiotracer extraction but no demonstrable excretion (A, *circle*), with resultant flattening of the renogram curve (B, *arrow*). There is decreased relative right renal function (calculated to be 41% for the right, 59% for the left) as measured at peak uptake at 2.5 minutes (B, *asterisks*). **(C)** Renogram curve from the baseline examination before captopril demonstrates normal excretory curves bilaterally (*arrow*) and symmetric parenchymal function (*asterisk*).

Differential Diagnosis

- ***Renovascular hypertension (RVH):*** Unilateral renal parenchymal dysfunction with captopril that normalizes without captopril is highly suggestive of this condition.
- *Chronic medical renal disease:* Abnormal renal parenchymal function would be seen both with and without captopril. It usually affects both kidneys.
- *Acute pyelonephritis:* This can demonstrate unilateral renal parenchymal dysfunction but would also not change with captopril. This is unlikely, given the history.

Essential Facts

- Hypertension is a common condition, most often with no identifiable etiology ("essential hypertension").
- When hypertension is present in a patient with a renal artery stenosis, particularly if it is of recent onset, refractory to medical treatment, or in a younger patient, the possibility that renovascular disease is the cause of the hypertension is increased.
- The most common cause of RVH is atherosclerotic disease. In younger patients, fibromuscular dysplasia is more common.
- In patients with RVH, the renin–angiotensin pathway is activated to maintain glomerular filtration pressures. However, systemic hypertension also results.
- Renal scintigraphy with an angiotensin-converting enzyme (ACE) inhibitor (e.g., captopril, enalapril) can confirm the diagnosis. Either DTPA (glomerular agent) or MAG3 (tubular agent) can be used with an ACE inhibitor.
- With MAG3, the worsening renal parenchymal appearance is due to delayed tubular washout (from decreased urine formation) of secreted tracer as the glomerular filtration rate drops. With DTPA, it is due to decreased tracer extraction as glomerular filtration pressures drop and the glomerular filtration rate decreases.
- A normal ACE-inhibited scan excludes the diagnosis of RVH. An abnormal scan is suggestive but must be confirmed by seeing improvement with no ACE inhibition.
- Although a qualitative change on renogram images/curves from normal to abnormal parenchymal function is very suggestive of RVH, several quantitative values can be used with the affected kidney:
  - A decrease in differential renal function of > 5%
  - A change in the 20-minute percentage of peak parenchymal activity of > 15%
  - An increase in time to peak activity of > 5minutes.

Other Imaging Findings

- Anatomic evaluation of the renal arteries can be performed with catheter angiography, CTA, or MRA. However, these will not indicate if the stenosis is physiologically significant.

✓ Pearls & ✗ Pitfalls

✓ Many patients have renal artery narrowing seen on anatomic imaging, and many have hypertension (usually essential). ACE inhibitor renal scintigraphy is the best way to prove that the renal stenosis is physiologically significant (the cause of the hypertension) and thus to predict which patients will improve with renal artery stenting.

✓ RVH is a very uncommon cause of hypertension in the general population (< 1%). Preselection of higher-risk patients is crucial before ACE renography is performed (e.g., young, refractory, sudden onset).

✗ Interpretation is much less sensitive and specific when there is poor baseline renal function, as a change in function may not be seen.

✗ A decrease in *bilateral* renal function with ACE inhibition may be due to bilateral RVH. However, this appearance is more commonly due to transient hypotension from ACE during the scan, which causes cortical retention mimicking bilateral RVH. Make sure that the patient is well hydrated, and monitor blood pressure to be sure that this is not the case.

✗ The early *angiographic* images (0–30 seconds) on ACE renogram are often normal with RVH, unless the stenosis is severe.

Case 47

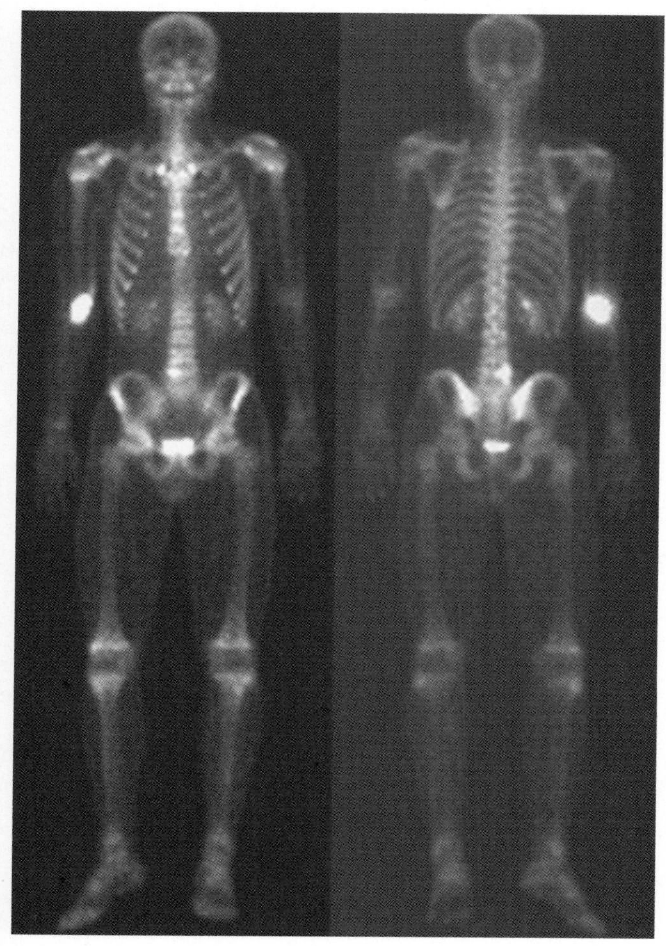

A

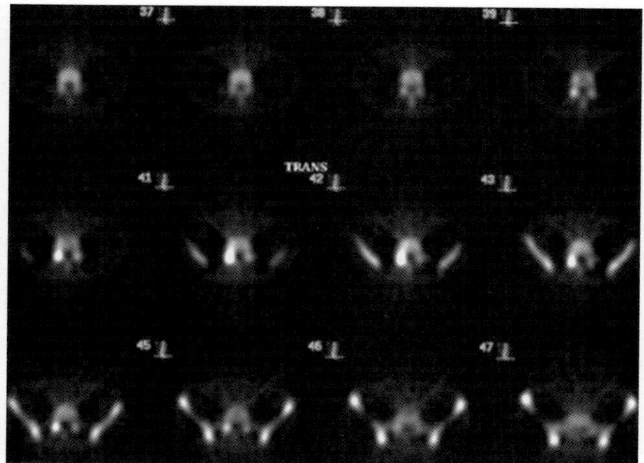

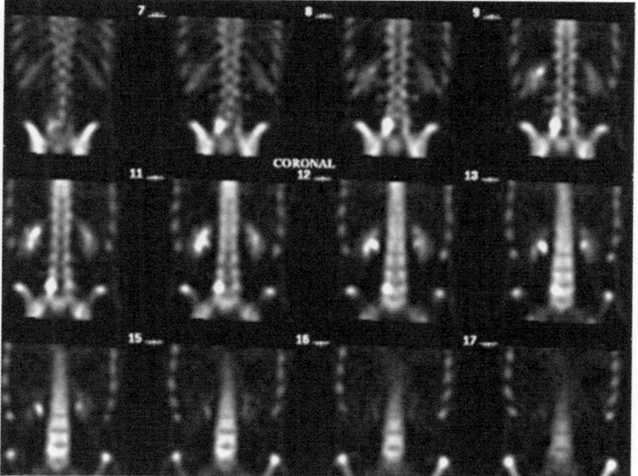

B

Clinical Presentation

A patient with low back pain. No specific documented trauma.

Imaging Findings

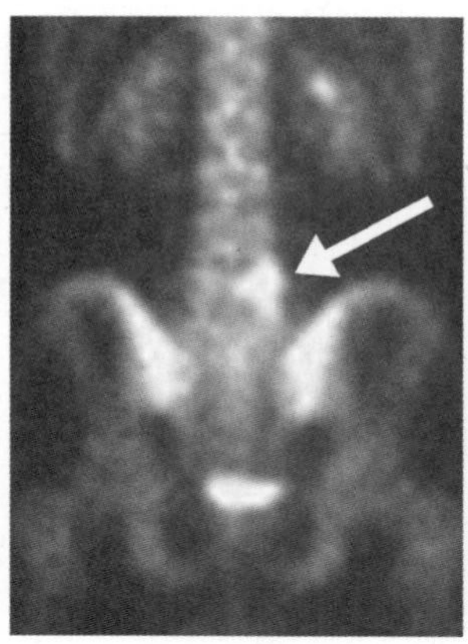

A

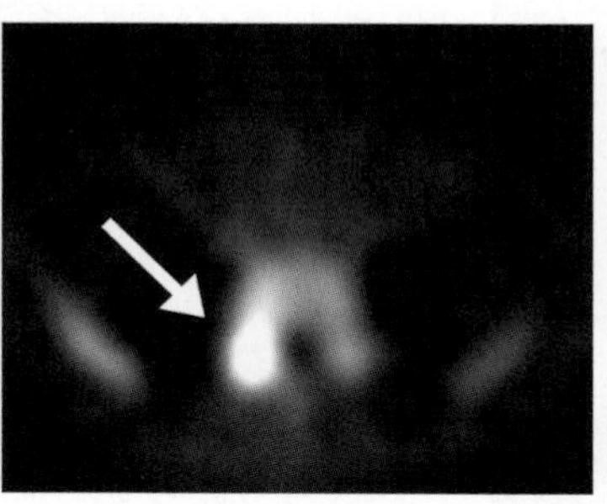

B

(A) Anterior and posterior whole-body bone scan demonstrates increased activity in the right posterior elements at L5 (*arrow*). Mild multifocal growth plate activity suggests a skeleton nearing maturity. Partial infiltration of the injected dose is noted at the right antecubital fossa. **(B)** Axial and coronal SPECT images further localize the focally increased activity to the right L5 pars interarticularis (*arrow*).

Differential Diagnosis

- ***Pars fracture:*** Increased uptake at the pars interarticularis makes this the most likely diagnosis in light of the history.
- *Osteoid osteoma:* This can also appear as focally increased uptake on bone scan but can be located anywhere, not just in the pars region. A history of night pain relieved by aspirin would be more suggestive.
- *Bone metastasis:* This more commonly involves the slightly more anterior pedicle and would be unusual without a history of malignancy.

Essential Facts

- Also known as pars defect or spondylolysis, pars fracture can be a congenital defect or an acquired stress fracture through the pars interarticularis.
- Seen in ~5% of the general population; 80% asymptomatic
- It is a common cause of low back pain, worsening with exercise, in young athletes involved in activities causing repetitive back stress (gymnasts, weight lifters).
- Most commonly seen in children and young adults, more commonly in females
- May or may not be associated with spondylolisthesis (vertebral slippage)
- Can be unilateral or bilateral, most often in the lower lumbar spine
- Treatment includes rest, anti-inflammatories, bracing, and physical therapy, with surgery for more severe cases or those with significant slippage.

Other Imaging Findings

- Plain radiograph can show a lucent line through the pars (the neck of the "Scotty dog") on oblique views. With unilateral defects, sclerosis can be seen on the contralateral side because of stress-induced remodeling. However, plain radiographic accuracy is not as high as that of bone scan.
- CT can show the fracture line with more sensitivity than plain radiograph but will not assess whether the defect is "active."
- MRI can show the fracture line and increased signal of marrow edema.

✓ Pearls & × Pitfalls

✓ Many people have back pain, and many people have pars defects. Bone scan can demonstrate if the defect is associated with active bony remodeling and thus the likely cause of the back pain.

✓ L5 is the most common location for a pars fracture, followed by L4.

× Osteomyelitis/diskitis is also a consideration for painful spine uptake on bone scan. However, increased activity is typically larger and is not localized to the pars—more common around the disk space.

× SPECT improves sensitivity and specificity over planar imaging. Ask for it if not provided.

Case 48

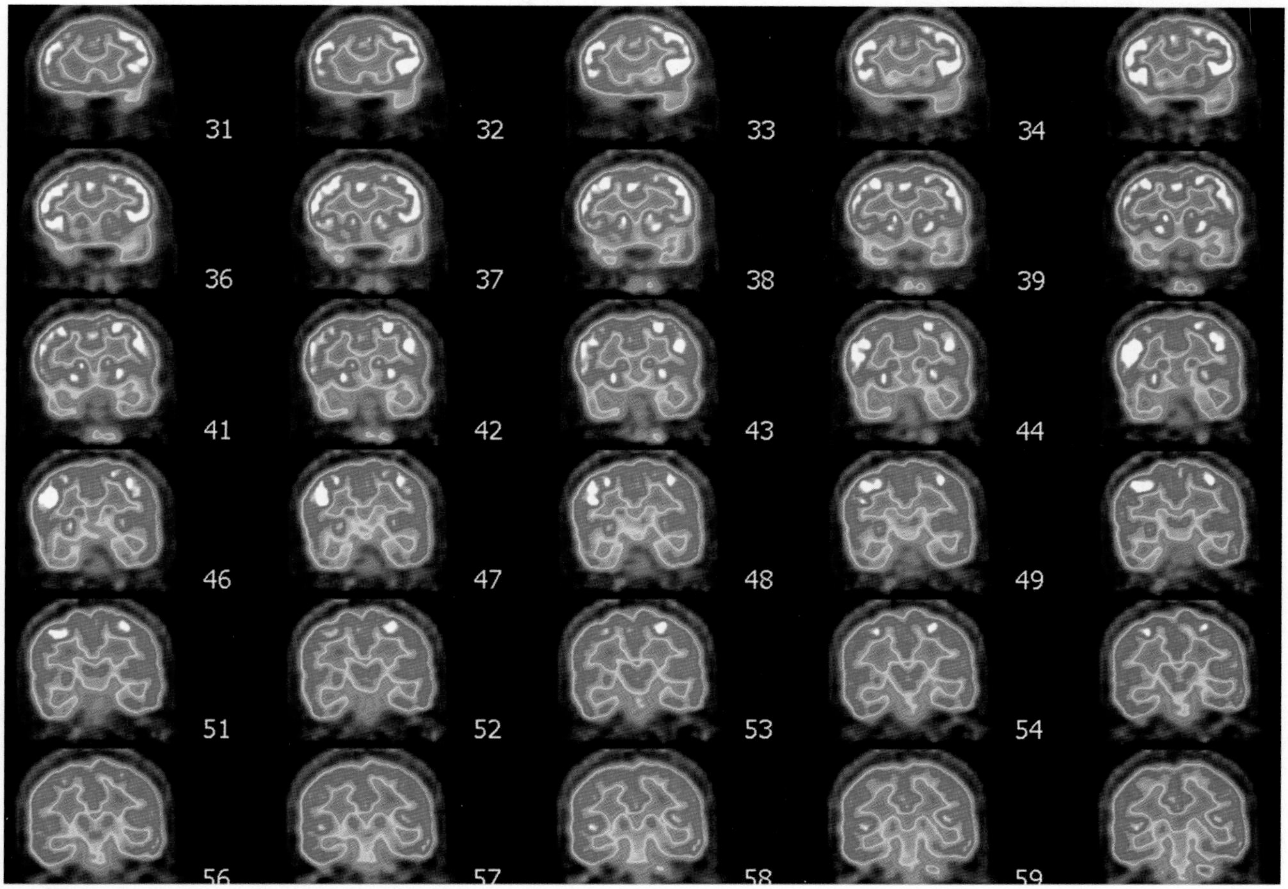

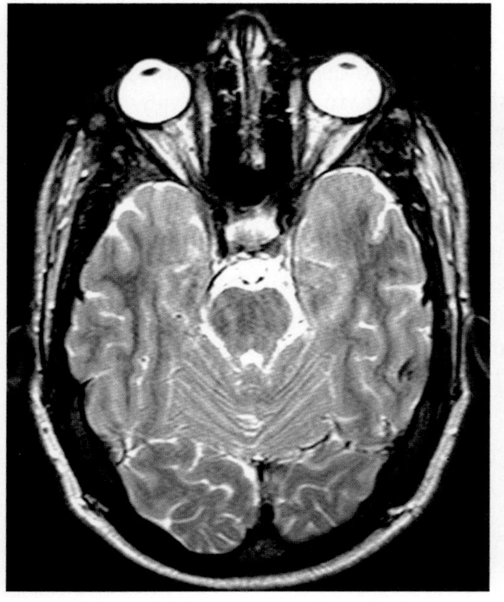

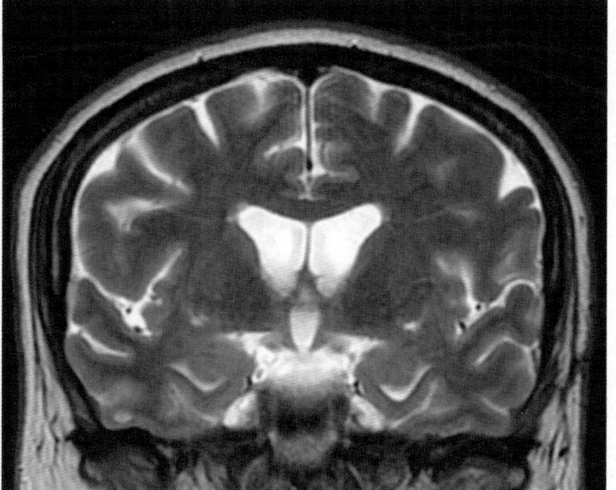

Clinical Presentation

A patient with a history of chronic seizures.

Imaging Findings

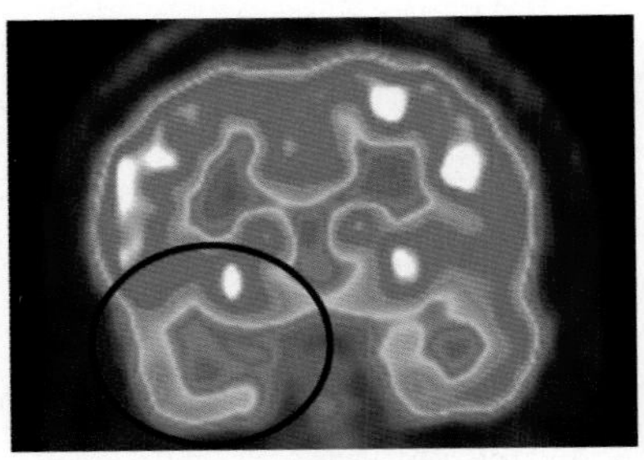

Coronal FDG-PET images of the brain (A in Clinical Presentation) demonstrate decreased metabolic activity at the right anterior temporal location (*circle*). T2-weighted axial and coronal MRI sections (B in Clinical Presentation) through the temporal lobes are unremarkable.

Differential Diagnosis

- ***Interictal seizure focus (right temporal lobe):*** This is the most likely etiology for the focal hypometabolism, particularly given the history and normal MRI appearance.
- *Low-grade glioma:* Low-grade tumors are usually low or non–FDG-avid and can also have this appearance on PET. Normal brain MRI makes this very unlikely, however.
- *Central nervous system infection:* This can be decreased on FDG-PET but is less likely, given the history.

Essential Facts

- Seizures can be generalized or partial and may be controlled with antiepileptic medications. They are also categorized as temporal lobe or extratemporal.
- The most common cause for partial seizures is mesial temporal sclerosis (MTS), an idiopathic disease of children and young adults characterized by hippocampal atrophy in the mesial temporal cortex.
- Most cases of MTS are refractory to antiepileptic medication. However, surgical anterior temporal lobectomy is usually successful in controlling the seizures.
- Brain FDG-PET can be used to confirm and localize MTS (right or left) before surgery. This is generally performed between (not during) seizures to localize a hypometabolic portion of the brain.
- Other etiologies for seizures include focal cortical dysplasia, cavernous malformations, and tumor.

Other Imaging Findings

- Brain perfusion SPECT with Tc99m-ECD or Tc99m-HMPAO can be used either during (hyperperfusion) or between (hypoperfusion) seizures. To increase the sensitivity of this technique further, a subtraction of these two studies can be performed.
- Brain CT is often normal in MTS but can detect other etiologies for the seizures, including tumor.
- High-resolution targeted brain MRI will often demonstrate hippocampal atrophy and increased T2 signal.
- Electroencephalography (EEG), standard or implanted, is also used to assist in identifying the ictal focus.

✓ Pearls & × Pitfalls

✓ Normal brain PET (metabolic) and brain SPECT (perfusion) have a similar distribution and imaging appearance. Generally, if the cerebellar uptake is similar to that of cerebral cortex, the examination is a perfusion SPECT. If the normal cerebellum is relatively decreased, it is likely FDG-PET.

✓ A hypometabolic seizure focus on PET may have an anatomic correlate on CT/MRI (e.g., gliosis, volume loss), or the anatomy may be completely normal.

✓ Remember that PET and SPECT demonstrate relative, not absolute, activity. The most intense pixel in the image is assigned 100% of the gray or color scale, and all other pixels are scaled down accordingly. Accurate absolute activity measurements generally require blood sampling.

× With seizure evaluation, brain PET is usually performed between seizures as the ictal event cannot be predicted and is brief. If the FDG actually is injected *during* a seizure, the ictal focus will be increased. Because of their longer half-life, SPECT (perfusion) agents can be used in conjunction with seizure induction methods, such as sleep deprivation, to more reliably produce an ictal event study.

Case 49

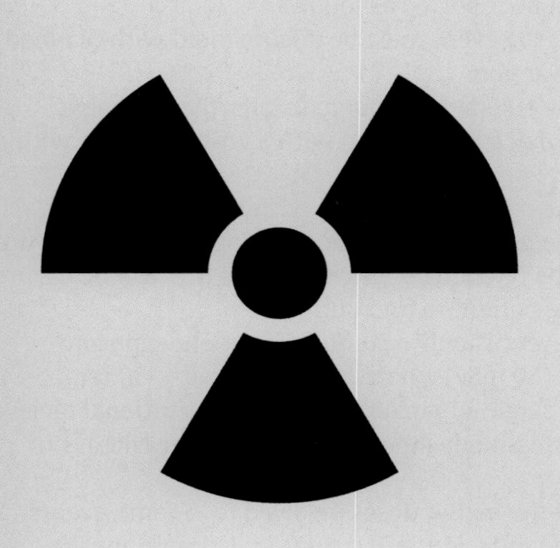

Clinical Presentation

A patient scheduled for a Tc99m-MDP bone scan was dosed with 100 mCi of radiotracer instead of the prescribed 20 mCi. The patient's estimated whole-body dose is 1.3 rem, and the highest organ dose is 5 rem to the bone. Is this event reportable?

Differential Diagnosis

What should be done now?

- ***This is a "recordable" event:*** Correct, because the administered dose differed from the prescribed dose by > 20%, but the total-body dose to the patient was < 5 rem (50 mSv) and the highest organ dose was < 50 rem (500 mSv). This event must be recorded locally, and documentation must be prepared that determines how this occurred and what steps have been taken to prevent it in the future. It does not have to be reported to the Nuclear Regulatory Commission (NRC), however.
- *This event must be reported to the NRC:* Incorrect. Reporting needs to occur only if the patient's whole-body dose was > 5 rem (50 mSv) or the highest organ dose was > 50 rem (500 mSv) when the administered dose differed from the written one by > 20%.
- *Nothing, as this is just a Tc99m-labeled agent:* Incorrect. If the administered dose differs from the written one by > 20%, it must be either recorded or reported, depending on the level of patient exposure to radiation.

Essential Facts

- The NRC no longer uses the term *misadministration. Medical event* is the current term.
- A medical event is an administration involving the wrong radiopharmaceutical, the wrong patient, the wrong route, *or* the wrong amount (differing by ≥ 20% from the dose prescribed the authorized user [i.e., physician with documented training in administering radiopharmaceuticals])
- The event is *reportable* if patient exposure from the administration is > 5 rem (50 mSv) whole-body dose or > 50 rem (500 mSv) single-organ dose. The medical event must be reported as follows:
  - Details of the event must be documented with planned course of action.
  - Notify the NRC by telephone no later than the next calendar day and follow up with a written report within 15 days.
  - Notify the *referring physician* within 24 hours.
  - Notify the *patient* unless the referring physician will do this, or the referring physician thinks this will be harmful for the patient to find out.
- A patient event is only *recordable* if patient exposure is < 5 rem (50 mSv) whole-body dose and < 50 rem (500 mSv) single-organ dose. Internal institutional review and risk assessment should be made but the NRC is not notified.
- Because of the higher doses involved (> 5 rem), events from therapeutic administrations will almost always be reportable. Diagnostic events may be reportable or recordable depending on the patient dose.

✓ Pearls & ✗ Pitfalls

✓ A written directive (signed prescription by an authorized user) is required for *all* therapeutic radiopharmaceuticals (e.g., iodine 131, samarium 153, yttrium 90) and for diagnostic doses of I131 > 30 µCi (*micro*curies).

✗ Some "agreement states" still use the ±10% rule rather than the NRC ±20% rule.

Case 50

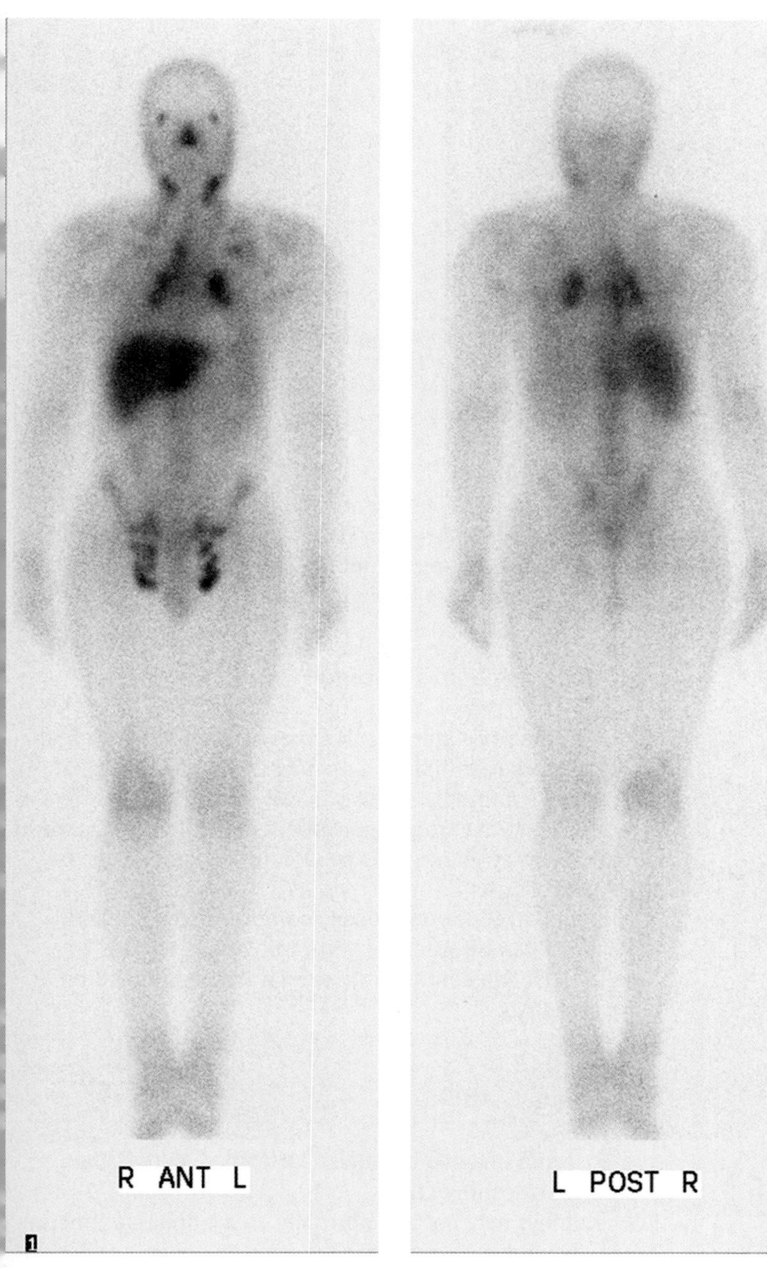

Clinical Presentation

A 24-year-old woman with cough and abnormal chest radiograph.

Imaging Findings

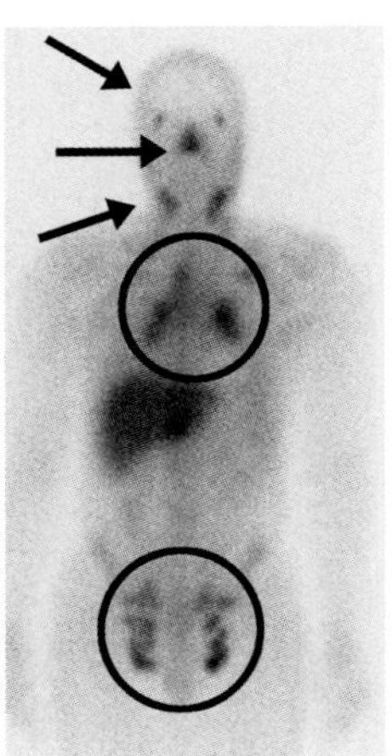

Standard delayed whole-body gallium scan demonstrates abnormal focal activity bilaterally in the hilar, paratracheal, and inguinal regions, compatible with lymph node uptake (*circles*). Focal tracer uptake is also seen in the lacrimal, nasal, and submandibular salivary regions (*arrows*). Normal gallium uptake is seen in the liver and bone marrow. Typically, the spleen demonstrates mild gallium uptake; however, this patient has had a splenectomy.

Differential Diagnosis

Gallium is a nonspecific agent, and abnormal uptake can be seen with infection, tumor, and granulomatous disease such as sarcoid.

- ***Gallium scan showing sarcoid:*** The symmetric uptake in a hilar and paratracheal lymph node distribution ("lambda" sign) as well as prominent lacrimal and salivary uptake favor sarcoid, even though the inguinal lymph node uptake is less typical and makes lymphoma another good possibility.
- *Tumor:* Lymphoma will demonstrate gallium uptake and may be indistinguishable from sarcoid. Typically with lymphoma, the hilar uptake will not be as symmetric as that seen with sarcoid.
- *Infection:* An infectious process such as coccidioidomycosis or tuberculosis can look similar in the chest. It would be less likely to also involve the pelvis.

Essential Facts

- Gallium is an iron analogue and binds to ferritin, lactoferrin, and transferrin.
- Normal gallium biodistribution includes liver, spleen, bone (marrow and cortex), salivary glands, and bowel.
- Gallium is a marker for some tumors (especially lymphoma and melanoma) as well as active inflammation (alveolitis, granuloma formation) because of uptake in macrophages, lymphocytes, and neutrophils.
- Sarcoid is a granulomatous disease of unknown etiology affecting children and adults (20–40 years of age most common), with a predilection for female black populations.
- Symptoms include fever, night sweats, weight loss, and cough, but patients may be asymptomatic. Patients may have elevated angiotensin-converting enzyme levels.
- Sarcoid can involve any organ but frequently has pulmonary mediastinal and/or parenchymal involvement
- Treatment is immunosuppressive; disease may spontaneously resolve or progress to fibrosis.

Other Imaging Findings

- Gallium uptake due to sarcoid can be seen in any organ, but symmetric hilar and mediastinal uptake (lambda sign) is commonly seen, as in this case.
- Intense uptake from involvement of the lacrimal, parotid, and salivary glands seen in sarcoid is described as the "panda" sign.
- Adenopathy and pulmonary parenchymal disease in sarcoid can be seen on chest radiographs or CT.
- FDG-PET can demonstrate similar findings to gallium in sarcoidosis.

✓ Pearls & × Pitfalls

✓ Gallium imaging is usually performed 48 to 72 hours after tracer injection.

✓ Kidneys may be seen normally on 24-hour gallium images; however, activity seen after 48 hours is abnormal.

✓ FDG-PET is increasingly supplanting gallium imaging for both tumor and inflammatory indications.

× Gallium is a very nonspecific tumor/infection/inflammation agent.

× Gallium may look superficially similar to labeled WBC scan. However, WBCs should not been seen in normal salivary glands or bowel (with indium 111 label), and with WBCs, the spleen is hotter than liver (see "Interpreting Whole-Body Scans").

Case 51

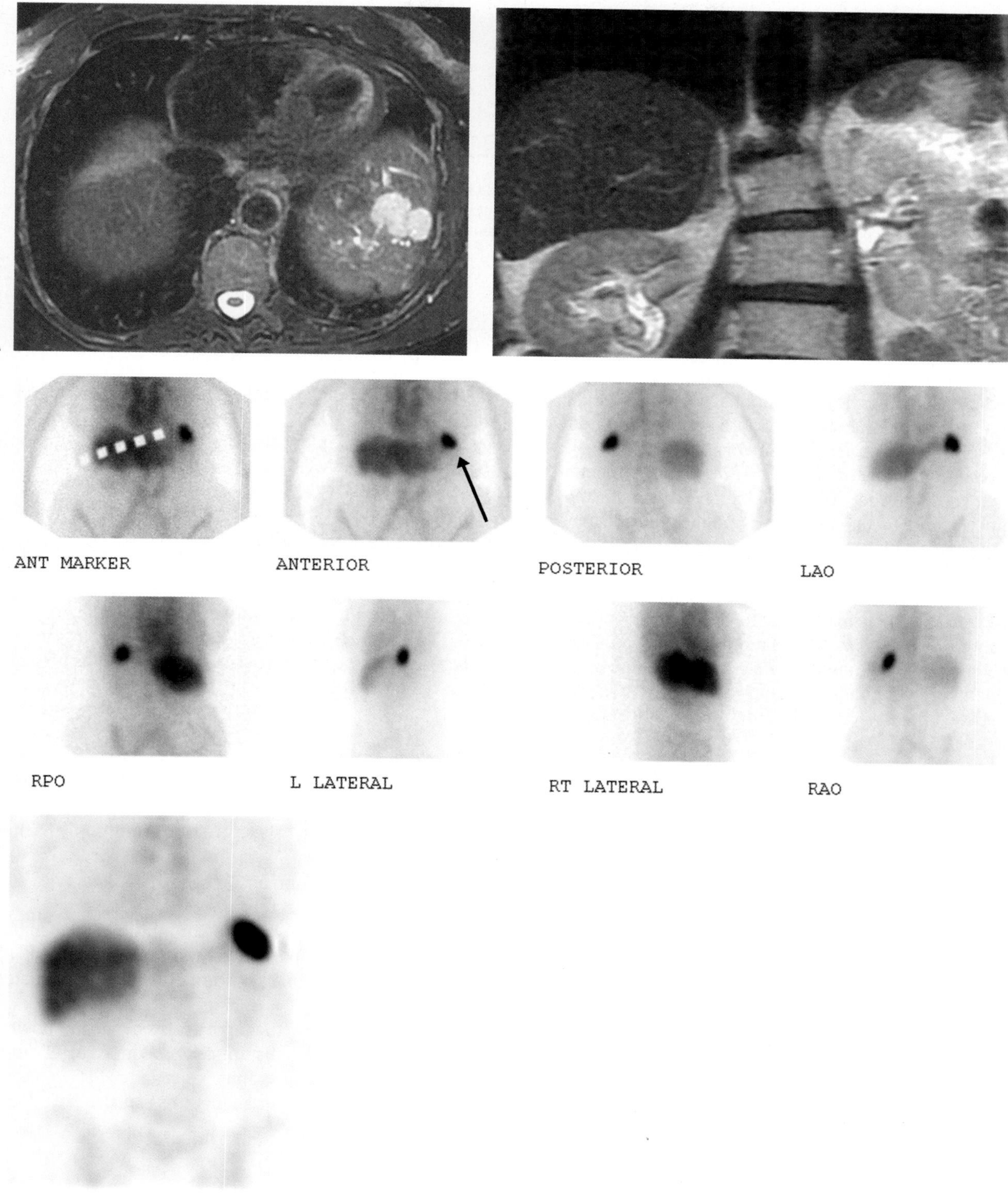

Clinical Presentation

A 67-year-old woman with an incidental mass detected in the left lobe of the liver on MRI. There is a remote history of a motor vehicle accident that resulted in an emergency splenectomy.

Imaging Findings

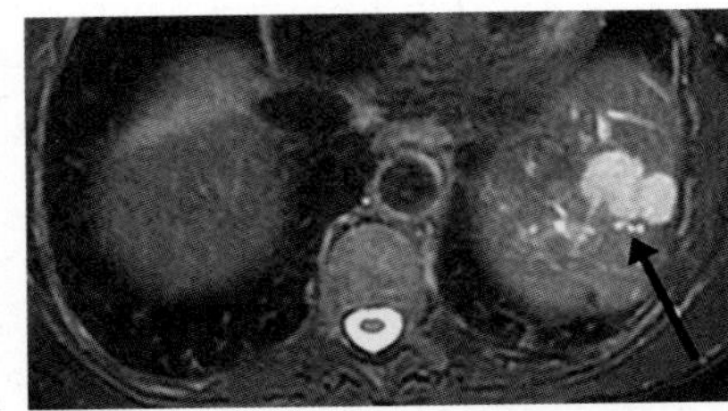

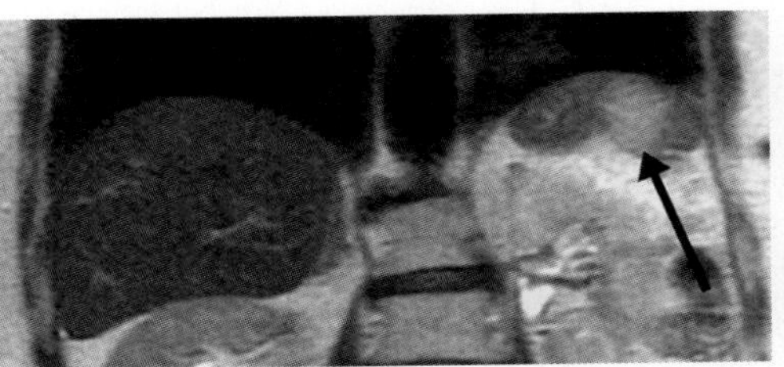

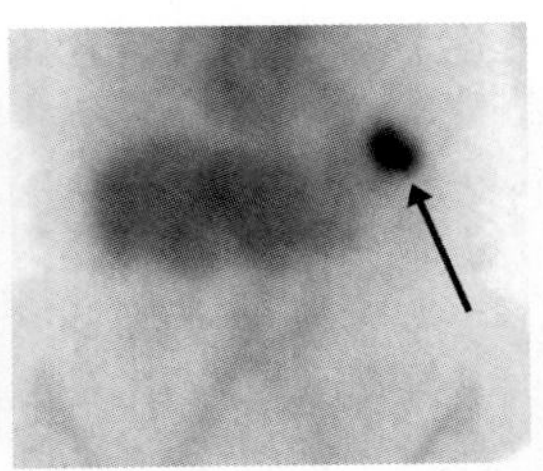

(A) Axial T2 fast spin echo MRI and coronal T2 single shot fast spin echo weighted MRI of the upper abdomen demonstrate a hyperintense lesion at the left lateral liver (*arrows*). **(B)** Multiple abdominal spot and coronal SPECT images through the abdomen demonstrate *mild* physiologic uptake in the blood pool, liver, and bone marrow with an intense focus in the left upper quadrant corresponding to the liver lesion (*arrow*).

Differential Diagnosis

- ***Heat-damaged RBC scan demonstrating splenosis:*** Mild blood pool and hepatic uptake makes a damaged RBC scan the most likely exam. The more intense focal uptake is most likely splenosis, given the history.
- *RBC scan (nondamaged) demonstrating a hepatic hemangioma:* Focal intrahepatic uptake of labeled RBCs is most commonly due to a hemangioma and must be considered. However, blood pool (e.g., cardiac chamber) activity would be hotter than liver with nondamaged RBCs.
- *SCOL scan demonstrating hepatic focal nodular hyperplasia (FNH):* SCOL also normally goes to liver, spleen, and bone marrow. However, it would be promptly cleared from the blood pool, and unlike on RBC scans, the degree of splenic tissue uptake is normally less than or equal to hepatic uptake. (FNHs *are* commonly hot on SCOL, however).

Essential Facts

- Splenosis is foci splenic tissue appearing outside the normal location of the spleen.
- It can be congenital (accessory splenule) or posttraumatic (including postsurgical), with vascularized tissue fragments implanting elsewhere.
- Ectopic splenic tissue is usually in the left upper quadrant adjacent to the spleen, but it can also be seen in the thorax if the diaphragm is violated or uncommonly can be intrahepatic (as this case) or intrapancreatic.
- Labeled RBC scintigraphy can be used to confirm that suspicious soft tissue is just benign splenic tissue or to assess if residual functioning splenic tissue is still present in patients with idiopathic thrombocytopenic purpura (ITP) who remain thrombocytopenic after splenectomy.
- Denaturing the RBCs with heat damage can increase the affinity for splenic tissue relative to the liver and blood pool.
- No treatment for splenosis is necessary unless symptomatic (e.g., refractory ITP).

Other Imaging Findings

- Anatomic imaging with CT/MRI can detect soft-tissue lesions but cannot confirm splenic tissue origin.
- SCOL will also go to splenic tissue and is used for these purposes, but the target to background is not as high as with damaged RBCs.

✓ Pearls & ✗ Pitfalls

✓ Twenty percent of the general population has accessory splenules at autopsy. These are most commonly located at the splenic hilum.
✓ Splenosis is a common occurrence in patients with a posttraumatic splenectomy.
✓ Ectopic splenules can be single or multiple and can be widely distributed, particularly after trauma.
✓ Congenital polysplenia syndrome can also be evaluated with RBC scan.
✗ Free pertechnetate artifact goes to stomach and bowel and can simulate splenic uptake. Anatomic correlation is useful for RBC scintigraphy (especially SPECT/CT).
✗ Splenic artery and other aneurysms can also have focal RBC uptake.

Case 52

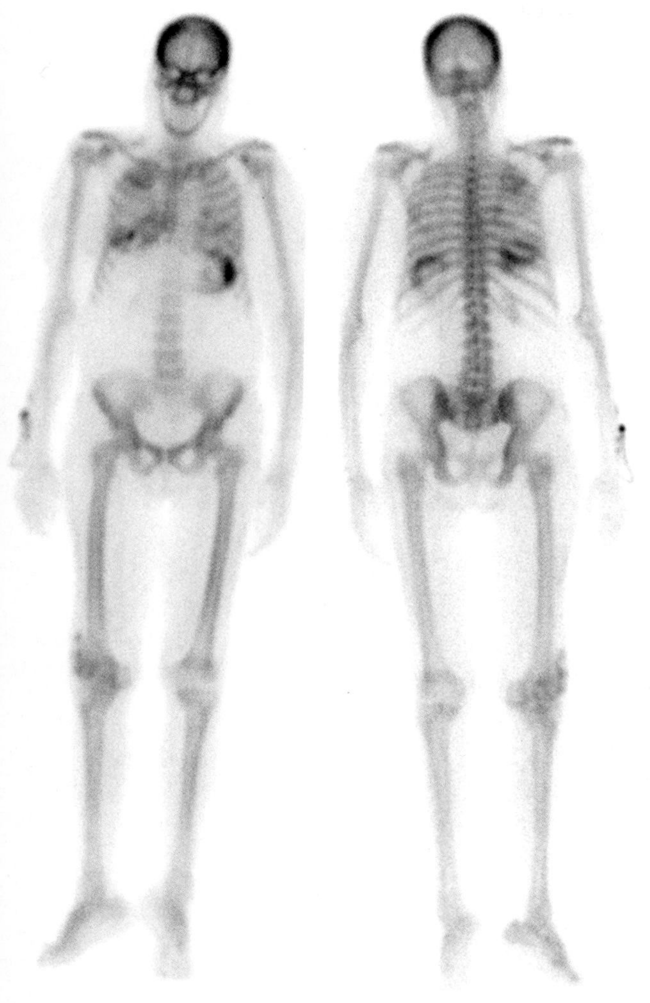

Clinical Presentation

A 49-year-old woman with abnormal blood chemistry. She is on dialysis.

Imaging Findings

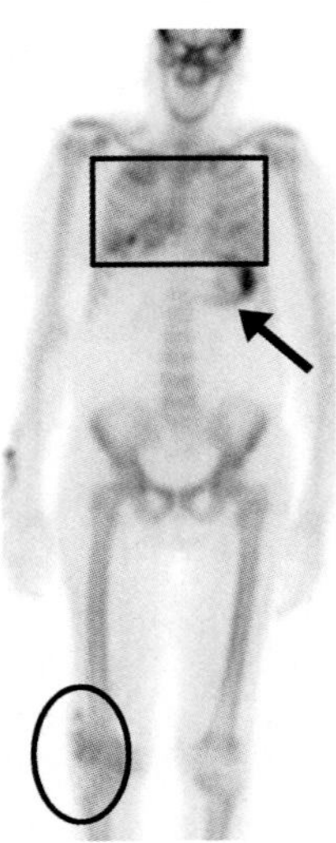

Anterior and posterior whole-body views from a Tc99m-MDP bone scan demonstrate abnormal soft-tissue accumulation of radiotracer in the stomach (*arrow*) and lungs (*box*) diffusely. There is faint, diffuse myocardial uptake as well. Soft-tissue uptake is also seen at the right knee (*circle*). No renal uptake is visualized, as can be seen with renal failure and dialysis. Periosteal "tram tracking" of the lower extremities suggests superimposed hypertrophic osteoarthropathy (see Case 13). Prominent mandibular and skull uptake is also seen.

Differential Diagnosis

- ***Hypercalcemia:*** Soft-tissue bone tracer accumulation in the stomach, lungs, and myocardium diffusely is essentially pathognomonic for this entity. (The right knee demonstrates secondary tumoral calcinosis.)
- *Mucinous soft-tissue metastases:* Several malignancies (particularly calcifying or ossifying) can demonstrate primary or metastatic soft-tissue uptake. However, the diffuse nature of the uptake in many organs seen here would be extremely unlikely.
- *Free pertechnetate artifact:* This can also demonstrate diffuse gastric uptake. However, it should also have thyroid/salivary uptake and would not have lung uptake.

Essential Facts

- Hypercalcemia has many causes; it is commonly associated with hyperparathyroidism (primary or secondary).
- In patients with hypercalcemia, calcium accumulates within organs that have a basic intracellular pH. Accordingly, diffuse gastric, pulmonary, and renal uptake may be seen (acid is exported, so tissue is basic intracellularly).
- Myocardial uptake can also be seen by related mechanisms.

Other Imaging Findings

- Severe renal osteodystrophy can result in increased osseous uptake on bone scan in the facial bones, maxillae and skull (as in this case), as well as increased periarticular uptake.
- Significant hyperparathyroidism and its related conditions, like hypervitaminosis D, can also result in a metabolic "superscan": diffusely increased skeletal uptake (head to toe) and decreased soft-tissue uptake, including in the kidneys.

✓ Pearls & × Pitfalls

✓ Always look at the soft tissues and kidneys on bone scan first to avoid missing important findings.

✓ With hypercalcemia, the increased renal uptake is in the parenchyma, as opposed to a normal bone scan, where the parenchyma is mild but the more central collecting system is very hot.

× If there is associated severe renal dysfunction, as in this case, renal uptake may not be visualized in hypercalcemia.

Case 53

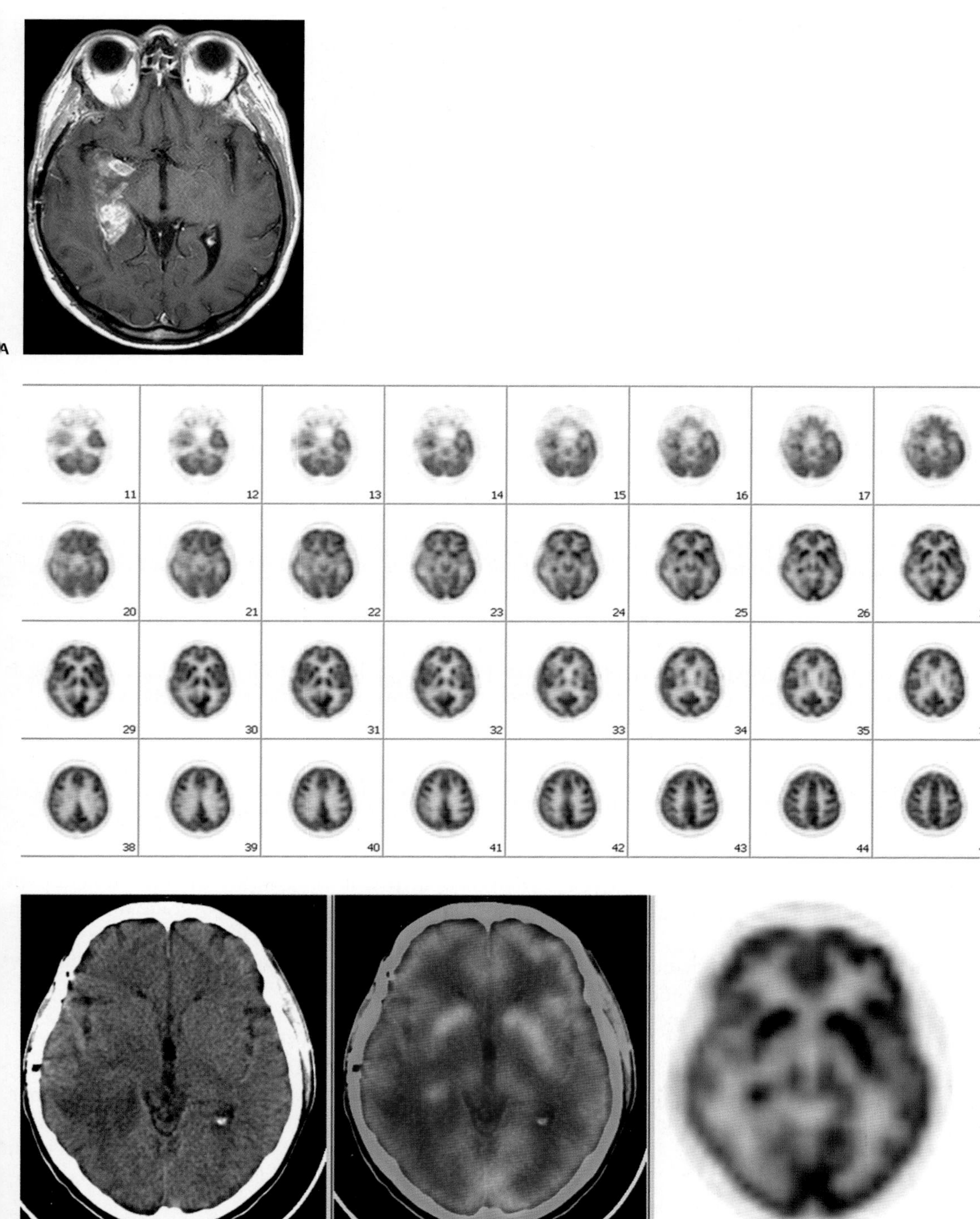

Clinical Presentation

A 48-year-old man with glioblastoma multiforme status post resection and radiation therapy presents for restaging.

Imaging Findings

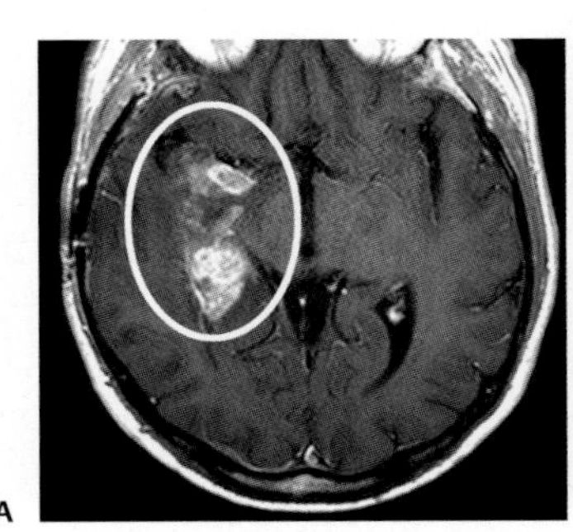

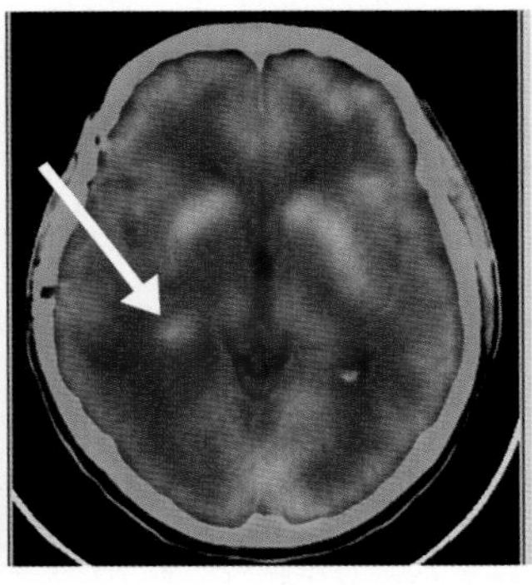

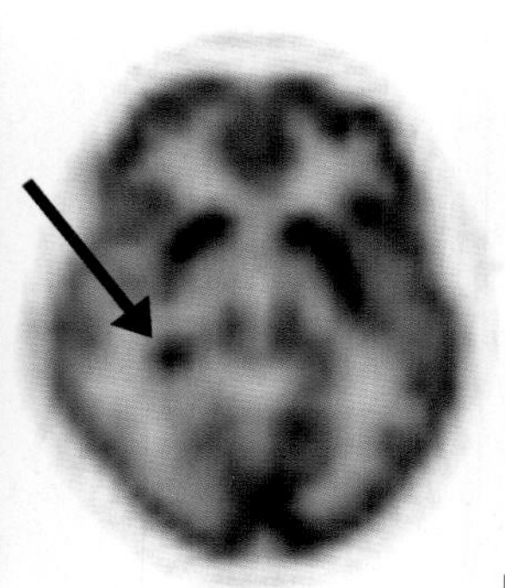

A B

(A) Axial T1 postcontrast brain MRI demonstrates abnormal enhancement in the medial right temporal lobe (*circle*). **(B)** Axial brain FDG-PET and a selected hybrid PET/CT image demonstrate increased radiotracer accumulation in the right temporal lobe, most prominently in the posterior medial aspect (*arrows*). This corresponds with the enhancing region on MRI. The CT portion shows low density in this area, indicating edema.

Differential Diagnosis

- ***Tumor recurrence:*** An enhancing lesion with increased FDG accumulation indicates recurrent tumor, given the history.
- *Radiation necrosis:* This will also enhance on CT/MRI but will not have significant FDG accumulation. (The enhancing portions on MRI that are not FDG-avid in this patient may indicate some superimposed radiation necrosis.)
- *Central nervous system infection:* This can also enhance and accumulate FDG but is less likely, given the history.

Essential Facts

- Treatment for brain tumors includes surgical resection and radiation therapy. Serial MRIs are performed for follow-up.
- However, both recurrent tumor and benign radiation necrosis can demonstrate enhancement on subsequent MRI because of a breakdown in the blood–brain perfusion barrier.
- FDG-PET can be useful to distinguish these conditions. Radiation necrosis does not have increased FDG uptake, whereas mid- to high-grade recurrent tumors will show increased uptake.

Other Imaging Findings

- CT and MRI will show enhancement for benign radiation necrosis and recurrent tumor. MRI is more sensitive, but neither is specific.
- Magnetic resonance spectroscopy is also used to help distinguish necrosis from recurrence.
- Thallium brain imaging has also been used to distinguish these conditions and has a better target-to-background ratio than FDG-PET for thallium-avid tumors (particularly if SPECT/CT is available with thallium imaging).
- Newer PET tracers, such as those that measure tumor cell proliferation (e.g., F18-fluorothymidine), are emerging as promising agents but are not yet routinely available.

✓ Pearls & × Pitfalls

✓ The degree of FDG uptake generally correlates with the grade of the tumor.

✓ FDG is very specific for recurrent tumors but not as sensitive for lower-grade tumors. Low-grade tumors may not demonstrate any FDG accumulation.

✓ Radiation necrosis will enhance on MRI but should have absent FDG accumulation.

× Gray matter and basal ganglia have intense FDG accumulation normally. A suspicious enhancing focus on MRI need not have FDG uptake approaching that of gray matter to diagnose recurrent tumor. Viable tumor uptake need only be greater than that of white matter (i.e., a lesion can demonstrate only mild FDG uptake but should still be considered likely tumor).

Case 54

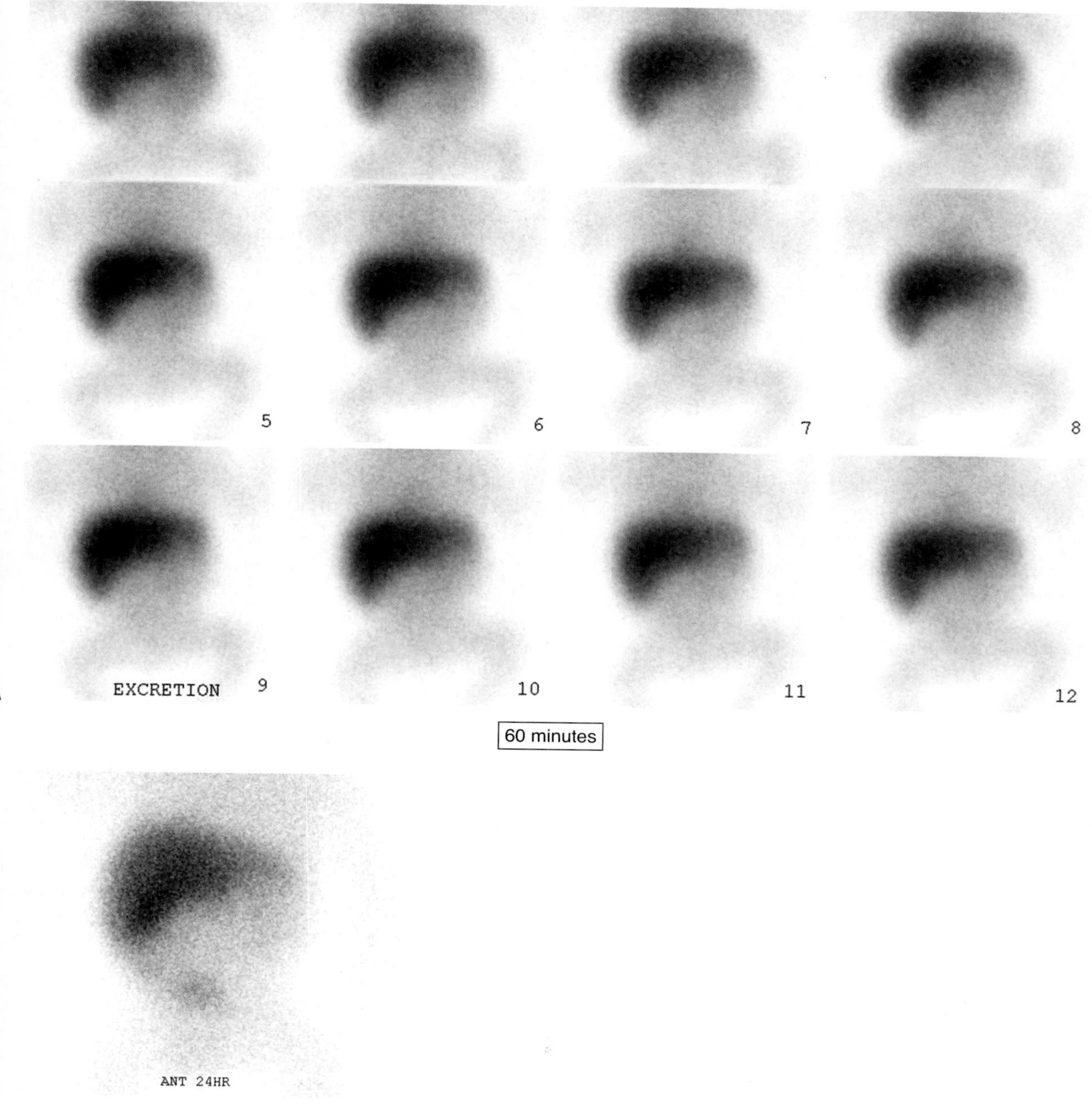

Clinical Presentation

A 2-month-old presents with jaundice and elevated direct bilirubin levels.

Imaging Findings

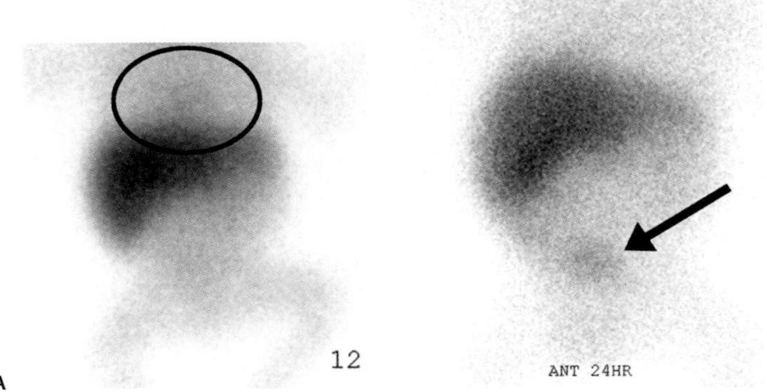

(A) Anterior images from a Tc99m-HIDA scan reveals prompt uptake of radiopharmaceutical into the liver. There is no evidence of biliary excretion after 1 hour. There is only mildly delayed blood pool clearance that can be faintly seen at 1 hour in the cardiac chambers (*circle*). **(B)** Twenty-four–hour delayed images reveal persistent uptake in the liver without any biliary excretion into bowel. Blood pool activity has cleared. Vicarious excretion of the radiopharmaceutical through the kidneys into the bladder is noted (*arrow*).

Differential Diagnosis

- ***Biliary atresia:*** Lack of any bowel activity, even at 24 hours, makes this the diagnosis of exclusion.
- *Neonatal hepatitis:* This will typically show some bowel activity by 24 hours, although it occasionally may not, if severe. It usually has more persistent blood pool activity (and the more the persistent the blood pool activity, the greater the severity of hepatic dysfunction).
- *Intrahepatic cholestasis:* Cholestasis can be caused by other disease processes, such as Alagille syndrome (non-syndromic bile duct paucity) or α_1-antitrypsin deficiency and would look similar to atresia. These entities are less common.

Essential Facts

- Biliary atresia is a congenital disease of unknown etiology in which prenatal biliary inflammation leads to fibrosis and atresia.
- It is the most common fatal liver disease of infants (1 in 10,000 live births) and has a slight female predilection.
- It typically presents by 1 month of age with persistent jaundice past 3 to 4 weeks and conjugated hyperbilirubinemia.
- The length and location of the atretic portion of the biliary tree are variable and difficult to ascertain before surgery.
- A Kasai surgical procedure (portoenterostomy) is curative, eliminating the atretic portion and bringing the duodenum closer to the liver.
- Surgery should be performed by 2 months to avoid permanent liver failure (success rate, 90%). By 3 months, the success rate drops to 20%. Unsuccessful surgical repair requires a liver transplant.
- Even with early surgery, many patients eventually go on to require a liver transplant later in life because of progressive biliary inflammation/fibrosis.
- A HIDA scan showing *any* definite bowel uptake (even on delayed images and only in the colon) excludes biliary atresia. Lack of bowel uptake is consistent with atresia but can be a false-positive due to severe hepatitis.
- To decrease false-positive studies, drugs such as phenobarbital (5 mg/kg for 5 days before HIDA) or ursodeoxycholic acid should be given to temporarily improve liver function for the exam.

Other Imaging Findings

- No other noninvasive imaging modalities are definitive.
- US is commonly used to assess the absence of a gallbladder (GB), but up to 25% of patients with atresia will have a GB present. An absent or a small, irregular GB plus a visualized fibrotic cord on US are suggestive, however.
- CT and MRCP can be attempted and can evaluate for other causes of cholestasis.
- ERCP or intraoperative cholangiography can be diagnostic, but both are invasive.

✓ Pearls & ✗ Pitfalls

✓ Always assess the size of the patient relative to the camera field of view (FOV). If, as in this case, the FOV includes most of the patient, it must be a small child because the largest gamma cameras are typically < 40 cm in the cranial–caudal length.

✗ Lack of bowel uptake by 24 hours is consistent with atresia but can still represent severe neonatal hepatitis. Presence of any bowel uptake excludes atresia.

✗ Do not confuse renal/urinary activity with bowel.

✗ Reasonable clearance of blood pool activity (by 30 minutes) but lack of biliary excretion is more typical of atresia. Very poor blood pool clearance of tracer is more typical of hepatitis but can also be seen with prolonged atresia (3 months) because of eventual liver failure.

✗ GB visualization does *not* exclude biliary atresia, as the GB is seen in 25% of patients with atresia. (And unlike adults undergoing HIDA imaging, neonates typically do not have to be fasting because cystic duct/GB patency is not the primary concern in these patients.)

Case 55

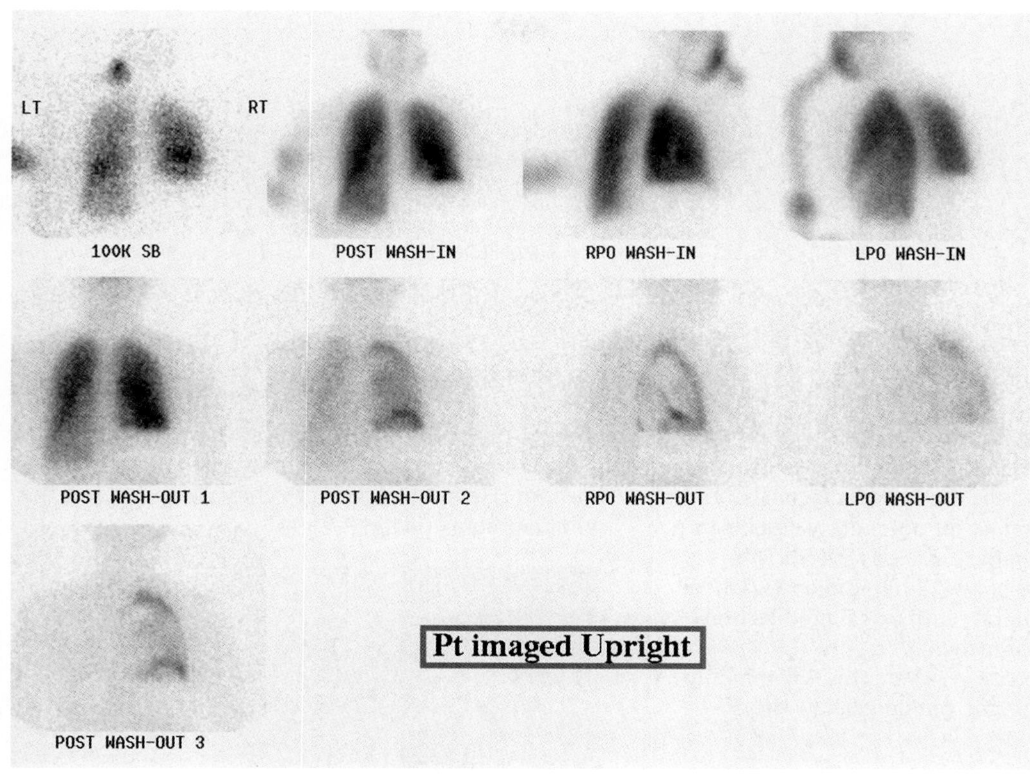

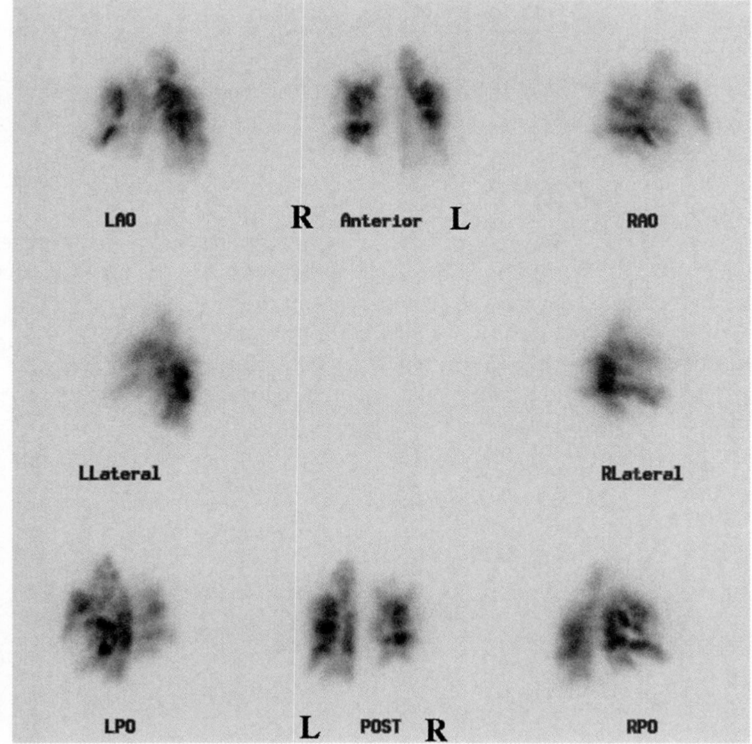

Clinical Presentation

A 55-year-old woman with persistent shortness of breath 3 weeks after lung biopsy. How best to account for the ventilation abnormalities?

Imaging Findings

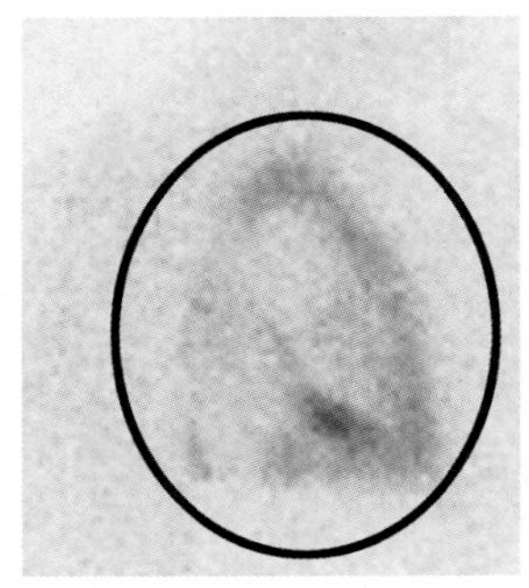

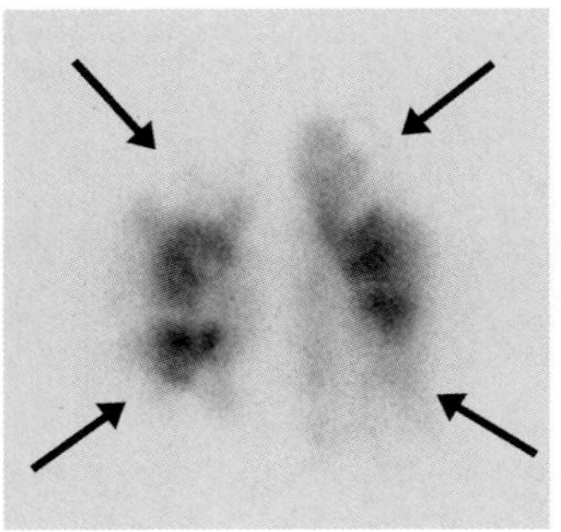

(A) Xenon 133 ventilation imaging demonstrates an elevated righ hemidiaphragm but no ventilation defects on single-breath/ear wash-in. However, on washout there is an unusual abnormal appea ance of radiotracer surrounding the right lung and also involving th major fissure (*circle*). **(B)** Tc99m-MAA perfusion imaging demonstrate multiple bilateral medium and large mismatched perfusion defect (*arrows*).

Differential Diagnosis

- ***Persistent right bronchopleural fistula:*** The eventual appearance of Xe133 gas in the pleural space surrounding the right lung makes this the correct diagnosis. (The study is also high probability for pulmonary embolism.)
- *Chronic obstructive pulmonary disease (COPD):* This is the most common cause of Xe133 retention on washout views but is usually bilateral (with apical predilection) and restricted to lung parenchyma.
- *Accumulation of xenon in a fatty liver:* This is commonly seen on washout on the right, but only below the diaphragm (see Case 9).

Essential Facts

- Bronchopleural fistulas are persistent communications between the bronchial tree and the pleural space.
- They most commonly occur following lung resection (complication rate of 2–3%) but can occasionally be seen following biopsy or other trauma that leads to pneumothorax.
- They can result in infections and failure to resolve the pleural space air, which raises the question of a persistent bronchopleural fistula.
- Xe133 ventilation imaging can demonstrate the presence of persistent fistulous communication.
- Treatment options include the administration of fibrin glue and surgery (minimally invasive or open).

Other Imaging Findings

- Chest x-ray or CT can demonstrate persistent pleural air but cannot demonstrate the bronchopleural communication. Here is this patient's chest x-ray showing the pneumothorax (*arrow*):

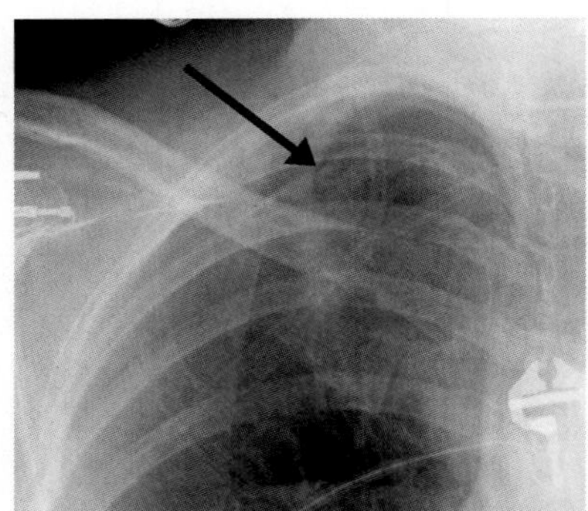

✓ Pearls & ✗ Pitfalls

✓ If xenon ventilation imaging is performed with a chest tube to suction, gas may not persist in the pleural space (but may be seen to exit the chest tube). Turning off suction can be useful in these cases.

✗ Although this study can be performed to both detect and localize a fistula, precise localization may not be possible.

Case 56

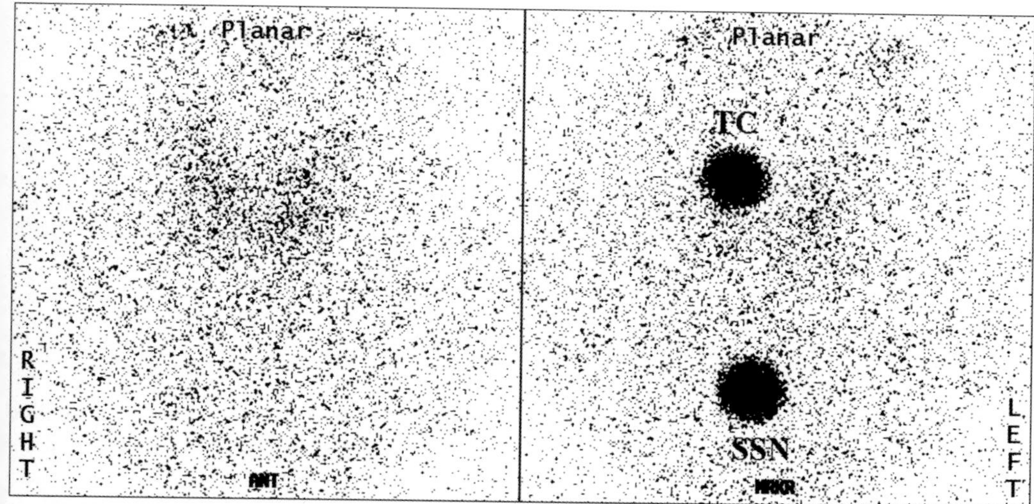

24-hr thyroid radioiodine uptake = 0.9%

Clinical Presentation

A 32-year-old woman with neck tenderness presents with palpitations and insomnia.

Imaging Findings

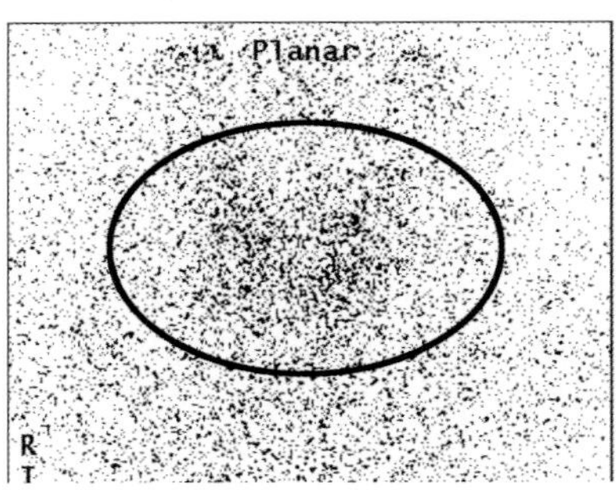

Anterior images from an iodine 123 thyroid scan with and without markers at the thyroid cartilage and suprasternal notch demonstrate uniformly markedly decreased thyroid activity (*circle*). This low uptake is confirmed on the uptake portion (normal, 10–30% at 24 hours).

Differential Diagnosis

- ***Subacute thyroiditis:*** In a thyrotoxic patient, markedly decreased thyroid radioiodine accumulation on thyroid uptake and scan is most commonly due to this entity.
- *Thyrotoxicosis factitia:* This entity, as well as amiodarone- or iodine-induced thyrotoxicosis and struma ovarii, can appear identical to thyroiditis on thyroid uptake and scan but are less common and usually do not include neck tenderness.
- *Graves disease:* This clinically presents very similarly to subacute thyroiditis (high T_4, low TSH, symptomatic hyperthyroidism) but is distinguished by markedly increased radioiodine accumulation on thyroid uptake and scan (see Case 2).

Essential Facts

- Subacute thyroiditis includes granulomatous (also known as de Quervain), silent (also known as lymphocytic or painless—seen in the elderly), and postpartum thyroiditis.
- De Quervain is most common, typically preceded by an upper respiratory viral infection that induces granulomatous inflammation of the gland, leading to the release of stored thyroid hormone into the blood, an increase in serum T_4, and a resultant suppression of TSH.
- Over the typical evolution of the condition following the initial hormone release, T_4 production eventually falls with an increase in TSH, with values returning to normal by 6 to 8 months.
- The disease is self-limiting, and treatment is supportive (no I131 therapy).

Other Imaging Findings

- US can show nonspecific increased blood flow on Doppler imaging during the acute phase and can also exclude a nodule that may be hyperfunctioning.
- Thyroid scan with pertechnetate also shows decreased activity. Other radiotracers, such as MIBI, thallium, and FDG, may, on other types of scans, incidentally show diffusely increased thyroid uptake due to the inflammation but are uncommonly used for this purpose.

✓ Pearls & × Pitfalls

✓ Other, less common causes of increased circulating thyroid hormone (with the exception of Graves disease) can have an identical appearance, with decreased thyroid uptake and scan: struma ovarii, thyrotoxicosis from amiodarone or iodine administration, and thyrotoxicosis factitia.

✓ Primary or secondary hypothyroidism can also cause decreased activity on thyroid uptake and scan but presents clinically as *hypo*thyroidism with low T_3/T_4.

✓ Hashimoto disease is a common cause of hypothyroidism, but thyroid scintigraphy is often not useful as the uptake can be increased or decreased depending on the phase.

× Widely metastatic thyroid cancer can rarely cause hyperthyroidism with decreased thyroidal iodine accumulation on thyroid (bed) uptake and scan.

× Primary thyroid cancer is *not* associated with local gland destruction and hypothyroidism; patients are usually euthyroid before diagnosis and treatment.

Case 57

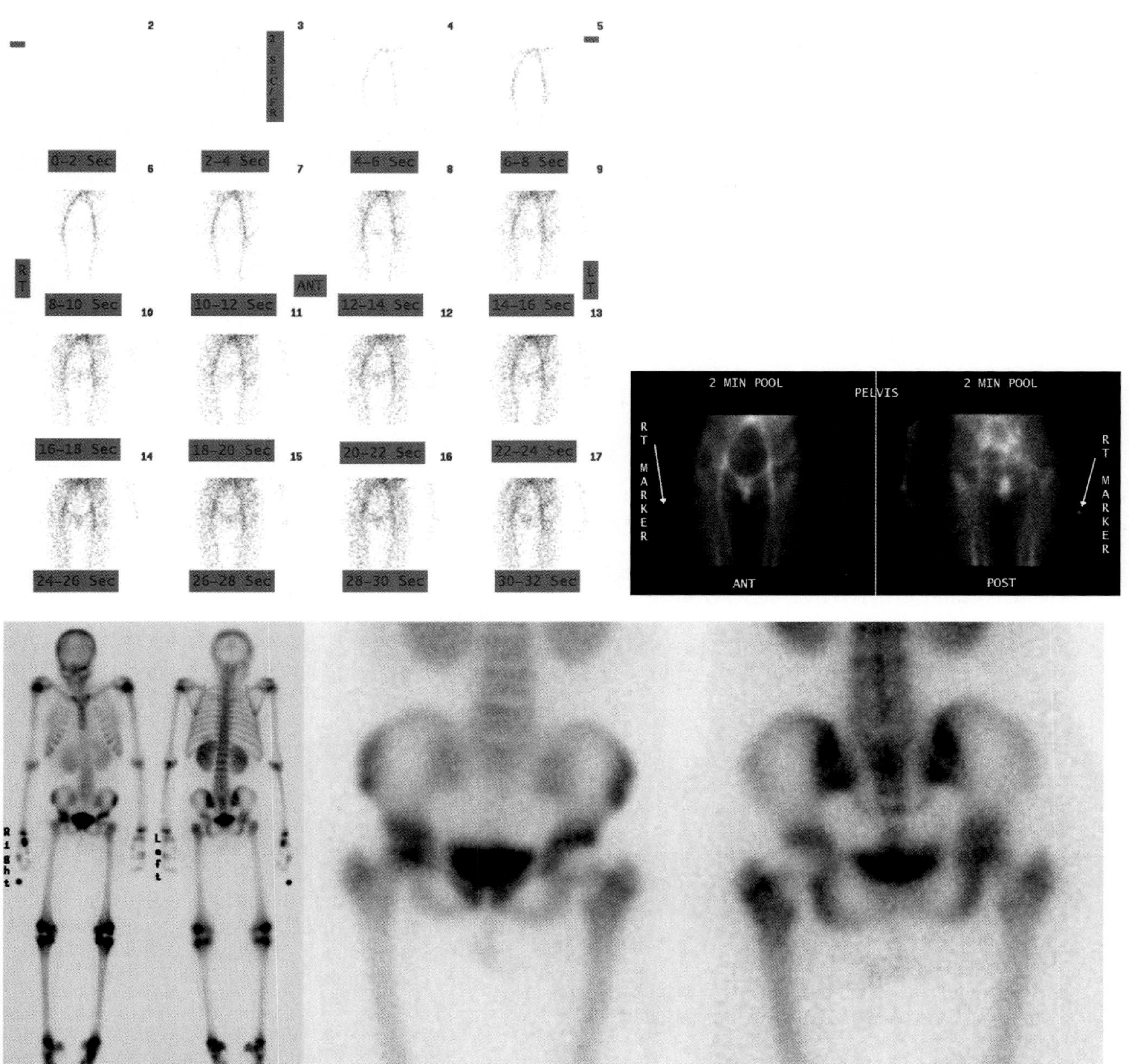

B

Clinical Presentation

A 15-year-old girl with acute left hip pain.

Imaging Findings

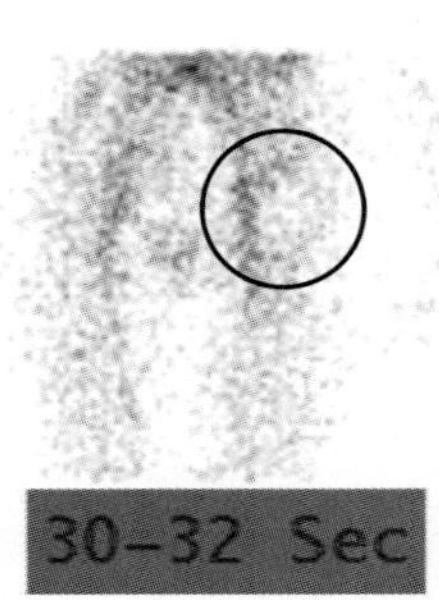

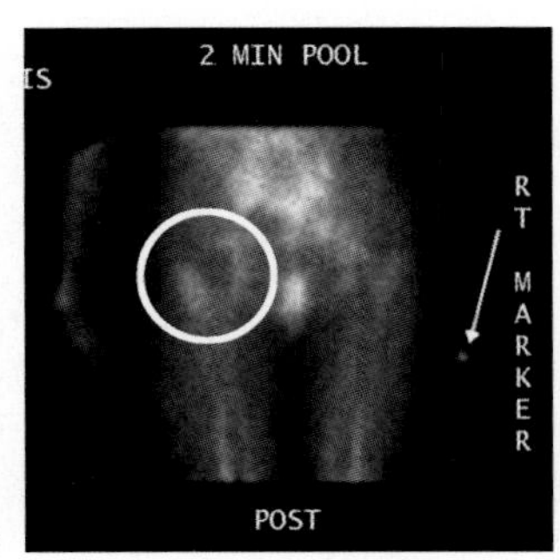

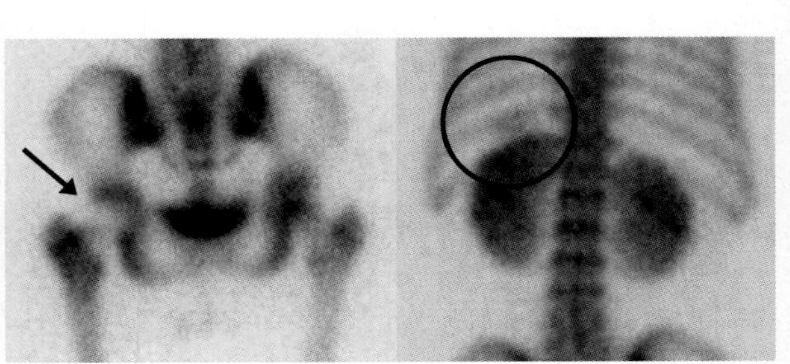

(A) Anterior pelvic angiographic images from a three-phase Tc99m-HDP bone scan show a subtle decrease in blood flow to the left hip (*circle*). **(B)** Anterior and posterior pelvic blood pool images reveal an asymmetric region of decreased activity in the left hip (*circle*). **(C)** Standard delayed whole-body and pelvic spot images demonstrate a concordant region of decreased uptake involving the left femoral head (*arrow*). Very subtle splenic soft-tissue uptake is also seen above the left kidney (*circle*). Symmetric tracer uptake is seen at the epiphyses, which is a normal finding in a child. Focal tracer activity in the right wrist is from injection site artifact.

Differential Diagnosis

- ***Acute avascular necrosis (AVN):*** Acute AVN will present with decreased activity on early and delayed phases of the bone scan.
- *Septic arthritis:* Typically, blood flow and pool will be increased because of hyperemia; however, increased pressure in the hip joint may cause decreased uptake.
- *Tumor:* Most tumors have increased delayed uptake. Lytic lesions can have decreased delayed uptake but should have preserved blood flow and pool.

Essential Facts

- AVN most commonly affects the epiphyses of long bones
- Common causes are trauma, steroids, sickle cell disease, vasculitis, alcohol abuse, radiation, and chemotherapy.
- Appearances on bone scan varies with age of infarct:
  - Acute/early AVN will demonstrate a photopenic defect on all three phases of the bone scan. This is typically seen within the first month after onset.
  - In subacute to chronic phases, the infarct can be mildly to moderately increased on delayed imaging as the bone heals.

Other Imaging Findings

- MRI can demonstrate nonspecific edema and joint effusion in early AVN and the more specific "double line" sign later. Here is the MRI from this same patient with early AVN showing both the nonspecific edema and effusion at the left hip (*circle*):

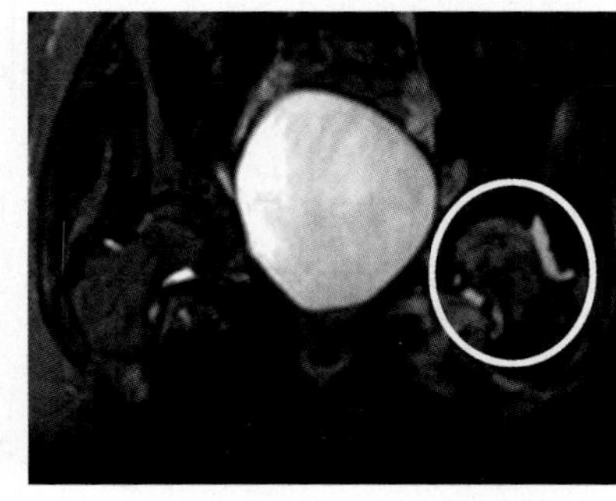

- Radiography and CT can show osseous sclerosis or collapse in the later stages of AVN but are not as sensitive.
- Splenic uptake on bone scan (as in this patient) suggests sickle cell disease (with splenic autoinfarction) as the underlying etiology of the AVN.

✓ Pearls & ✗ Pitfalls

✓ In small children, high-resolution pinhole images may be required to visualize the femoral head on bone scan.
✓ External-beam radiation will also cause decreased osseous uptake on bone scan; however, this is not seen acutely and may take 3 to 4 months.
✓ Bone marrow imaging with Tc99m-SCOL is more sensitive than bone scan in detecting areas of AVN/infarct, but AVN cannot always be distinguished from osteomyelitis.
✓ The combination of splenic uptake and osseous lesions (increased or decreased) on bone scan suggests sickle cell disease (and bone infarcts).
✗ A dysplastic femoral head may mimic AVN on scintigraphy.
✗ In diseases such as lupus, AVN of the hip is often bilateral; diagnosis may be difficult because of the symmetric appearance of increased or decreased uptake on bone scan.
✗ In children, the epiphyses are normally increased, and in the later stages of AVN, it can be difficult to differentiate a site of abnormal uptake from a site of physiologic uptake. Look carefully for asymmetry.
✗ Metallic attenuation artifact such as coins in the pocket may mimic a cold defect on bone scan.

Case 58

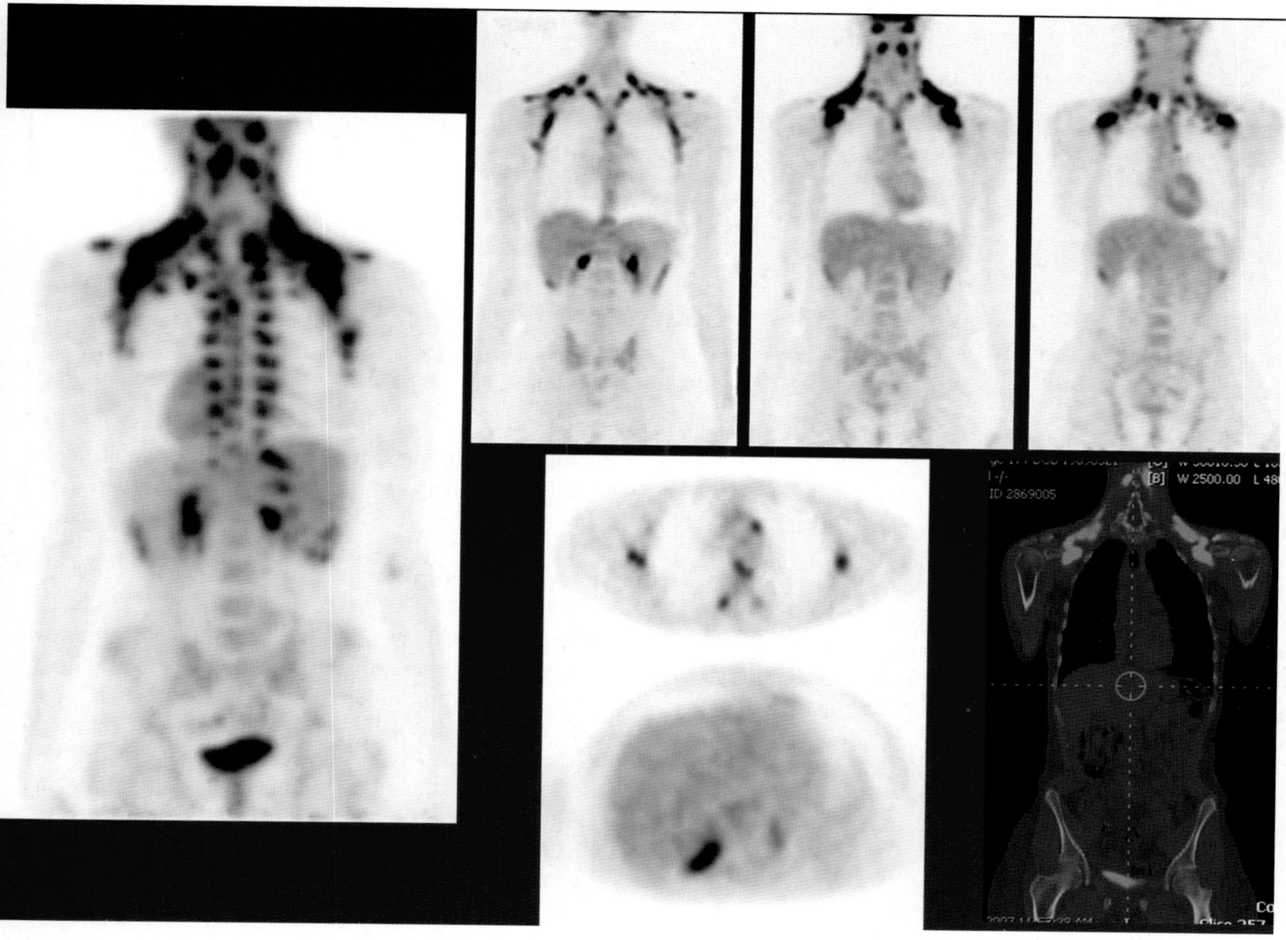

Clinical Presentation

A 28-year-old woman with a history of malignancy presents for restaging.

Imaging Findings

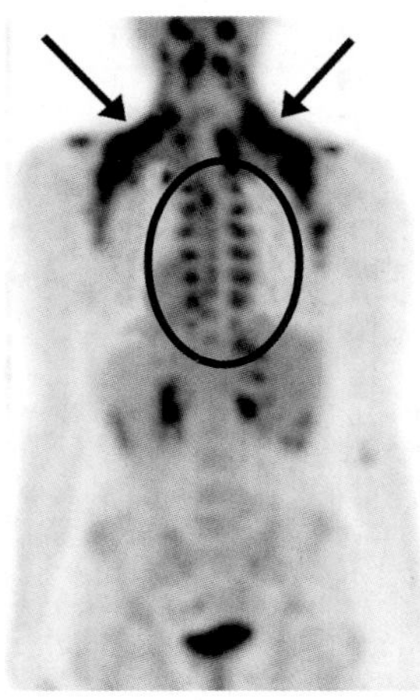

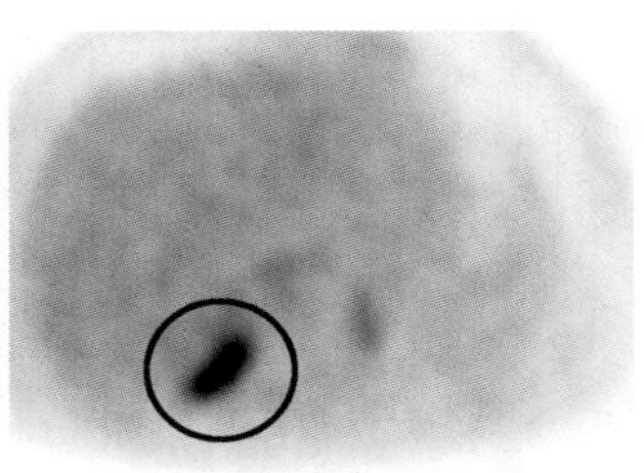

Posterior MIP and additional selected axial and coronal images from a whole-body FDG-PET/CT demonstrate symmetric, markedly increased glucose metabolism in the neck, shoulders (*arrows*), and paraspinal regions (*oval*), as well as in the superior mediastinum and right upper abdomen (*circle*).

Differential Diagnosis

- ***Brown adipose tissue (BAT) hypermetabolism:*** Characteristic, symmetrically increased activity in the neck, shoulders, upper mediastinum, and paraspinal locations makes this the most likely diagnosis.
- *Non-Hodgkin lymphoma:* This can appear similar, with abnormal activity in the neck and upper thorax, but is not typically this symmetric and does not involve the paraspinal region diffusely.
- *Myositis:* This can appear with similarly increased uptake in isolated muscle groups but is rarely this extensive or symmetric.

Essential Facts

- BAT, also called brown fat or uptake in the supraclavicular area (USA) fat, is a common cause of incidental benign although intense FDG uptake.
- Unlike the more common white fat, brown fat has a high mitochondrial density and sympathetic innervation, and it plays a role in metabolic hormonal pathways and heat generation.
- Although BAT is present in all humans, BAT hypermetabolism is more commonly seen in younger women and during colder temperatures.
- The appearance is important to recognize and distinguish from tumor uptake, such as that in lymphoma and head and neck cancer.

Other Imaging Findings

- BAT uptake will almost always correlate with fat density on the CT portion, as in this patient:

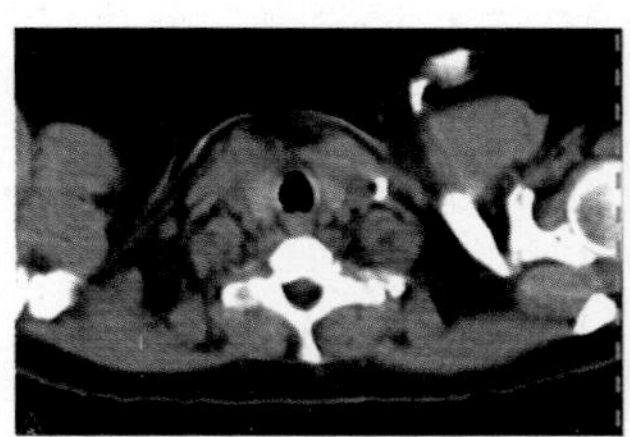

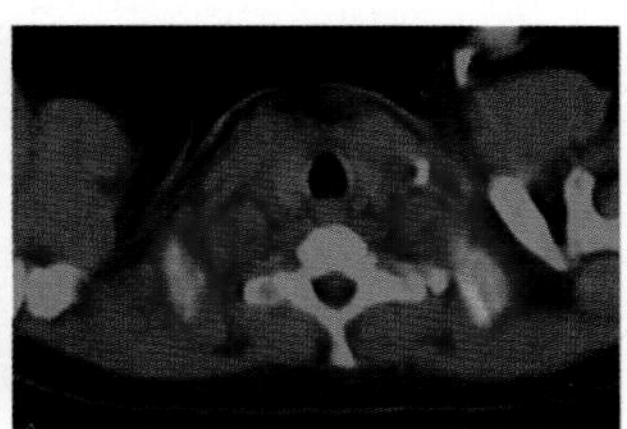

- BAT increased uptake can occasionally be visualized on an MIBG scan owing to the sympathetic innervation.

✓ Pearls & × Pitfalls

✓ A reduction in BAT uptake has been reported with various patient preparations for the FDG-PET exam: drugs (diazepam, propranolol), diet (low carbohydrate/high fat), and vigorous patient warming before injection.

✓ Although usually typically located symmetrically in the neck, shoulders, mediastinum, and paraspinal regions, BAT can occasionally be seen below the diaphragm, including asymmetrically in the upper abdomen (as in this patient's right renal fossa).

× Benign BAT and pathologic tumor uptake can coexist. Symmetric neck and supraclavicular tumor can mimic BAT. Be certain that all presumptive BAT uptake corresponds to fat density, not lymph node or other soft-tissue density (except linear muscle activity, which is also physiologic), particularly in patients with lymphoma or head and neck carcinoma. Here is a different patient with lymphoma simulating BAT (*circles*):

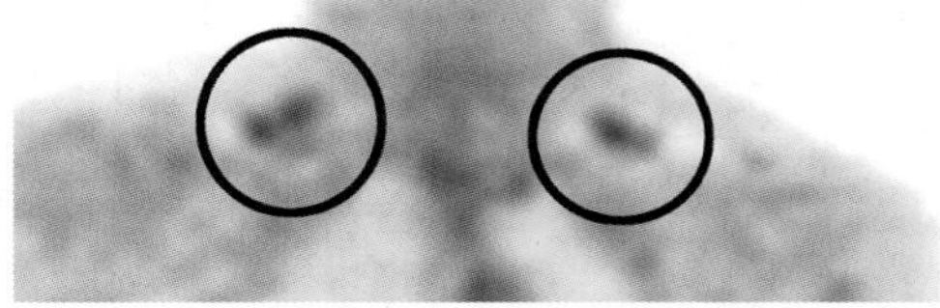

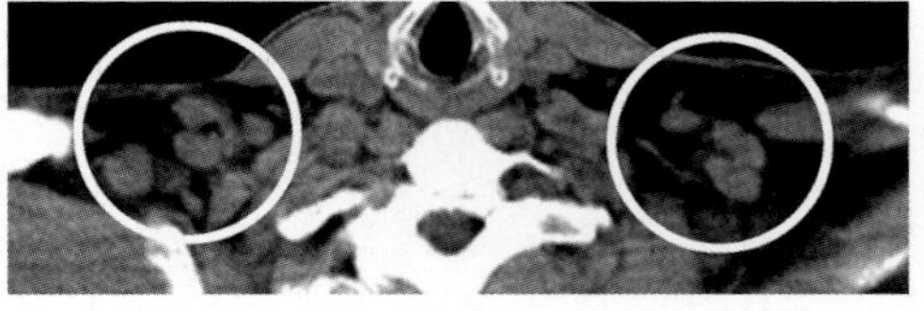

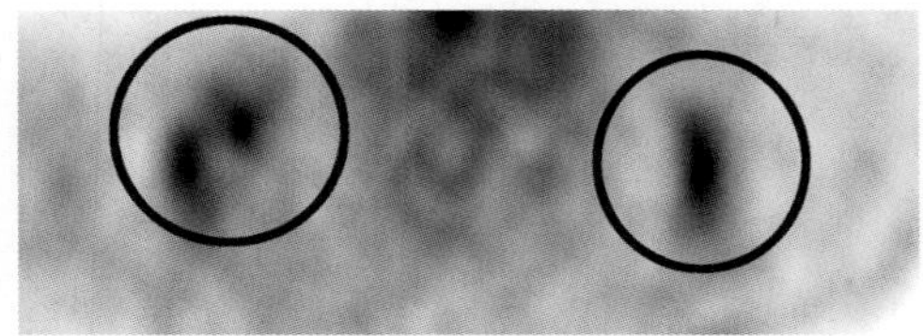

Case 59

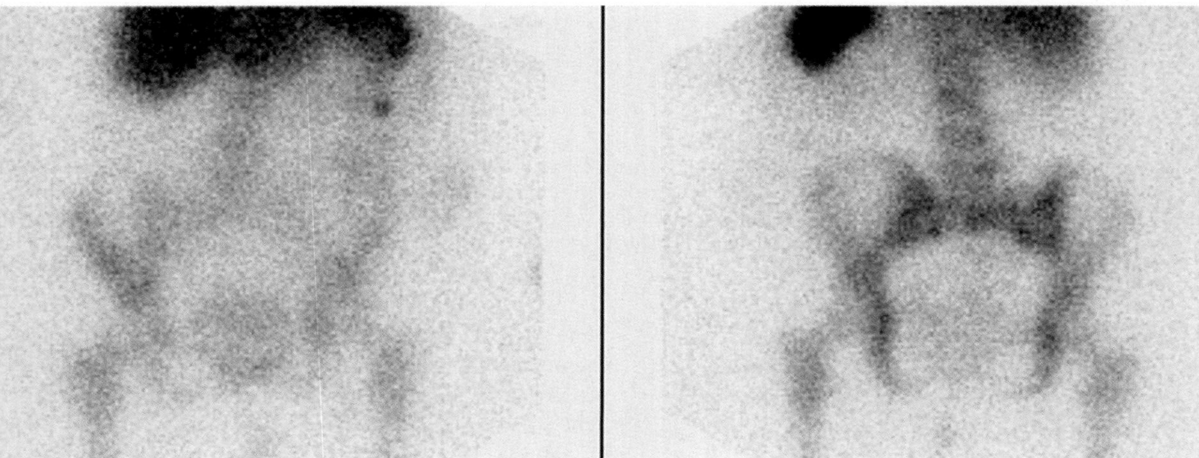

Clinical Presentation

An 80-year-old woman with fever of unknown origin. She is on gastrostomy tube feeds.

Imaging Findings

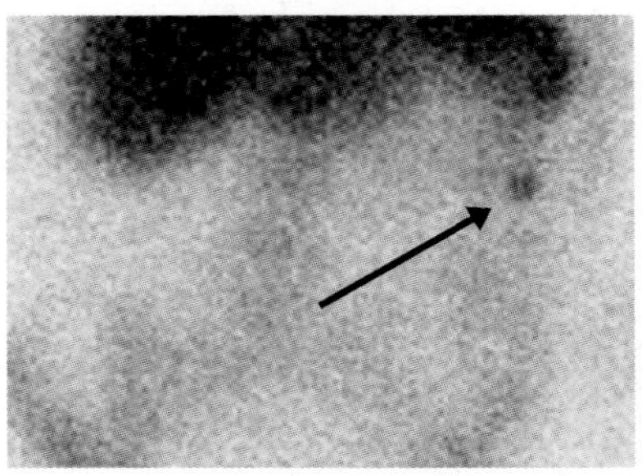

Physiologic uptake confined to the spleen, liver, and bone marrow (most intense in the spleen, as seen on posterior view) makes this most likely a labeled leukocyte exam. Lack of significant normal bowel excretion makes indium 111–oxine the likely radiolabel (over Tc99m-HMPAO). A small increased focus is seen in the anterior left upper quadrant (*arrow*).

Differential Diagnosis

- ***Expected physiologic WBC accumulation surrounding gastrostomy tube tract:*** Given the history, this is the most likely etiology for the findings.
- *Abdominal infection:* This is conceivable, although clinically important infections are typically more intense.
- *Physiologic intraluminal excretion in bowel:* This does occur with Tc99m-HMPAO–labeled WBCs after 4 hours, but not with In111-oxine label. Also, this uptake would be more diffuse.

Essential Facts

- Labeled autologous WBC imaging is often used as a primary management pathway for several indications, including occult fever, leukocytosis of unknown origin, suspected abdominal abscess, and prosthetic complications (e.g., aseptic loosening vs. infection).
- WBCs may be labeled with In111-oxine or Tc99m-HMPAO. The Tc99m label allows for a higher administered dose (and thus superior image quality) and earlier imaging (1–4 hours vs. 24–72 hours for In111).
- However, Tc99m is a weaker label, and elution into bile ducts, bowel, and the genitourinary system (all by 3–4 hours) can complicate interpretation, particularly on more delayed imaging.
- Regional uptake equal to or greater than that in liver is suggestive of significant infection/inflammation.
- However, physiologic "healing" uptake will also occur at several sites, particularly stomas and skin incisions for catheter insertions and recent surgery.
- Mild uptake at these sites suggests expected (noninfected) inflammation.

Other Imaging Findings

- Gallium 67 is also useful for infection/inflammatory imaging (and tumors) and may be better in more chronic and vertebral infections.
- FDG-PET is gaining acceptance as a good infection/inflammatory imaging tool.
- Bone scan is a good way to detect osteomyelitis unless the underlying bone is abnormal to begin with (like joint prosthesis or neuropathic diabetic foot), in which case WBC imaging can be helpful.
- CT and MRI have become mainstays for infectious/inflammatory imaging, particularly for pulmonary infections and abdominal abscesses. SPECT/CT can be useful with WBC scintigraphy. Here is this patient's CT showing the gastrostomy tube insertion in the left upper quadrant (*circle*):

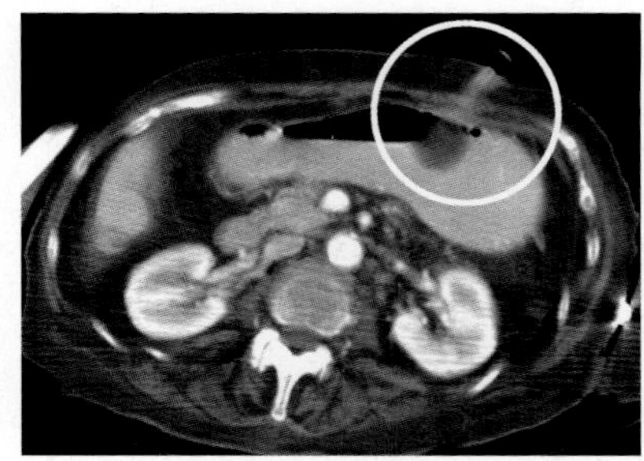

✓ Pearls & × Pitfalls

- ✓ Patient leukocyte counts should be > 3000/mm^3 for proper labeling.
- ✓ Tc99m-HMPAO–labeled WBCs should be imaged by 1 to 2 hours after injection to avoid normal gastrointestinal and genitourinary uptake; for In111, 24- to 48-hour imaging is performed. Lung imaging, if needed, should be performed *after* 4 hours with either label (normal diffuse lung uptake is seen earlier because of slow clearing through the pulmonary vasculature).
- ✓ Surgical wounds have normal mild WBC uptake for 1 to 2 weeks. If intense, however, suspect superinfection.
- × Swallowed labeled WBCs from mild sinusitis or pulmonary disease can simulate abnormal gastrointestinal uptake. Look at the head and chest images for a source.
- × Renal transplants normally have significant WBC accumulation, and diffuse uptake does not necessarily indicate infection.
- × Tumors are a rare cause of false-positive WBC accumulation (but they usually do *not* accumulate WBCs).

Case 60

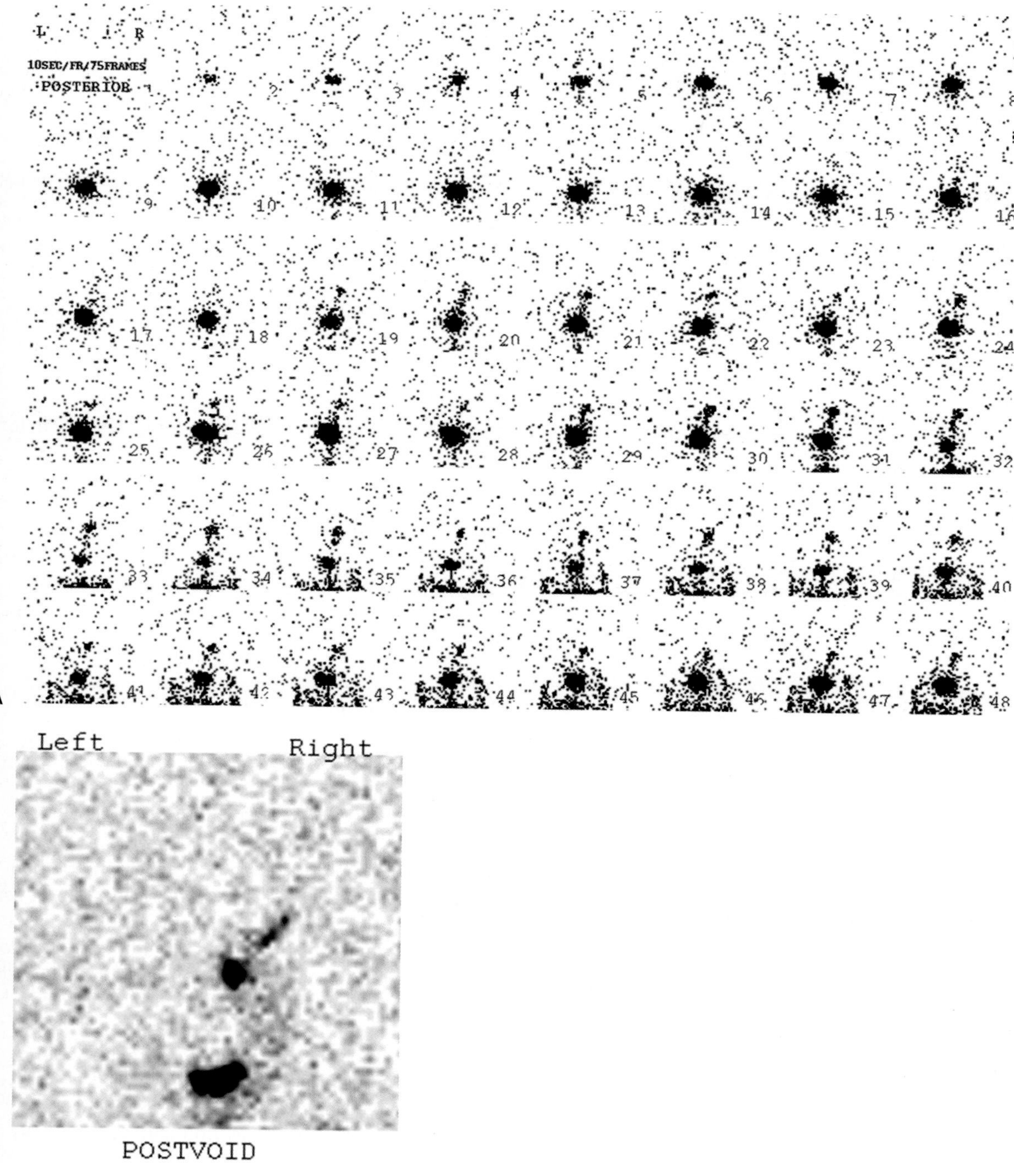

A

B

Clinical Presentation

A 1-year-old girl presents after recent urinary tract infection.

Imaging Findings

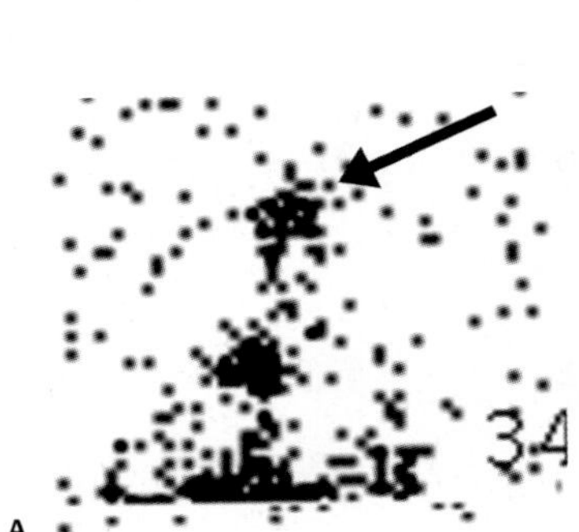

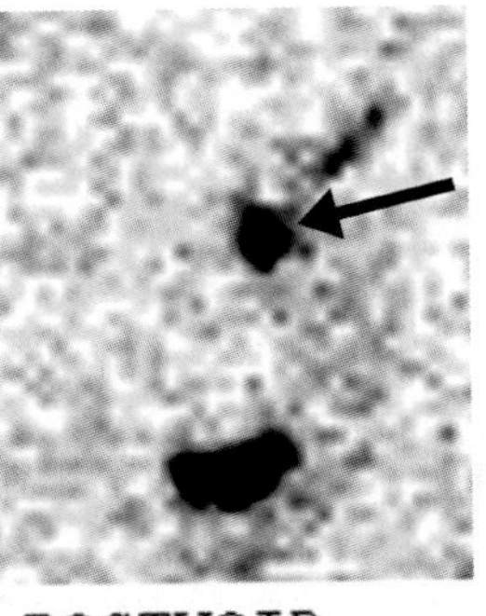

(A) Direct radionuclide cystography was performed with 0.5 mCi of Tc99m-pertechnetate. Dynamic posterior images reveal abnormal radiotracer appearing above the bladder on the right (*arrow*), increasing during the voiding phase. **(B)** A static posterior postvoid image demonstrates retention of radiotracer above the bladder on the right (*arrow*).

Differential Diagnosis

- ***Vesicoureteral reflux (VUR):*** Activity should not be seen above the level of the bladder and if present indicates reflux.
- *Urinary contamination artifact:* This is commonly seen but appears *below* the bladder, from leakage around the bladder catheter.
- *Urinary leak:* This is much less likely and would appear outside the expected location of the bladder and collecting system.

Essential Facts

- VUR is seen in 35 to 40% of children with urinary tract infection.
- Resolves spontaneously in most children
- Occurs in 35 to 45% of asymptomatic siblings
- Contrast-enhanced fluoroscopic cystography is recommended as the first procedure in males as this permits better anatomic evaluation (e.g., assessment for posterior urethral valves).
- When reflux is seen, note should be made of the volume of fluid instilled.
- Follow-up evaluation can be performed to determine if the volume required to cause reflux has increased, which indicates a better chance of spontaneous resolution.
- The International Reflux Study Committee grading system:
  - Grade I: reflux into ureter only
  - Grade II: reflux reaches the renal pelvis; no dilatation of the collecting system; normal fornices
  - Grade III: mild or moderate dilatation of the ureter, with or without kinking; moderate dilatation of the collecting system; normal or minimally deformed fornices
  - Grade IV: moderate dilatation of the ureter with or without kinking; moderate dilatation of the collecting system; blunt fornices, but impressions of the papillae still visible
  - Grade V: gross dilatation and kinking of the ureter, marked dilatation of the collecting system; papillary impressions no longer visible; intraparenchymal reflux

Note that these criteria are for *fluoroscopic* contrast voiding cystourethrogram (VCUG). Radionuclide cystography typically classifies reflux as mild, moderate, or severe, as the study does not provide enough anatomic resolution for more detailed grading.

Other Imaging Findings

- Contrast-enhanced fluoroscopic cystography is useful for a better anatomic evaluation of the bladder and male urethra.

✓ Pearls & ✗ Pitfalls

✓ A patient's estimated bladder volume can be calculated as follows:
- Volume (mL) = (Age [y] + 2) × 30

✓ Radionuclide cystography has significantly lower patient radiation exposure and a greater sensitivity than does contrast-enhanced fluoroscopic cystography. It can detect < 1 mL of reflux.

✓ As a result, in many institutions the initial VCUG is fluoroscopic to define the anatomy, with scintigraphy used on follow-up exams.

✗ Sensitivity of radionuclide VCUG is decreased for very mild reflux occurring only adjacent to the bladder because of intense bladder activity.

✗ Leakage of radiotracer from the catheter/bladder can obscure images and make it difficult to see small amounts of reflux.

✗ Radiotracer absorbed through the bladder wall, if inflamed, may be excreted by the kidneys and cause a false-positive exam.

Images courtesy of Dr. Lionel Zuckier, Department of Radiology, University of Medicine and Dentistry of New Jersey, Newark, NJ.

Case 61

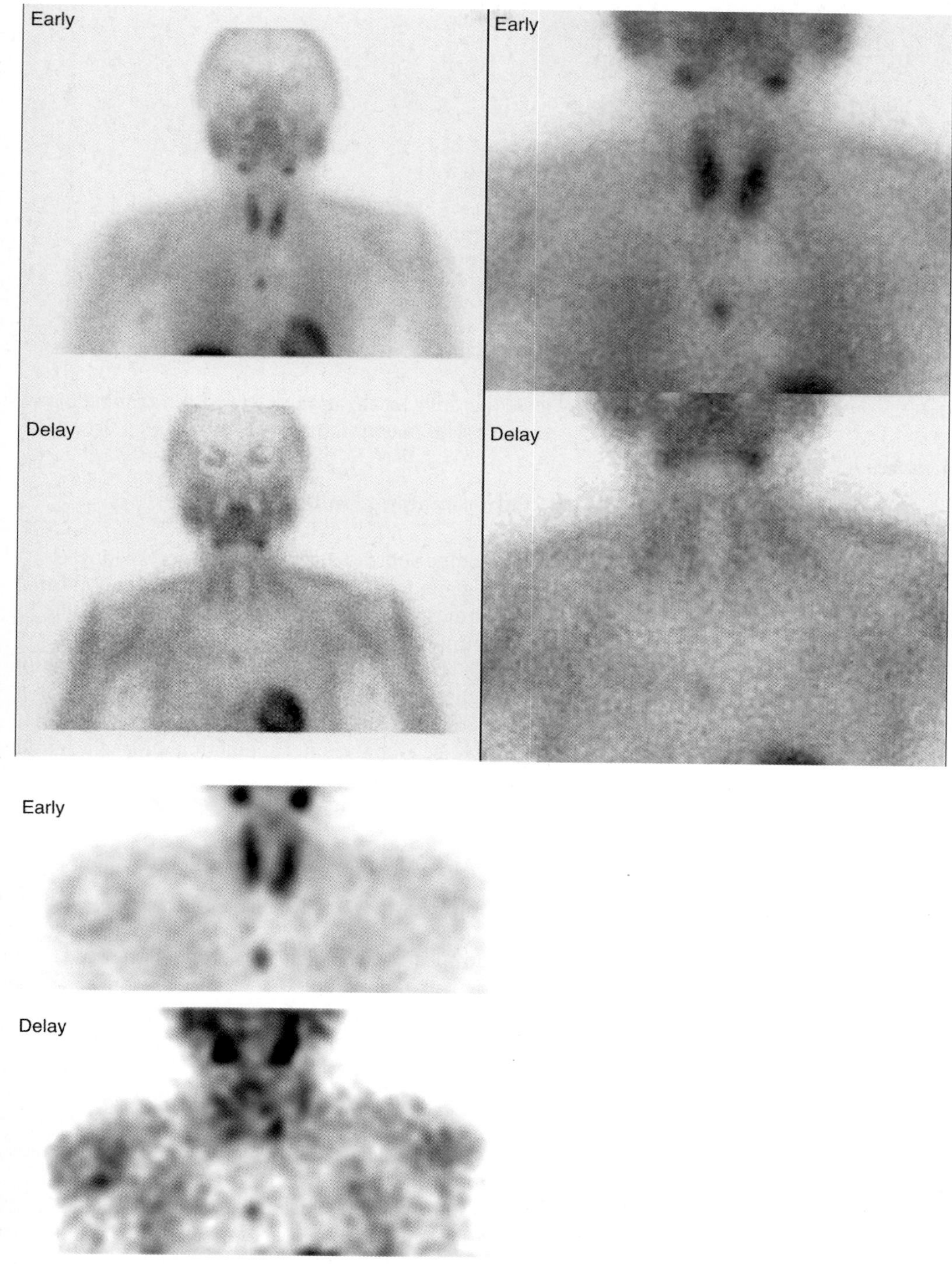

Clinical Presentation

A 52-year-old man with hypercalcemia. Images were acquired 20 minutes and 3 hours after injection.

Imaging Findings

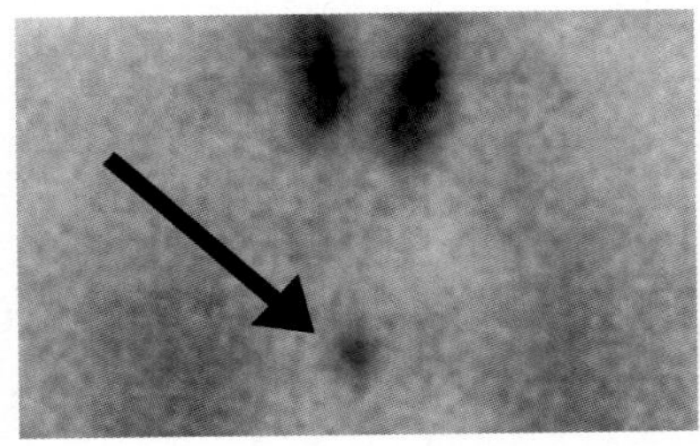
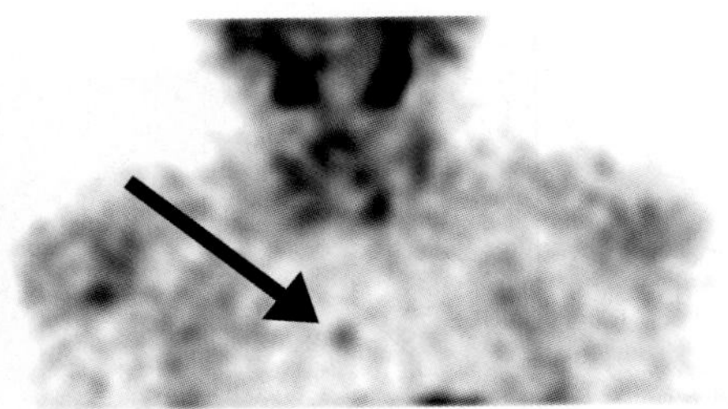

(A) Early planar images demonstrate physiologic radiotracer uptake in salivary, lacrimal, thyroid, and myocardial tissue, making Tc99m-MIBI or -TETRO the most likely agent (parathyroid scan). An abnormal mediastinal focus is seen on early images (*arrow*); it persists mildly on delayed images. Normal thyroid activity washes out on the delayed planar images. **(B)** Early and delayed selected coronal SPECT slices demonstrate the abnormal mediastinal focus (*arrow*). Again, the thyroid is largely washed out on delay.

Differential Diagnosis

- ***Ectopic parathyroid adenoma:*** An abnormal mediastinal focus is most likely this diagnosis, particularly given the history.
- *Mediastinal tumor:* MIBI and TETRO are nonspecific tracers, and a number of metastatic and primary lesions, including lymphoma, could have this appearance.
- *Pulmonary infection/inflammation:* Again, these are nonspecific tracers, and an active process could have focal activity.

Essential Facts

- Hyperparathyroidism can be primary (autonomous hyperfunction of gland[s]), secondary (physiologic gland hyperfunction to compensate for low calcium with renal failure), or tertiary (also in renal failure but in which a parathyroid gland[s] becomes autonomous).
- Patients with elevated parathyroid hormone and elevated serum calcium typically have primary hyperparathyroidism.
- Primary hyperparathyroidism is most commonly due to parathyroid adenoma (85–90%), less often hyperplasia (10%), and rarely parathyroid carcinoma ($< 1\%$).
- Although most adenomas are typically located at the upper or lower thyroid, 5 to 10% can be ectopic, frequently located in the mediastinum or occasionally higher in the neck.
- Treatment for parathyroid adenoma is surgical resection of abnormal gland(s). Ethanol or radiofrequency ablation is also utilized.
- Tc99m-MIBI or -TETRO early and delayed imaging is the most common scintigraphic method; tracer binds to increased mitochondria in abnormal parathyroid glands and enters normal thyroid early then washes out of thyroid late.
- Scintigraphic preoperative imaging (for localization and diagnosis) has become standard, particularly with minimally invasive techniques, often in conjunction with intraoperative localization with a gamma probe following repeat tracer injection the day of surgery.

Other Imaging Findings

- Dual-isotope subtraction of a tracer specific for the thyroid gland from a tracer that also binds to abnormal parathyroids is another imaging option. Historically, thallium/pertechnetate was used with mixed results, although today, (early) MIBI/I123 subtraction is possible with higher accuracy.
- Parathyroid US to look for a hypoechoic perithyroidal lesion can be employed in conjunction with scintigraphy; CT or MRI is less commonly useful, although SPECT/CT is an emerging possibility.

✓ Pearls & ✗ Pitfalls

✓ An ectopic adenoma can occur anywhere from the carotid sheath in the high neck through the lower mediastinum. Imaging should be performed from the upper neck through the lower cardiac border.

✓ The sensitivity of parathyroid scintigraphy is much higher for an adenoma (90%) than for hyperplasia (50%).

✓ Hyperfunctioning parathyroid tissue does not always persist on delayed imaging; any focus seen on early images should be treated as suspicious despite potential washout.

✓ SPECT increases exam accuracy. If only one SPECT image is acquired, it should be performed *early* to use normal thyroid as a landmark (and avoid potential lesion washout).

✗ Stasis of swallowed salivary activity in the esophagus can mimic abnormal accumulation. Repeat imaging after the patient drinks water can be useful to distinguish.

✗ Ectopic thyroid tissue or asymmetric salivary activity can mimic a parathyroid adenoma. Mapping the patient's normal salivary and thyroid activity with Tc99m-pertechnetate can be useful if a concern.

Case 62

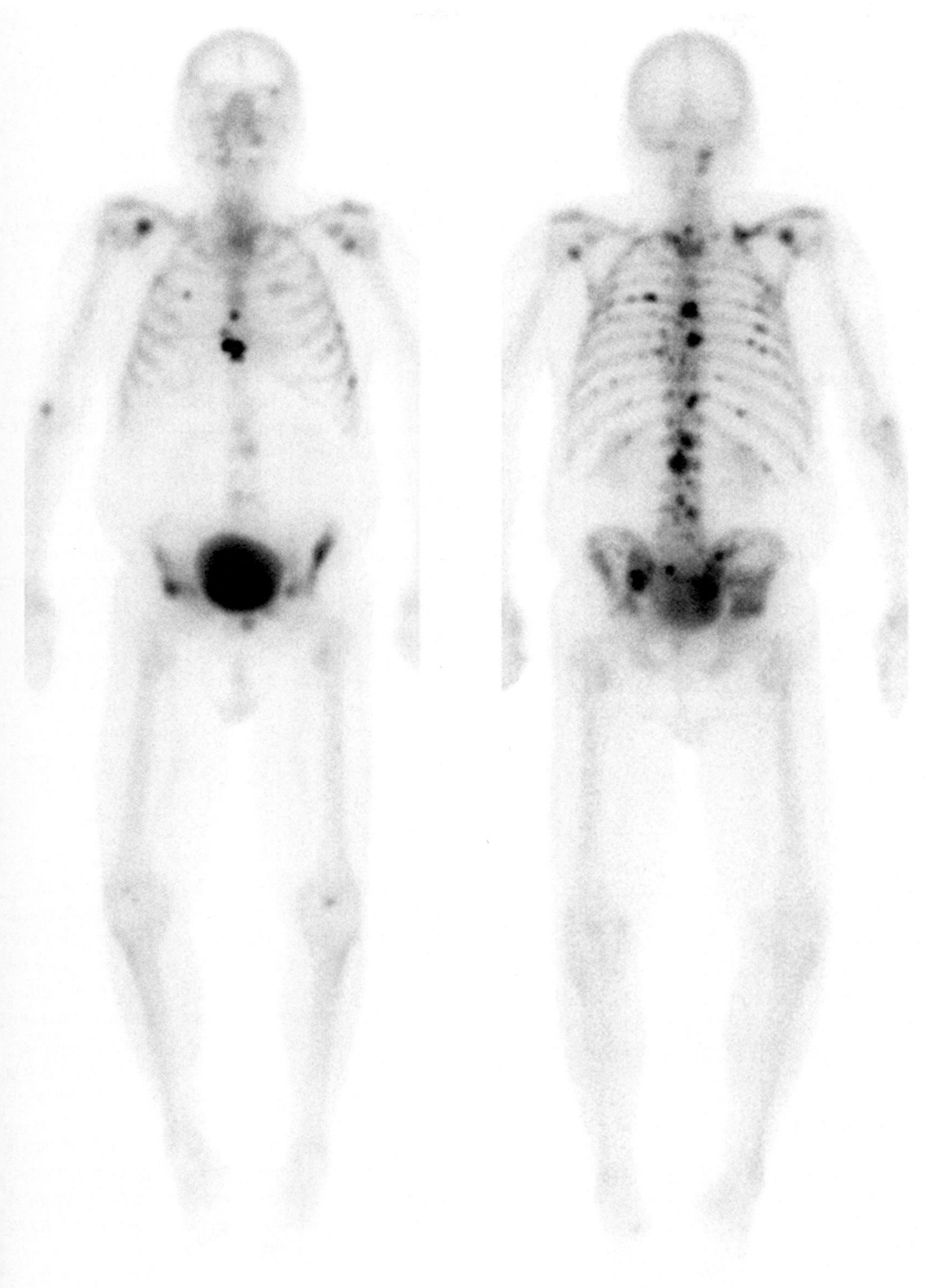

Clinical Presentation

A 57-year-old man with a history of prostate cancer and diffuse body pain.

Imaging Findings

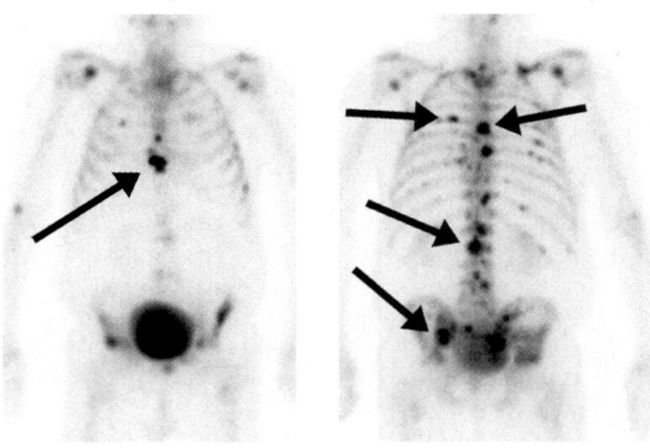

Three-hour–delayed anterior and posterior whole-body bone scan demonstrates too numerous-to-count osteoblastic lesions in the axial and proximal appendicular skeleton (*arrows*).

Differential Diagnosis

- ***Diffuse osteoblastic metastases:*** This pattern of uptake is most consistent with diffuse osseous metastatic disease. Note that there is minimal abnormal uptake in the appendicular skeleton (beyond red marrow distribution).
- *Multifocal Paget disease:* This can also demonstrate multiple lesions. However, these need not be confined to the axial skeleton and typically appear as long-segment lesions that, in the extremities, start at the bone ends (see Case 17).
- *Multiple bone lesions associated with a metabolic disorder:* Occasionally, hyperparathyroidism or other metabolic conditions can give the appearance of multiple bony lesions that can be apparent on bone scan. However, the lack of significant uptake in the peripheral appendicular skeleton argues against this possibility.

Essential Facts

- Bone scans are most often used to assess for osteoblastic metastatic disease. Tc99m-HDP and Tc99m-MDP are equivalent.
- Bone scan is 50 to 80% more sensitive than plain film.
- Bone scans are standard to assess for metastatic lesions associated with prostate, breast, and lung cancers. These cancers have a significantly higher percentage of osteoblastic than osteolytic lesions. In prostate cancer, nearly all lesions are osteoblastic in nature.
- The vast majority of osseous metastatic lesions are within the axial and proximal appendicular skeleton (red marrow distribution).
- Osteolytic lesions such as renal cell carcinoma and multiple myeloma are much less sensitively detected on bone scan. Consider other modalities, such as FDG-PET/CT.

Other Imaging Findings

- Bone scan SPECT is more sensitive and specific than planar images for metastases, particularly in the spine (and without additional radiation). Consider obtaining if planar imaging is equivocal.
- CT is more sensitive than plain films. However, it is not as sensitive as bone scan (for blastic lesions) and cannot as readily characterize interval change.
- MRI is nearly as sensitive as bone scan, with much higher anatomic resolution. However, the lack of efficient whole-body MRI limits it to more regional problem solving.
- FDG-PET, especially when combined with CT, is particularly useful for identifying metastatic bony lesions before chemotherapy and for identifying recurrence. FDG is not optimal for purely osteoblastic and/or low-grade metastatic lesions (like prostate cancer). FDG images the lesion itself (as opposed to surrounding bone increased turnover) and can also assess soft tissues.
- NaF18-PET images increased bone turnover (like conventional bone scan) but takes advantage of PET physics, with improved tomographic resolution. Early data have been very encouraging, with significantly higher sensitivity than traditional bone scan for identifying bony metastasis.

✓ Pearls & ✗ Pitfalls

✓ An equivocal lesion on bone scan followed by a negative plain film is even *more* suspicious for metastasis (as benign findings like fracture and degenerative joint disease are usually seen on x-ray). If a lesion is not seen on plain films, more advanced imaging is recommended.

✓ Ninety percent of patients with bone metastasis present with multiple lesions. Ribs have the highest frequency of metastasis, followed by the spine. However, a *solitary* rib lesion has only an approximately 10% probability of metastasis.

✗ If the patient is clinically better 2 to 6 months following chemotherapy but the bone scan looks worse, consider the *flare phenomenon,* in which healing lesions temporarily become more osteoblastic. Additional short-term follow-up may be required.

✗ Do not forget to look at the soft tissues, such as in the liver and breast, for tumor uptake (primary or metastatic), which can occasionally be seen with a variety of tumor types on bone scan.

✗ When bone metastases become extremely widespread, they may become uniformly confluent appearing as a metastatic superscan.

Case 63

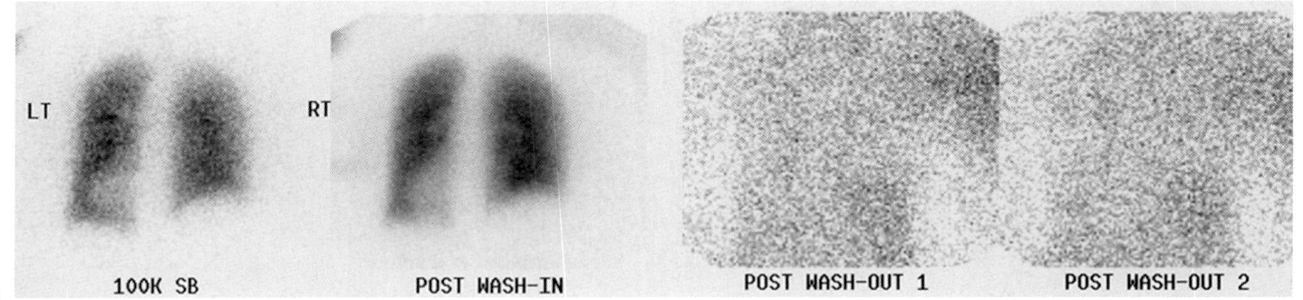

A

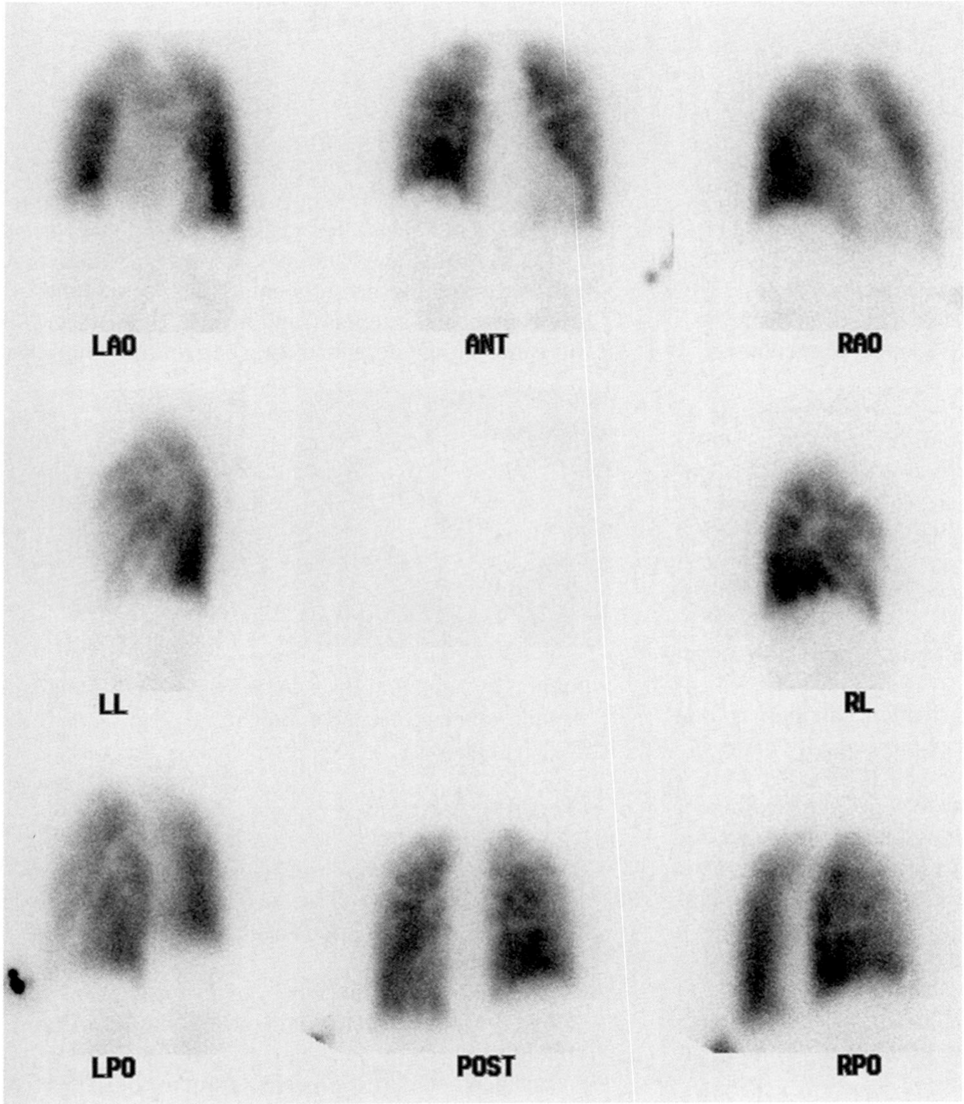

B

Clinical Presentation

A 64-year-old woman with breast cancer presents with shortness of breath.

Imaging Findings

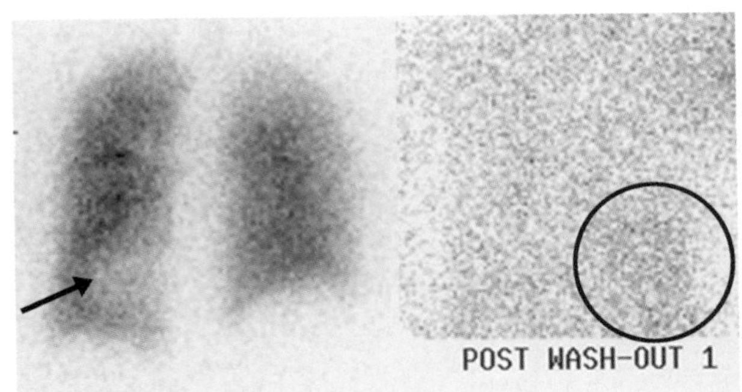

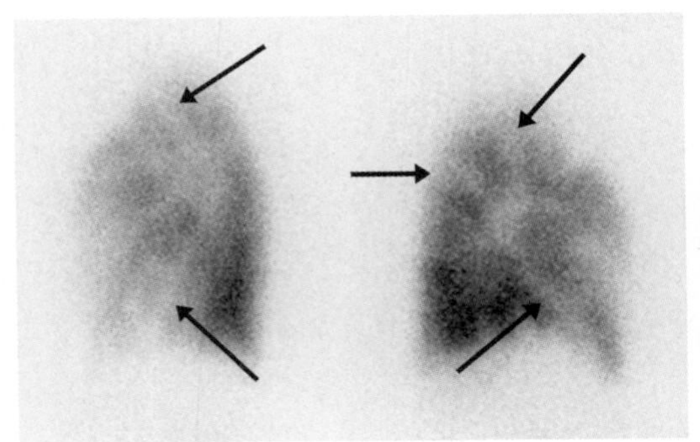

(A) Sequential Xenon 133 ventilation images demonstrate focal decrease in single-breath ventilation at the left lung base (*arrow*), but with the remaining distribution uniform. There is no abnormal retention. Faint accumulation of tracer is seen on washout in a fatty liver (*circle*) below an elevated right hemidiaphragm (see Case 9). **(B)** Tc99m-MAA images demonstrate multiple linear perfusion defects outlining the periphery of most segments: the "segmental contouring" sign or "contour mapping" sign (*arrows*).

Differential Diagnosis

- ***Diffuse tumor microemboli (TM):*** Multiple linear mismatched perfusion defects outlining the periphery of most segments make this the correct diagnosis.
- *High probability for venous thromboembolic disease:* This will also have multiple mismatched perfusion defects, but these will be larger, wedge-shaped segmental and subsegmental defects.
- *Pleural fluid in the fissures:* This can also demonstrate a linear perfusion defect at the periphery of a lobe. However, this is seen only along a fissure and is matched on the ventilation images.

Essential Facts

- Tumor cells that invade the systemic venous system can become microembolic.
- Lung, breast, colon, and stomach adenocarcinomas most commonly form TM, but TM can be seen with many other malignancies.
- Clinically, TM present similarly to venous thromboembolism, with pleuritic chest pain, dyspnea, hypoxemia, and right heart strain. Lung biopsy may become necessary to distinguish and avoid unnecessary anticoagulation or inferior vena cava filter.
- Unlike venous pulmonary embolism (PE), which demonstrates mismatched wedge-shaped subsegmental and segmental perfusion defects, defects from TM are smaller, linear, and much more peripheral, outlining the contour of most segments.
- TM defects are not considered true metastatic disease unless there is subsequent invasion and spread into the lung interstitium.
- TM therapy is typically aimed at treating the primary tumor, although the prognosis is poor.

Other Imaging Findings

- Chest x-ray or CT is often normal but can show enlargement of the right heart (left image) and pulmonary arteries. If there is subsequent "lymphangitic spread," there may be hazy thickening along the interlobar septa of the bronchovascular bundles (right image). Here is the CT of this same patient demonstrating both of these findings:

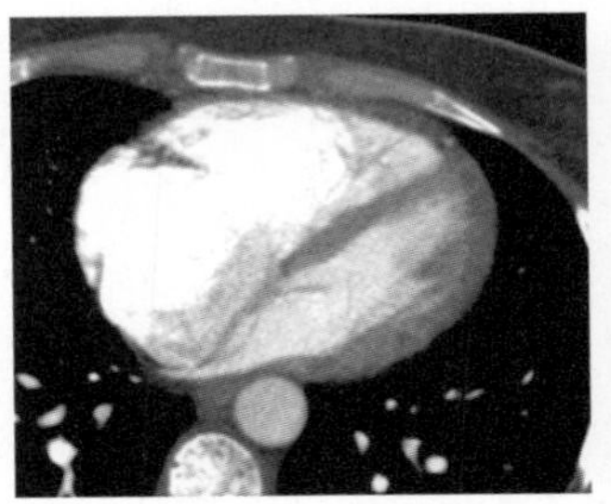

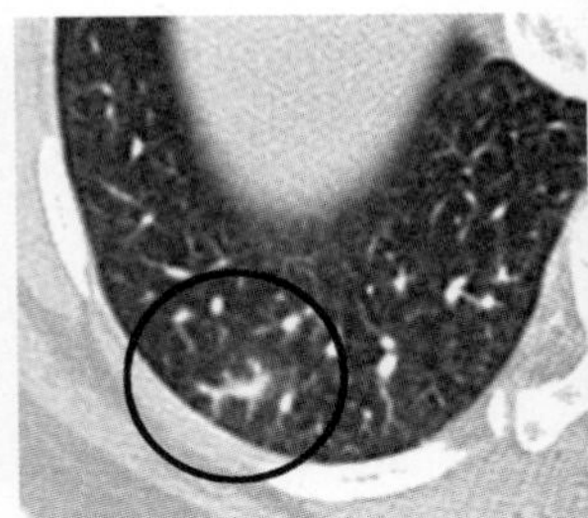

- Pulmonary angiography is not sensitive for TM but can exclude venous thromboembolism.

✓ Pearls & × Pitfalls

✓ Any microembolic disease, including fat and talc microemboli and small-vessel vasculitis, can demonstrate similar segmental contouring; TM are the most common, however.

✓ Remember that the periphery of a segment runs both along the pleural surface *and* more centrally within the lung.

× A mismatched perfusion defect from venous PE is typically wedge-shaped, getting larger toward the lung periphery. Larger tumor emboli can occasionally occlude more proximal pulmonary arteries, appearing similar to typical venous thromboemboli.

Case 64

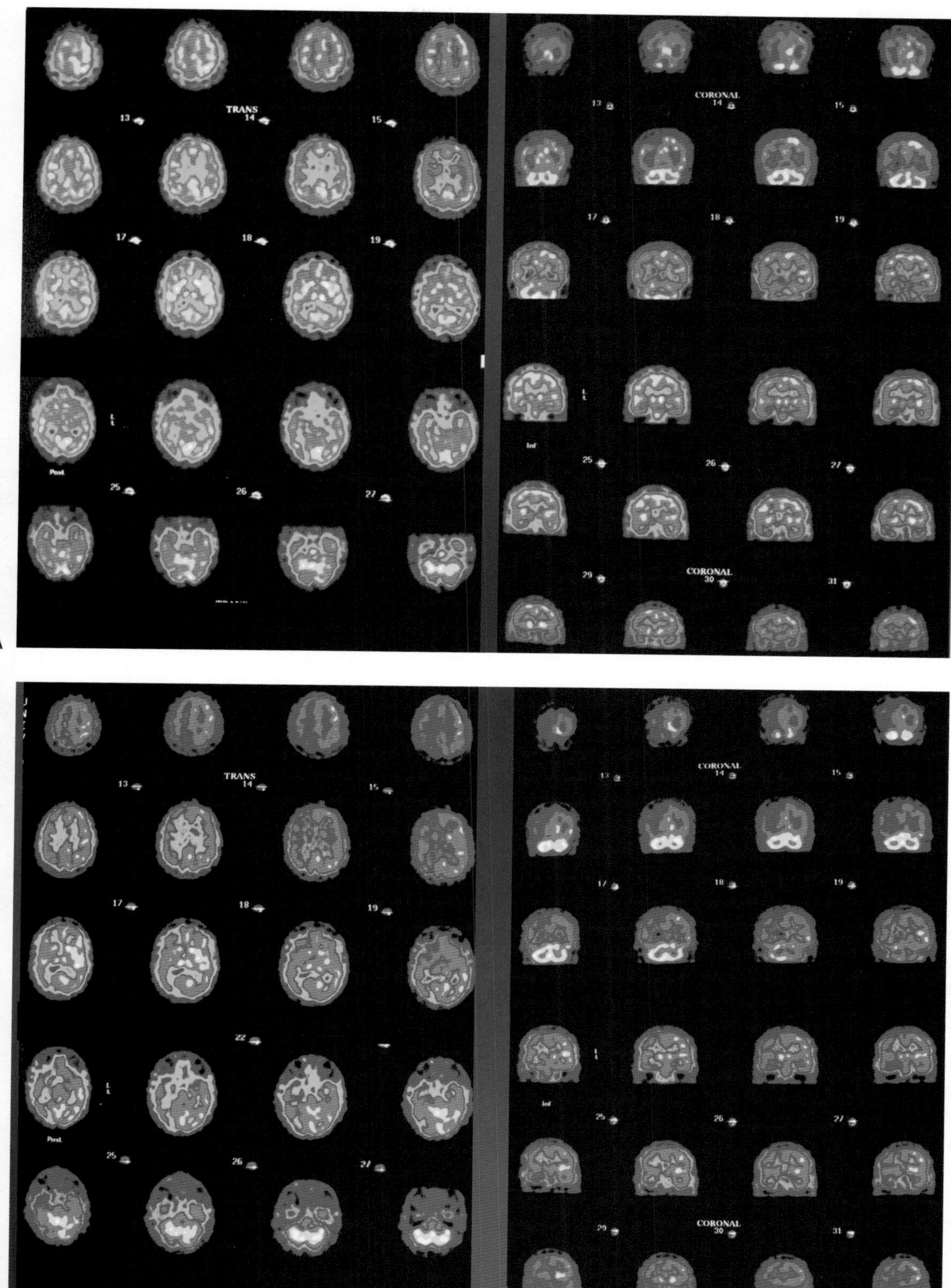

Clinical Presentation

A 64-year-old man with transient ischemic attacks. The exam was acquired before **(A)** and after **(B)** a pharmacologic intervention.

Imaging Findings

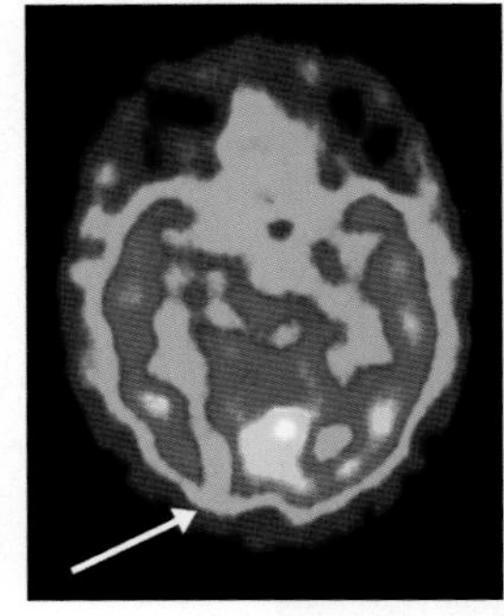

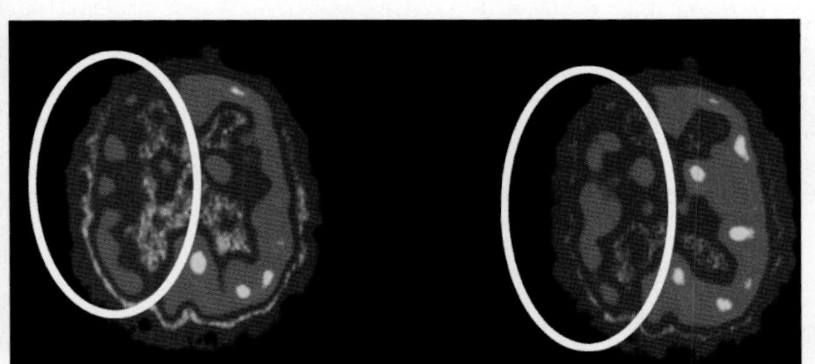

(A) Axial and coronal brain perfusion SPECT images obtained with Tc99m-HMPAO demonstrate a small cortical defect in the right posterior temporal–occipital location (*arrow*). The remainder of the perfusion is normal. **(B)** Axial and coronal brain perfusion SPECT images following acetazolamide administration demonstrate markedly decreased perfusion to most of the right cerebral hemisphere (*circles*).

Differential Diagnosis

- ***Diminished cerebral vascular blood flow reserve:*** A significant decrease in relative right hemispheric blood flow after acetazolamide makes this the most likely diagnosis (plus a small right posterior infarct).
- *Right cerebral seizure (ictal and interictal appearance):* Although perfusion SPECT can be used to localize an ictal focus, the ictal SPECT should have increased, not normal, uptake. And although the interictal focus would have decreased flow, the affected area is usually much smaller.
- *Large right hemispheric infarct:* A large perfusion defect would be present on the *baseline* images.

Essential Facts

- Acetazolamide (Diamox; Teva Pharmaceuticals USA, North Wales, PA) is an antihypertensive carbonic anhydrase inhibitor that causes systemic and cerebral vasodilation.
- Similar to cardiac adenosine, acetazolamide can be used in conjunction with perfusion brain SPECT to perform a pharmacologic cerebral "stress test" and identify territory at risk for stroke (diminished cerebral vascular flow reserve).
- Patients with significant "reversible defects" can be treated with internal carotid artery (ICA) revascularization (e.g., endarterectomy, stents) or even external carotid artery–ICA bypass.
- Perfusion defects at baseline before acetazolamide indicate regions of existing infarct.

Other Imaging Findings

- CT or magnetic resonance perfusion mapping may achieve similar levels of sensitivity.
- Perfusion SPECT can also be performed following temporary neurointerventional unilateral ICA balloon occlusion to assess for adequate cross-filling via the circle of Willis before possible permanent ICA occlusion for several surgical conditions.

✓ Pearls & ✗ Pitfalls

✓ Any cerebral cortical perfusion scintigraphic agents can be used with acetazolamide, including HMPAO (Ceretec) and ECD (Neurolite).

✗ Brain SPECT, like cardiac SPECT, demonstrates relative, not absolute, perfusion. The right-sided perfusion after acetazolamide in this patient is diminished *relative* to the normally dilating contralateral vessels. The abnormal side cannot dilate significantly, but absolute flow is not decreased (unless there is an uncommon "steal phenomenon").

Case 65

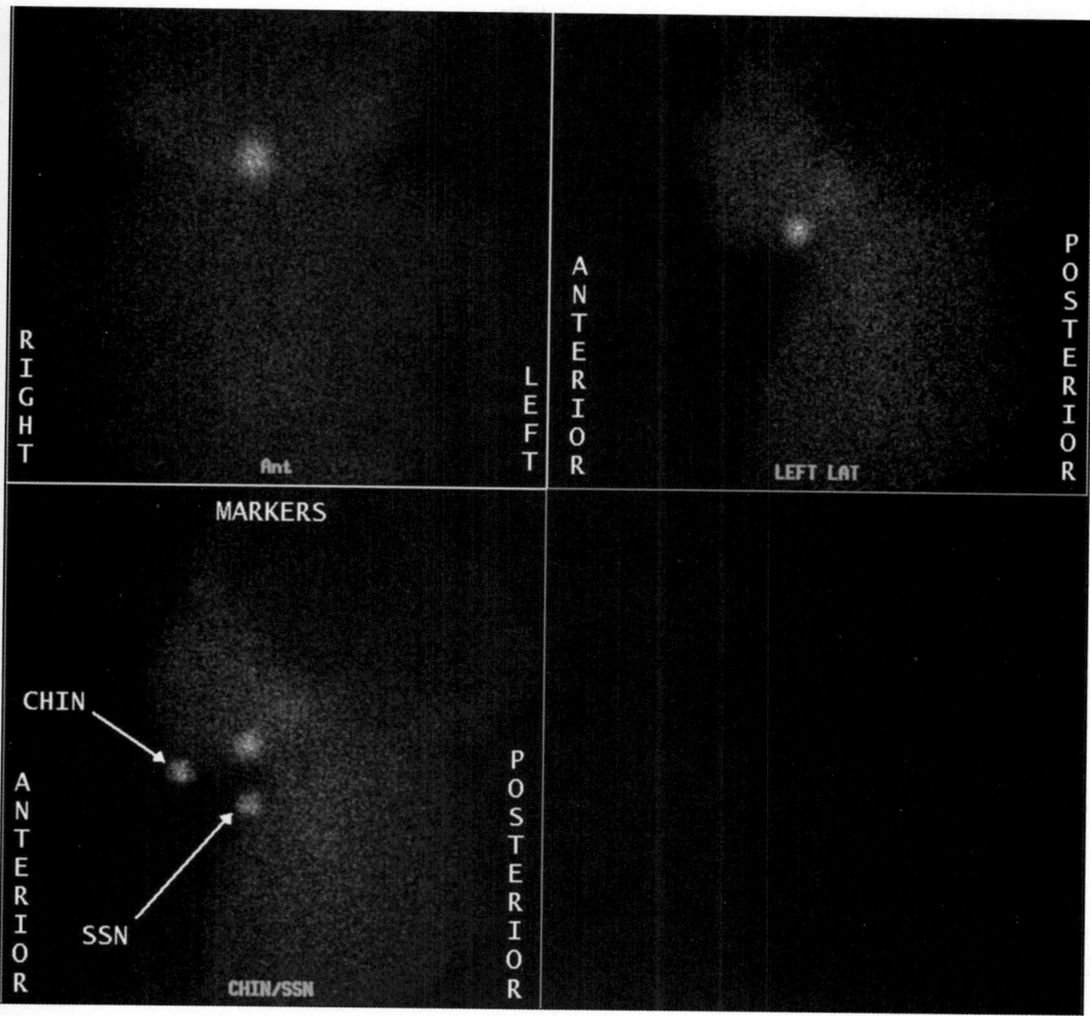

Clinical Presentation

A young child presents with hypothyroidism.

Imaging Findings

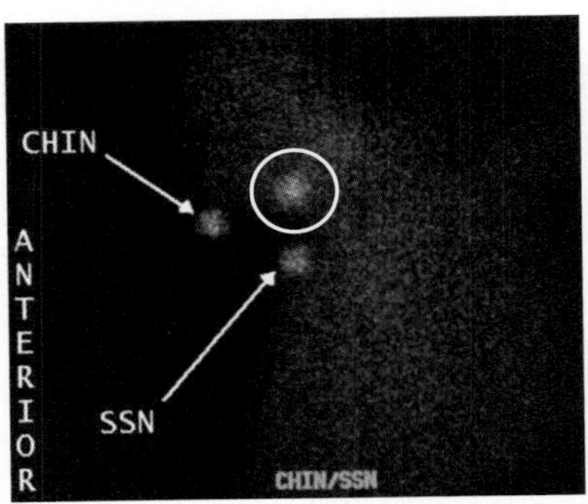

Anterior and lateral views from an iodine 123 scan demonstrate a focus of activity in the region of the tongue base (*circle*) and no activity in the thyroid bed. Markers have been placed on the chin (*CHIN*) and suprasternal notch (*SSN*).

Differential Diagnosis

- ***Lingual thyroid:*** A focus at the tongue base with lack of uptake in the expected thyroid bed is diagnostic.
- *Hyperfunctioning thyroid adenoma:* This can also appear as a solitary focus with nonvisualization of the remainder of the (suppressed) gland, but it is located in the thyroid bed and typically in clinically euthyroid or hyperthyroid adults (see Case 23).
- *Ectopic goiter:* Although it can extend superiorly, it more commonly extends to the mediastinum and is rarely this focal (see subsequent images from another patient). This is typically seen in euthyroid adults.

Essential Facts

- Lingual thyroid is caused by failure of descent of the embryologic thyroid anlage from the posterior tongue.
- Usually diagnosed in children, significantly more commonly in girls
- Patients are often hypothyroid as the gland may function poorly.
- Patients may be asymptomatic when the mass is small but can present with obstruction to breathing or swallowing with larger lesions, which can exceed 4 cm.
- Treatment options for the mass effect include I131 ablation, gland suppression with thyroid hormone administration, and surgical resection ± reimplantation.

Other Imaging Findings

- I123 is the radionuclide of choice given its high specificity and high target-to-background ratio. However, pertechnetate imaging can also be used. I131 is a less commonly used option.
- Unenhanced CT can be very suggestive, given the higher attenuation of this iodine-rich structure. Neck US may also be used.
- I123 can be useful for evaluating for other ectopic tissue, such as mediastinal or cervical goiter or struma ovarii. Here are images from another patient. CT shows a partially calcified mediastinal mass (*circle*). I123 scan shows it to be functioning thyroidal tissue in a substernal goiter. (Markers on suprasternal notch and xiphoid process.)

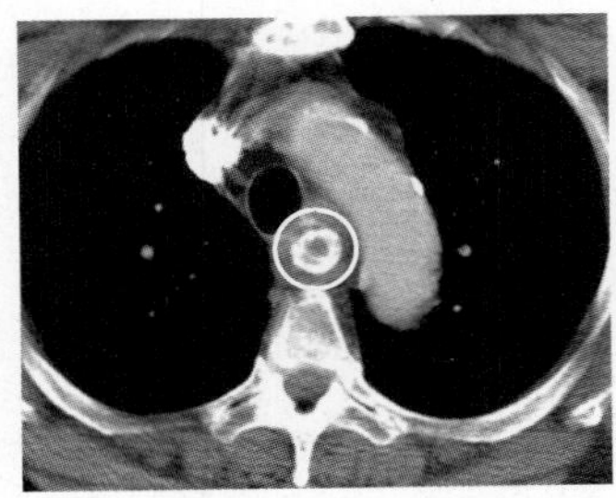

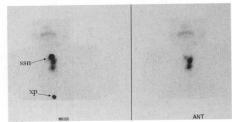

✓ Pearls & ✗ Pitfalls

- ✓ Thyroid scintigraphy can be useful to survey for other functioning thyroidal tissue before surgical excision of a lingual thyroid (most such patients do *not* have additional thyroid tissue in the thyroid bed or elsewhere).
- ✓ Other, less common locations for thyroid embryologic ectopy (< 10%) include the submandibular glands, trachea, and cervical lymph nodes.
- ✓ Parathyroid tissue is uncommonly present in a lingual thyroid.
- ✓ Thyroid carcinoma can rarely originate from a lingual thyroid.
- ✗ Biopsy of a suspected lingual thyroid should be considered with caution, given the risk for hemorrhage and precipitation of thyroid storm.
- ✗ Any disease that can affect the normal thyroid can affect a lingual thyroid.

Case 66

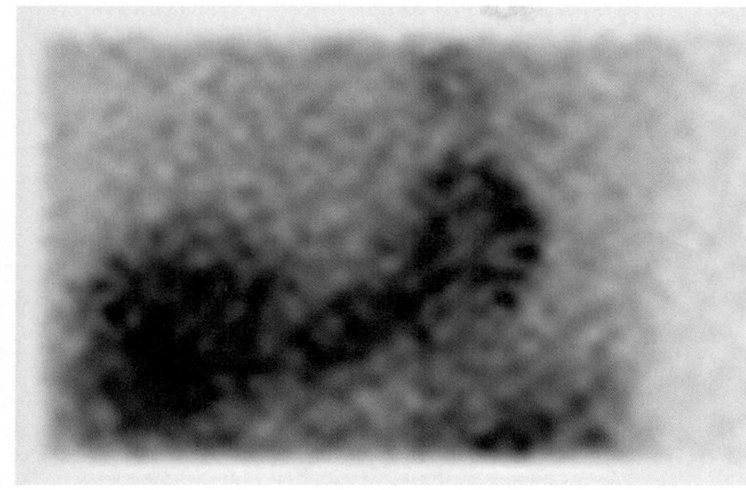

A

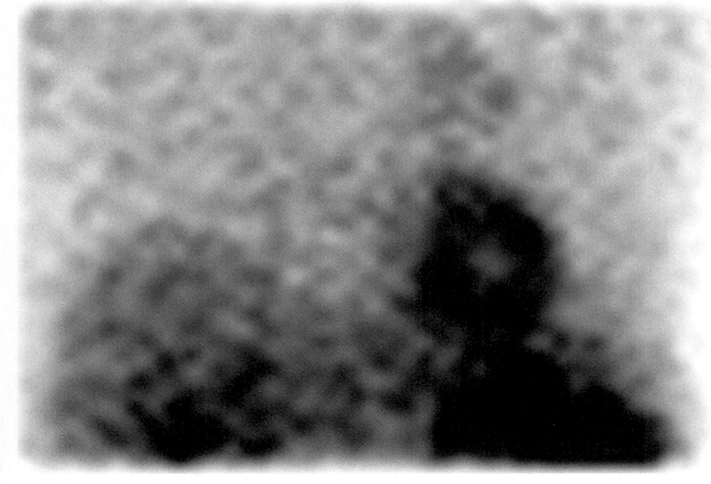

B

Clinical Presentation

A 72-year-old man with chest pain undergoes rest–stress myocardial perfusion scintigraphy.

Imaging Findings

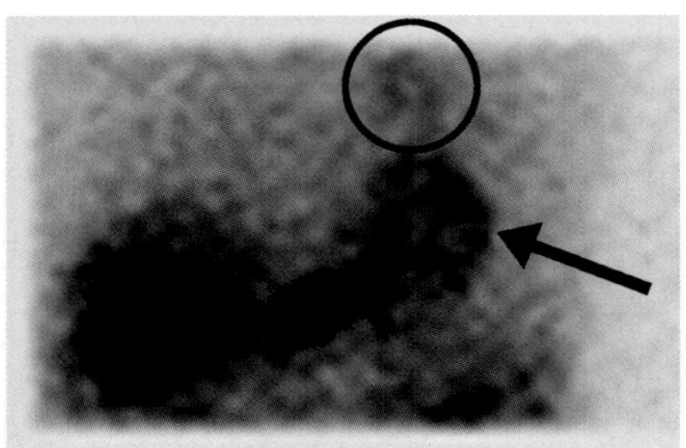
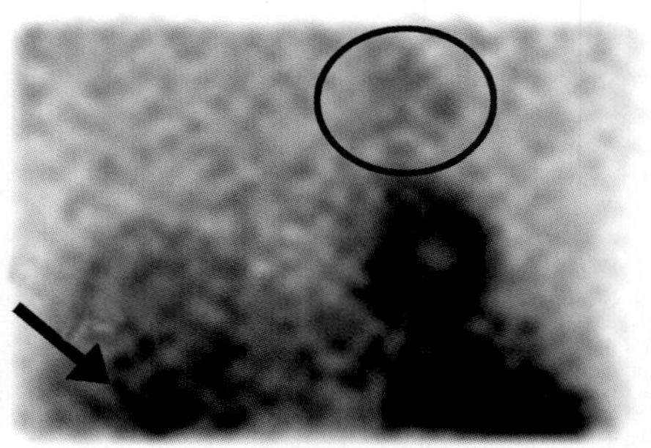

(A) Anterior projection of the raw data from a resting myocardial perfusion scan with thallium 201 demonstrates normal uniform uptake throughout the liver and left ventricular myocardium (*arrow*). However, an abnormal focus of activity is seen more superiorly in the left paramediastinal location (*circle*). **(B)** Anterior projection of the raw data from the stress myocardial perfusion portion with Tc99m-TETRO demonstrates normal uniform uptake throughout the liver and left ventricular myocardium. Also note the normal biliary/gallbladder (GB) excretion (*arrow*) that is seen with TETRO and MIBI, but not with thallium. An abnormal focus of activity is again seen more superiorly in the left paramediastinal location (*circle*).

Differential Diagnosis

- ***Thoracic malignancy:*** Primary or metastatic cancer (including bronchogenic carcinoma and lymphoma) is the diagnosis of exclusion for focal abnormal thoracic uptake on thallium, TETRO, and/or MIBI scan.
- *Pulmonary inflammatory process:* Pneumonia or an inflammatory process such as sarcoidosis can also show avidity for these tracers.
- *Benign mediastinal neoplasm:* An ectopic mediastinal parathyroid adenoma or other benign lesion could also have this appearance. However, malignancy is the diagnosis of exclusion.

Essential Facts

- Myocardial perfusion scintigraphy is commonly performed with thallium, used at rest, and TETRO or MIBI, used at stress and often rest.
- Thallium is a K^+ channel analogue taken up by cells with intact membranes. TETRO and MIBI bind to mitochondria.
- In addition to imaging myocardial perfusion, these three tracers are also nonspecific markers of infection/inflammation/neoplasm.
- When these studies are interpreted, the raw data should be surveyed, and any abnormal focus in the field of view (i.e., thorax, breasts, and upper abdomen) should be further investigated.
- Lung cancer, lymphoma, and breast cancer are some of the more commonly encountered incidental lesions.
- Similar incidental lesions can be seen on a parathyroid scan, which uses the same tracers.
- Some pathologic processes may be hot on thallium only and some on TETRO/MIBI only, whereas some will be hot on both (and some on neither).

Other Imaging Findings

- Chest radiography or CT of the chest or abdomen is typically the next step for further evaluation of a suspicious lesion. Mammography can be performed for breast lesions. Here is this patient's chest CT demonstrating the incidental lung carcinoma (*circle*):

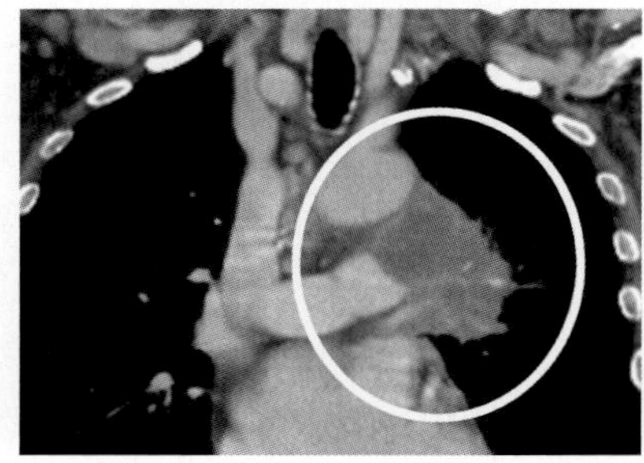

✓ Pearls & × Pitfalls

✓ MIBI and TETRO are very similar tracers and can be thought of as interchangeable for most practical purposes.

✓ With myocardial perfusion scintigraphy, source images should be first inspected to assess for patient motion and potential attenuation artifacts (like breast), and for a broad overview of the cardiac appearance (chamber sizes, wall thickness, gross perfusion defects).

✓ Other extracardiac findings that can be seen on the raw images include abnormal fluid (pericardial, pleural, abdominal—all cold defects) and biliary findings like GB filling (possible with TETRO/MIBI).

Case 67

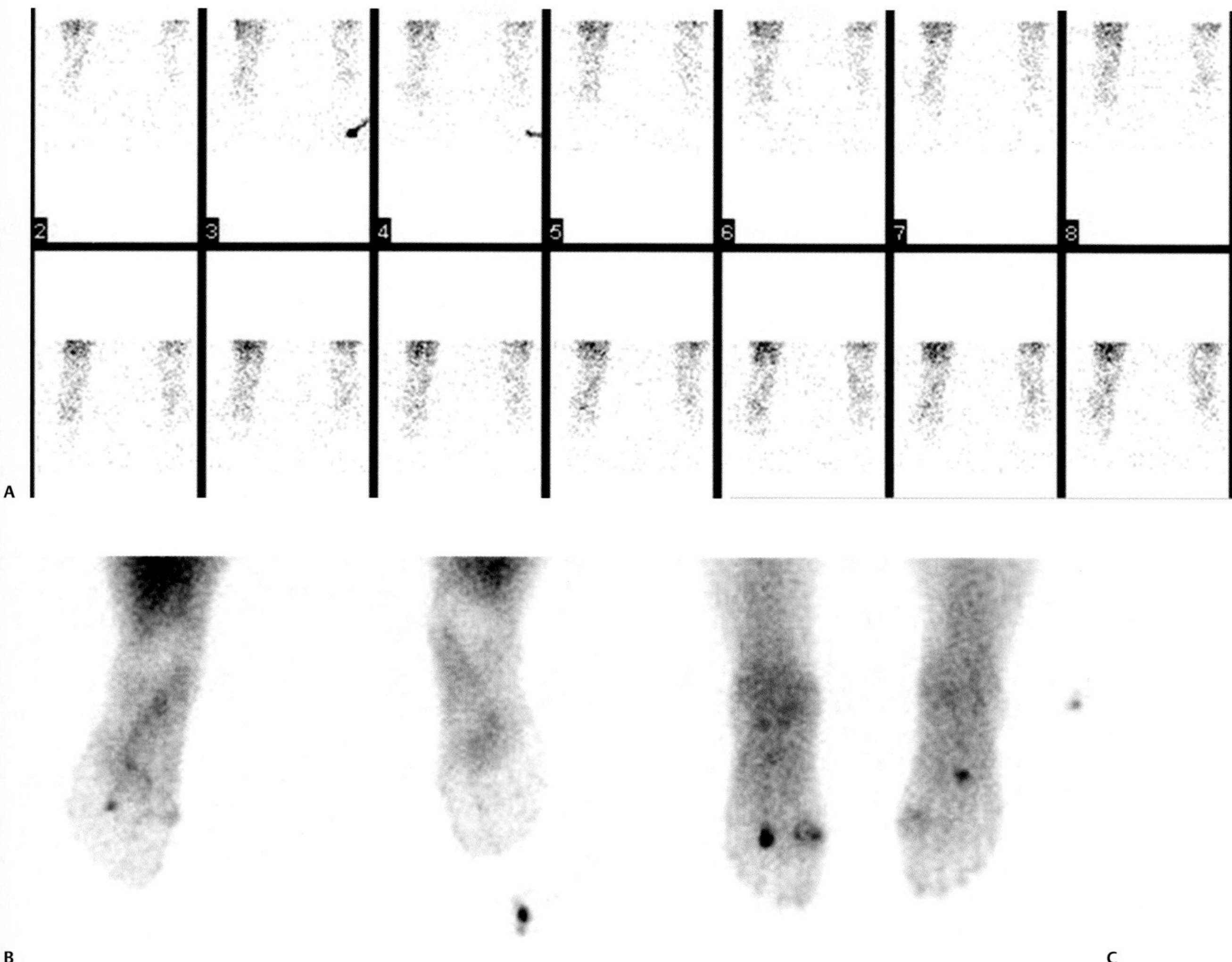

A

B

C

Clinical Presentation

A 72-year-old woman with a history of diabetes and a nonhealing wound in the plantar aspect of the left foot.

Imaging Findings

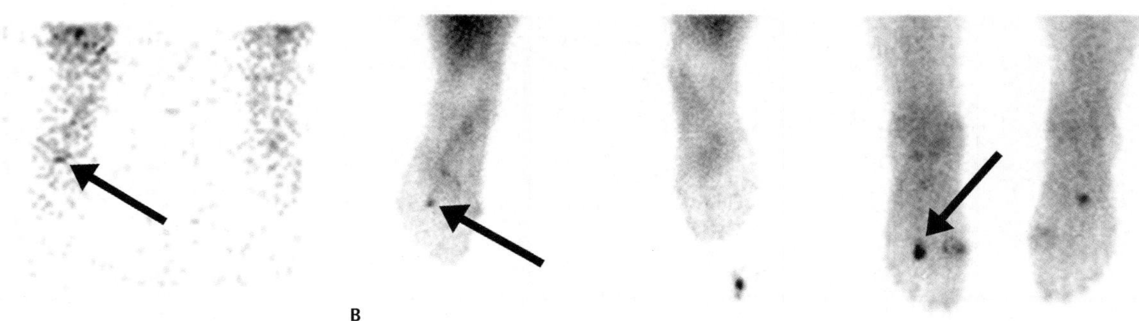

(A) Plantar flow images reveal mild, diffuse increase in activity involving the left foot. Slightly increased focal activity is seen in the region of the third metatarsal (*arrow*). **(B)** Plantar blood pool images reveal focal increase in activity in the region of the left third metatarsal (*arrow*). **(C)** Plantar delayed images reveal intense focal uptake at the left third distal metatarsal (*arrow*). Less pronounced uptake is seen at the left first metatarsophalangeal joint and in the right midfoot (regions where uptake was not significantly increased on the earlier phases and where it is likely related to degenerative changes).

Differential Diagnosis

A three-phase positive bone scan can be seen with fracture (stress or completed), infection, or even tumor.

- ***Osteomyelitis:*** Focal three-phase positive uptake is the diagnosis of exclusion, given the history.
- *Neuropathic joint/fracture:* This can also be positive on three-phase bone scan and cannot be differentiated by bone scan alone.
- *Cellulitis:* This will be hot on blood flow and blood pool, but with no significant uptake on delayed imaging.

Essential Facts

- Osteomyelitis most commonly affects children or immunocompromised adults.
- *Staphylococcus aureus* is the most common organism.
- Can result from hematogenous or regional spread (e.g., from adjacent cellulitis or hardware)
- The long bones (especially in children), spine, and pelvis are the most commonly affected; diabetic foot involvement is also common.
- Treatment options include prolonged intravenous antibiotics and debridement, with amputation for severe cases.
- Although a three-phase positive bone scan is not specific for osteomyelitis, a negative bone scan essentially rules out the diagnosis.
- With therapy, the blood flow and blood pool abnormalities will resolve within 2 months; however, increased delayed activity can persist for 1 to 2 years, especially in weight-bearing bones.
- Gallium 67– and indium 111–WBC scans are better for monitoring response to treatment.

Other Imaging Findings

- Radiographs can reveal osseous destruction and periostitis.
- MRI has sensitivity similar to that of bone scan for evaluating infection but is more specific (e.g., for fracture).

✓ Pearls & × Pitfalls

✓ Cellulitis may present with increased blood flow and blood pool. However, delayed images should not reveal focal activity in bone.

✓ Labeled WBC imaging has similar sensitivity and better specificity for diagnosing acute osteomyelitis.

✓ Dual In111-WBC and Tc99m-bone scan imaging is often the most accurate for diabetic foot evaluation. Cellulitis is hot on WBC only, fracture or neuropathic joint is hot on bone scan only, and osteomyelitis is focally hot on both. (More recently, labeled WBC SPECT/CT can determine if the WBC abnormality localizes to bone, in lieu of an additional bone scan.)

× Bone scan specificity for osteomyelitis is significantly decreased if there has been surgery or hardware placement. (Use WBC/SCOL scintigraphy for painful prosthetic joint evaluation.)

× In diabetics, vascular insufficiency in the lower extremities may delay bone uptake. A fourth-phase image performed at 24 hours may help determine if abnormal uptake is increasing within bone versus soft tissue (better target-to-background ratio).

Case 68

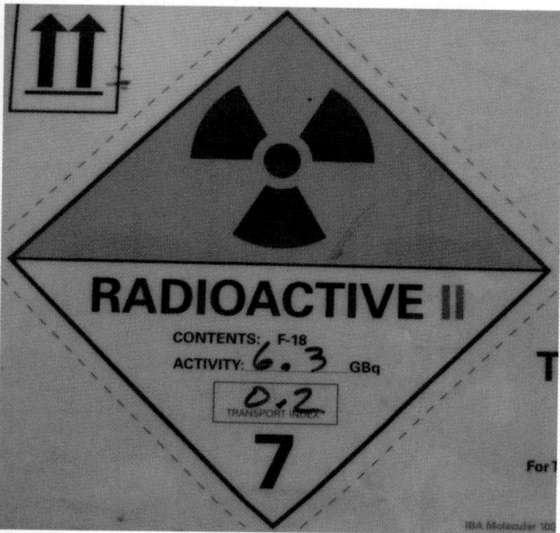
RADIOACTIVE II
CONTENTS: F-18
ACTIVITY: 6.3 GBq
0.2
TRANSPORT
7

Clinical Presentation

A package arrives in the nuclear medicine department marked with a Yellow II radiation label. What needs to be done?

Differential Diagnosis

What needs to be done?

- ***Inspect the package and monitor for external radiation and surface contamination:*** Correct, see subsequent discussion.
- *Lock the package in the hot laboratory and notify the radiation safety officer (RSO):* Incorrect.
- *Immediately open the package and log the contents:* Incorrect.

Packages marked with a radioactive White I, Yellow II, or Yellow III label should be received expeditiously and monitored for external and surface contamination.

Essential Facts

- Radioactive packages must be checked in within 3 hours of delivery during working hours. If the clinic is closed, packages must be checked in within the first 3 hours of the next working day.
- The U.S. Department of Transportation defines radiation levels as follows:
  - White I: $<$ 0.5 mrem/h at package surface and zero at 1 m
  - Yellow II: $<$ 50 mrem/h at surface *and* $<$ 1 mrem/h at 1 m
  - Yellow III: $>$ 50 mrem/h at surface *or* $>$ 1 mrem/h at 1 m
- The delivery company, RSO, and Nuclear Regulatory Commission (NRC) must be notified by telephone if:
  - Activity is $>$ 200 mrem/h (2 mSv/h) at surface or $>$ 10 mrem/h (0.1 mSv/h) at 1 m.
  - Removable surface contamination for γ-/β-emitters is $>$ 22 disintegrations per minute/cm^2.
- Packages containing radioactive gases do not need to be monitored.

Procedure

- Wear gloves to prevent contamination of hands.
- Inspect the package for signs of external damage/leaking. If there is significant damage, stop and notify the RSO.
- Monitor the package for external radiation levels at the surface and at 1 m.
- Monitor the package for external radiation contamination. Wipe 300 cm^2 of the package surface and assay the wipe.
- Remove the packing slip.
- Open the outer packaging and look for any specific instructions by the manufacturer.
- Open the inner packaging and confirm that the contents match the packing slip.
- Inspect the radioactive material container for signs of damage. If there is question of damage, wipe the container and assay for signs of removable contamination.
- Monitor the packaging material for signs of contamination and deface all radioactive labels before discarding.
- Make a record of the package receipt. Records must be maintained for 3 to 5 years (NRC says 3 years; in agreement states, can be longer).

✓ Pearls & ✗ Pitfalls

✓ Radioimmunoassay kits are shipped as White I.
✓ Radiopharmaceuticals are shipped as Yellow II.
✓ Generators are shipped as Yellow III.
✓ Each licensee must have a written procedure for accepting and opening radioactive packages.
✗ If a delivered radioactive package is significantly damaged, the driver should not be allowed to leave, and the RSO should be called to determine if the delivery vehicle requires inspection.
✗ Packages must be surveyed within 3 hours of receipt during business hours or, if received after hours, within the first 3 hours of the next working day.
✗ After business hours, an individual must be designated to receive radioactive packages. Packages should not be left unattended, even in a designated area.

Case 69

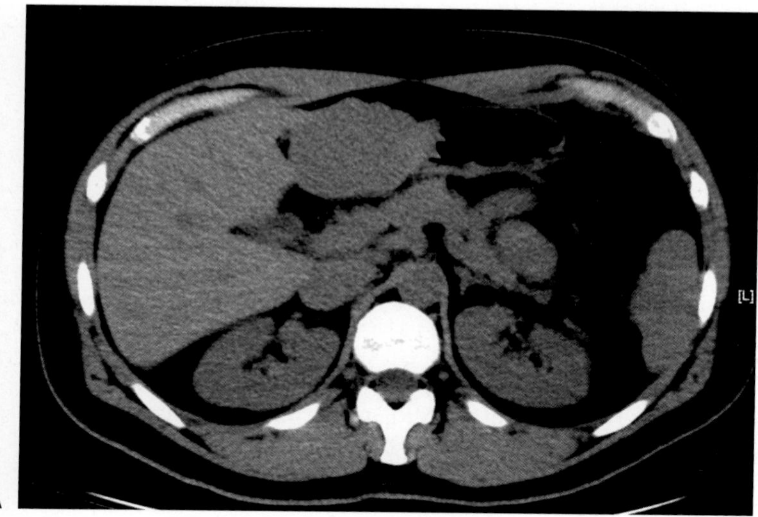

A

Clinical Presentation

A 34-year-old woman with left upper quadrant pain.

Further Work-up

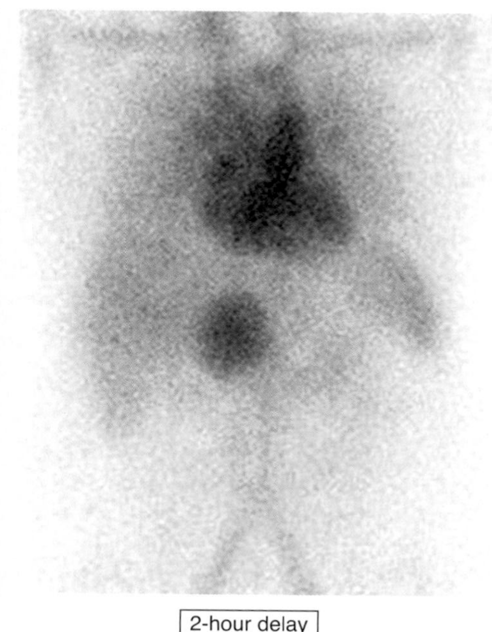

B

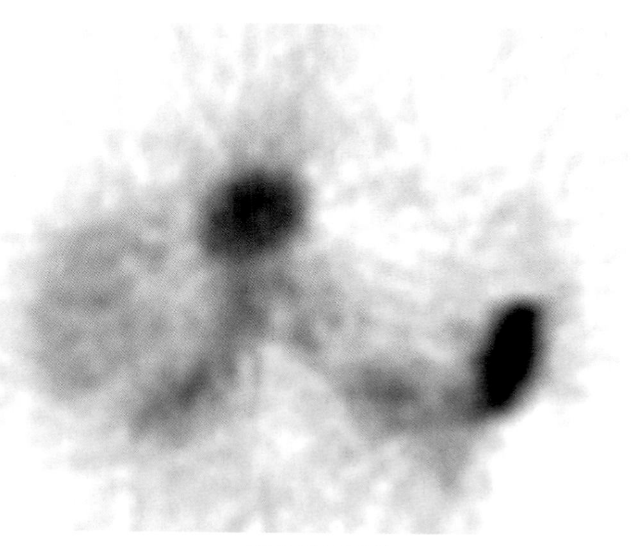

C

Imaging Findings

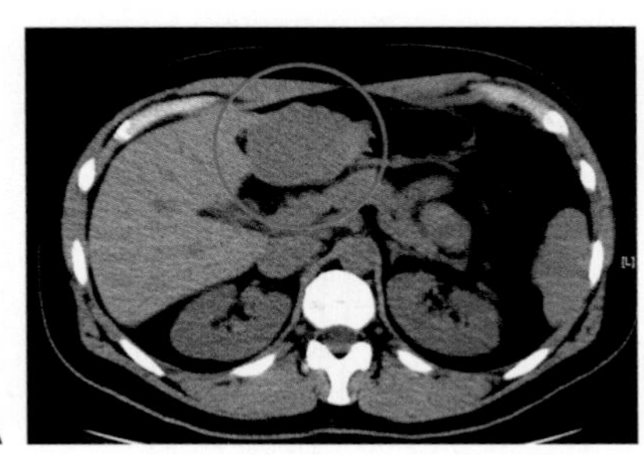
A

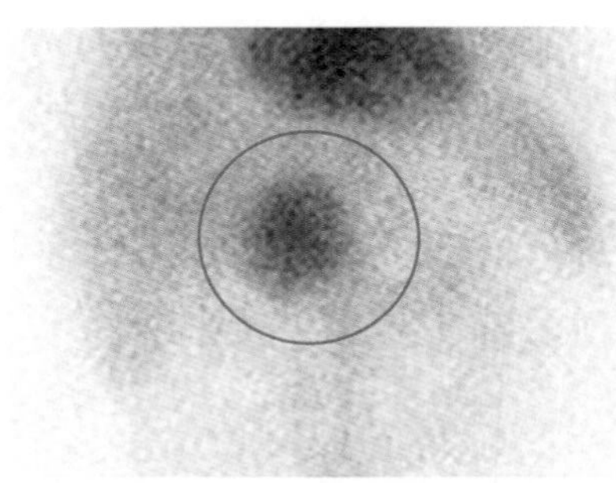
B

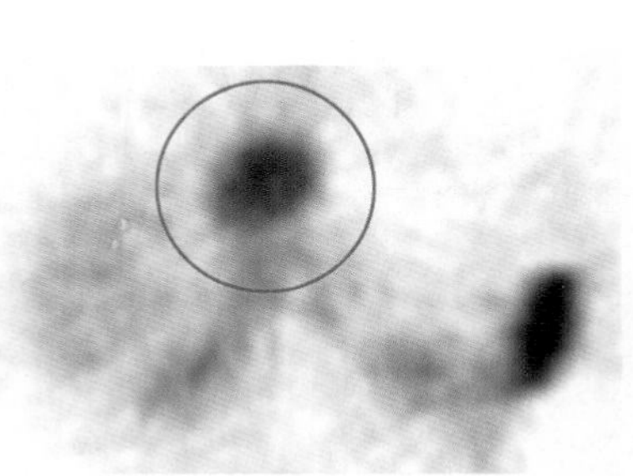
C

(A) Noncontrast CT demonstrates a hypodense mass in the medial segment (segment 3) of the left lobe of the liver (*circle*). **(B,C)** Two-hour–delayed anterior planar and axial SPECT images of the abdomen from a Tc99m-RBC scan demonstrate a corresponding focus of increased activity (*circles*).

Differential Diagnosis

- ***Cavernous hemangioma:*** Focally increased RBC accumulation on delayed blood pool imaging is virtually pathognomonic for this entity.
- *Angiosarcoma:* This can reportedly have the same appearance but is exceedingly rare.
- *Focal nodular hyperplasia:* This is the second most common benign tumor of the liver but is cold on an RBC scan (often hot on SCOL and HIDA).

Essential Facts

- Cavernous hemangiomas are the most common benign liver tumors (and second overall only to hepatic metastatic disease). Estimated prevalence ranges from 0.5 to 20% of the population.
- Hemangiomas arise from the endothelial cells that line the blood vessels. They can be multiple in up to 50% of patients.
- In adults, there is a female-to-male ratio of 5:1. In children, there is no gender predominance.
- They are usually asymptomatic and incidentally found but need to be distinguished from more worrisome lesions.
- They require no therapy.

Other Imaging Findings

- On multiphasic contrast CT, cavernous hemangiomas are hypodense before contrast, show peripheral "puddling" early in the contrast phase, and then eventually fill in by 30 minutes (follows blood pool contrast). Here are the early and delayed CT images from this same patient:

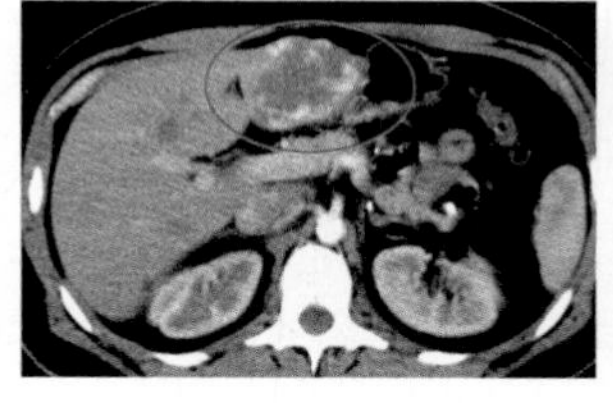

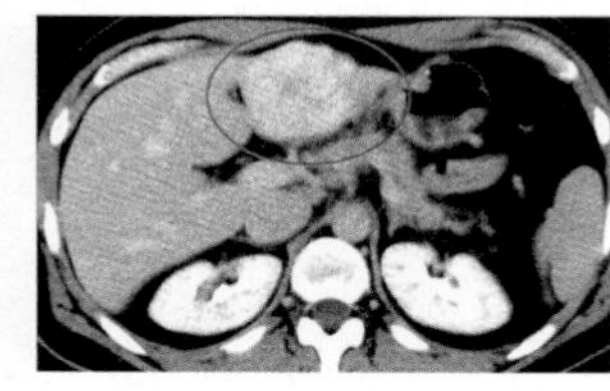

- On noncontrast MRI, hepatic hemangiomas are very bright on T2 ("light bulb" sign). If contrast is given, enhancement features are similar to those on CT.
- On US, these are homogeneously hyperechoic masses. Up to 75% may have posterior acoustic enhancement, but this feature is not specific.
- Hemangiomas are not FDG-avid on PET.

✓ Pearls & × Pitfalls

✓ RBC scintigraphy is the most specific imaging modality for diagnosing hepatic hemangiomas.

✓ Only 1- to 2-hour–delayed imaging (usually planar and SPECT) is required for RBC scintigraphy of a potential hemangioma. Angiographic and immediate blood pool imaging is not necessary (but would usually show no increased blood flow and decreased early pool).

✓ If angiosarcoma is considered a possibility, the angiographic phase can be performed (would be increased).

✓ Do not confuse the early or delayed blood pool phase of RBC imaging for the angiographic phase. On the RBC blood pool phase (early or late), persistent tracer is seen most intensely in blood pool organs: cardiac chambers, larger vessels (arteries *and veins*), diffuse spleen (red pulp), and occasionally the penis (corpora cavernosa).

✓ On angiographic-phase imaging (with labeled RBCs or any other tracer), tracer *moves* down the *arterial* tree.

× Some otherwise hot hemangiomas can be centrally photopenic on RBC scan because of central thrombosis/fibrosis. Do not let this alter the diagnosis.

× Although highly specific, RBC scintigraphy is not highly sensitive for detecting small hemangiomas. A hepatic lesion should be at least 1 to 1.5 cm before attempts are made to characterize it with SPECT (or > 3 cm if only planar imaging is being used).

× If there are multiple hepatic lesions, carefully analyze each individually on RBC scan before determining that they are all benign hemangiomas.

Case 70

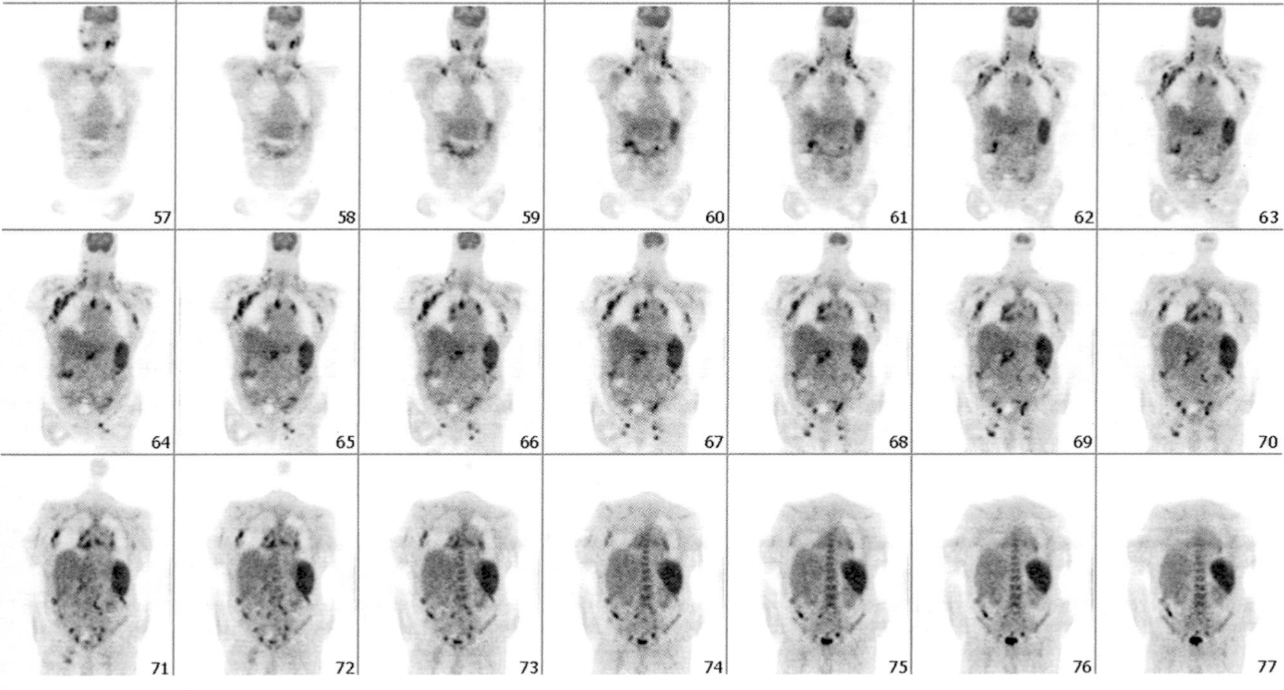

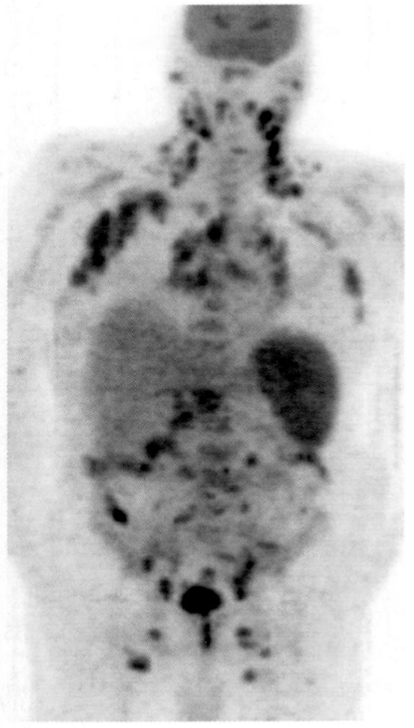

Clinical Presentation

An 84-year-old man with weight loss.

Imaging Findings

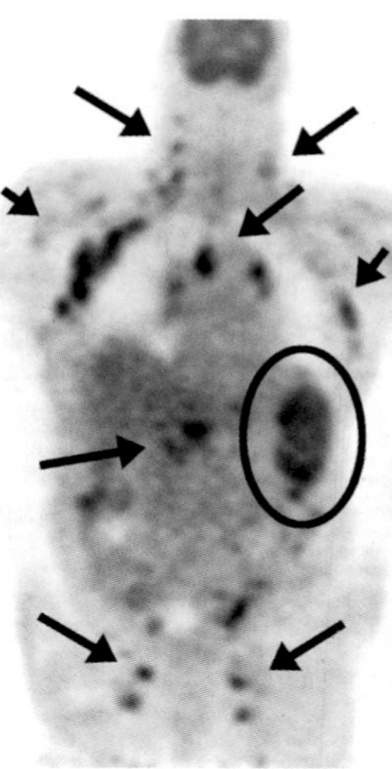

Coronal and anterior MIP images from a whole-body exam demonstrate normal brain gray matter, making this mc likely an FDG-PET. Multiple abnormal foci are seen corresponding to lymph node stations in the neck, chest, abdome and pelvis (*arrows*), as well as diffuse abnormal splenic uptake (*circle*).

Differential Diagnosis

- ***FDG-PET demonstrating lymphoma:*** Widespread symmetric hypermetabolic lymph nodes as well as diffuse splenic involvement make this the most likely etiology.
- *FDG-PET demonstrating sarcoidosis:* This is more commonly confined to the chest but can appear more diffusely and symmetrically, as in this case. It would be a more likely consideration in a younger female.
- *FDG-PET demonstrating diffuse metastatic disease from another primary neoplasm:* This can occasionally be this diffuse, such as with melanoma, but the symmetric involvement and diffuse splenic involvement would be less likely.

Essential Facts

- FDG is a nonspecific neoplasm and infection/inflammation imaging agent similar to gallium (which was previously used to image lymphoma and other tumors).
- Both Hodgkin and non-Hodgkin lymphomas are usually intensely FDG-avid. PET cannot reliably differentiate between lymphoma types. The level of uptake within the lymph node (SUV_{max}) on initial staging exams often corresponds to the aggressiveness of the lymphoma.
- Some low-grade lymphomas have low FDG avidity, including mucosa-associated lymphoid tissue (MALT), small lymphocytic lymphoma, primary cutaneous anaplastic large T-cell lymphoma, and splenic marginal zone lymphoma. FDG-PET will generally not be useful for following these lymphomas.
- For FDG-avid tumors, PET is also a valuable tool to determine response to therapy.
- Typically, follow-up PET scans are performed several weeks after chemotherapy and 2 to 3 months after radiation therapy to most accurately assess the response and to avoid false-positive inflammatory uptake.

Other Imaging Findings

- Diagnostic CT of the neck through pelvis with contrast is used in conjunction with PET for the most accurate (re)staging for both lymph node and splenic evaluation.
- If brain involvement is a concern, FDG-PET is of limited value, given the normal brain (gray matter) distribution Brain MRI is best for this indication.

✓ Pearls & × Pitfalls

✓ Lymphoma should be a consideration for patients with more diffuse involvement of the lymph nodes beyond what is expected from a primary neoplasm (e.g., breas lung primaries with hot pelvic nodes). There is a highe incidence of secondary lymphoma in patients previously treated for another neoplasm.

✓ With lymphoma, it is important to identify which nod stations are involved and if they are on both sides of th diaphragm.

✓ Although focal splenic lesions are usually obvious, diffuse involvement can be subtle. The spleen should not normally be diffusely increased above liver.

× FDG-PET is specific but insensitive for marrow involveme with lymphoma, and bone marrow biopsy may still be indicated despite a negative PET for marrow disease. How ever, if positive, PET can guide marrow biopsy location.

× Once granulocyte colony-stimulating factors (G-CSF) are started, increased FDG uptake can be seen diffusely throughout the bone marrow and spleen, limiting evaluation of these organs. PET should be performed with the patient off these agents (5–7 days for the shorter-acting ones).

× Both G-CSF (splenic) and benign brown fat (particularly supraclavicular) uptake can mimic uptake from lymphoma. Be sure to consider both of these condition and correlate with history and CT.

Case 71

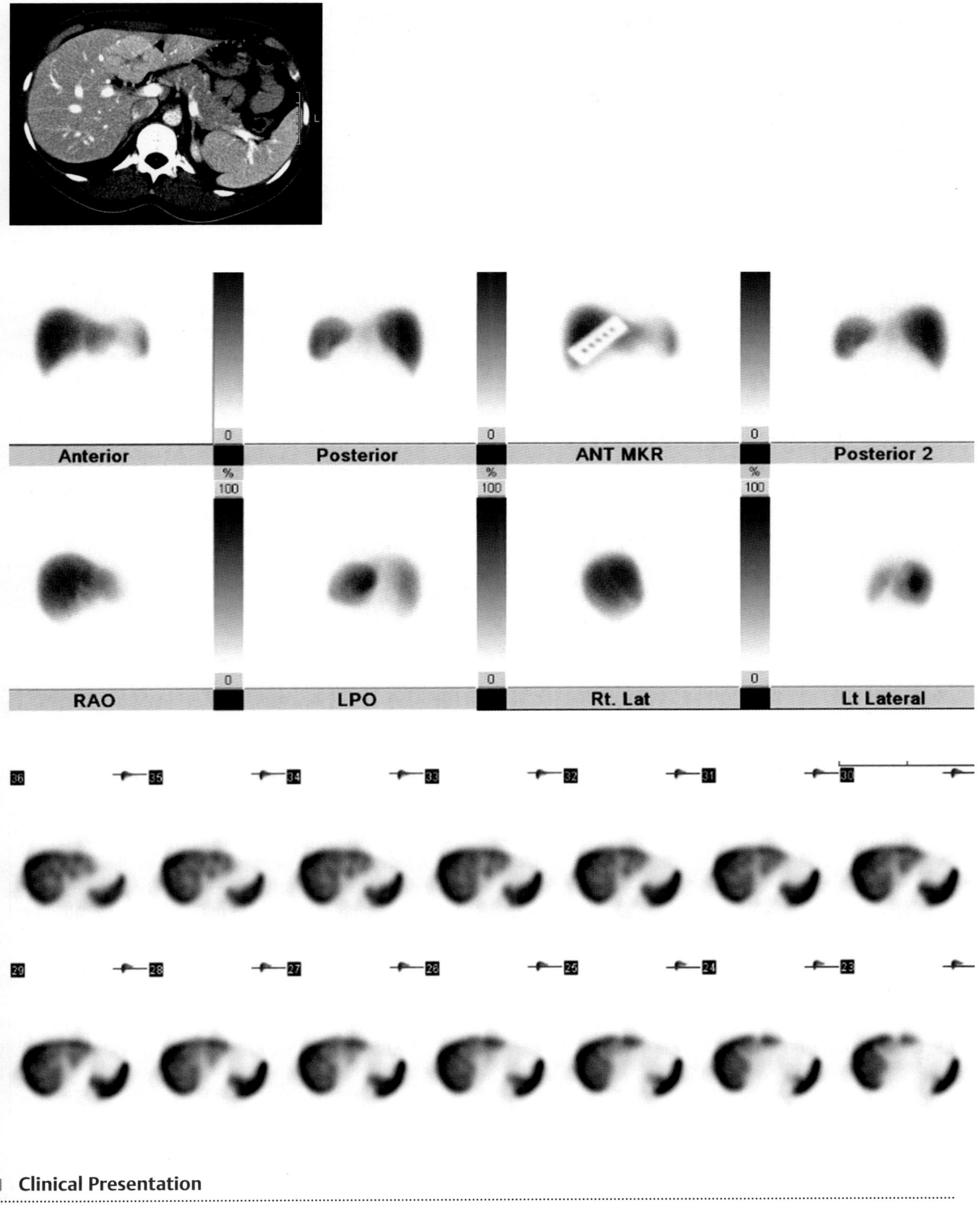

Clinical Presentation

32-year-old woman with a left lobe liver lesion seen on CT, performed to evaluate abdominal pain.

Imaging Findings

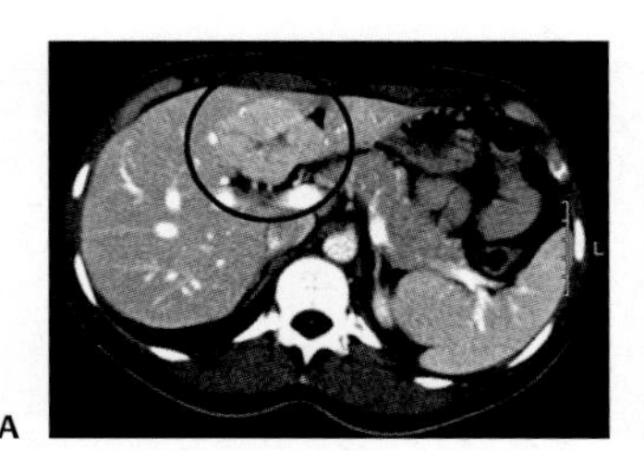

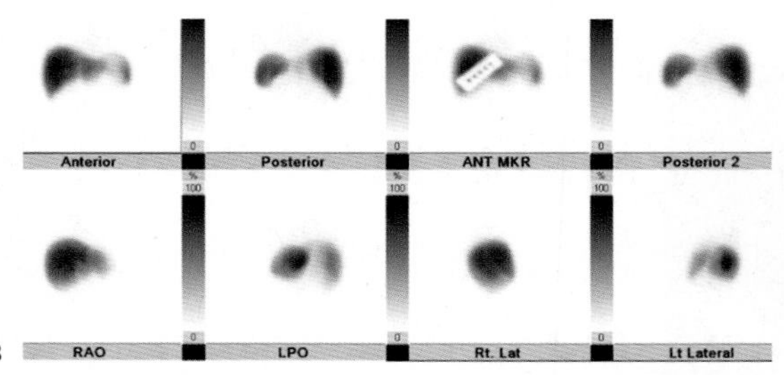

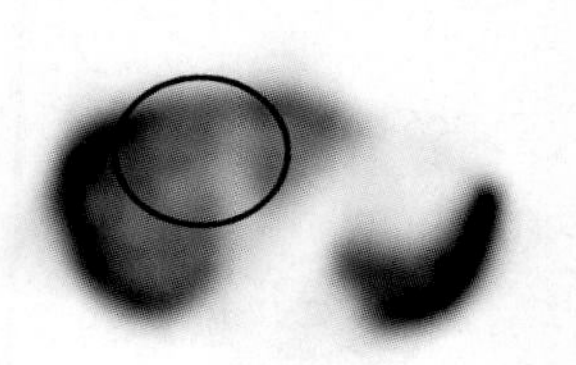

(A) Axial CT image reveals an enhancing mass in the left lobe of the liver with a central scar (*circle*). **(B)** Planar images from a Tc99m-SCOL scan reveal homogeneous tracer uptake in the liver and spleen. No colloid shift is seen. No focal abnormalities are seen in the left lobe of the liver. **(C)** Transverse SPECT images reveal the region corresponding to the CT abnormality has significant Tc99m-SCOL accumulation, similar although slightly less compared to the remainder of the liver (*circle*).

Differential Diagnosis

- ***Focal nodular hyperplasia (FNH):*** This contains Kupffer cells and thus usually demonstrates uptake similar to or greater than that in surrounding liver. In a young, asymptomatic patient, this is the most likely diagnosis.
- *Regenerating nodule:* This also contains Kupffer cells and thus shows normal tracer uptake. It is associated with cirrhosis and would not have a central scar on CT.
- *Hemangioma:* This is a common hepatic lesion and can have a central scar on CT, but it should be cold on SCOL. A tagged RBC study would be the most specific test to confirm this diagnosis.

Essential Facts

- FNH is the second most common benign hepatic mass (after hemangiomas).
- FNH is a congenital hamartomatous lesion containing Kupffer cells, hepatocytes, bile ducts, and blood vessels.
- More than three-quarters are solitary and are most commonly found in the right lobe.
- FNH is usually asymptomatic and found incidentally, requiring no specific therapy.
- SCOL uptake in the liver is due to the presence of Kupffer cells.
- On SCOL scan, FNH can demonstrate uptake similar to that in surrounding liver (60%), increased uptake (10%), or decreased uptake (30%). This is due to the variable number of Kupffer cells in the lesions.

Other Imaging Findings

- HIDA imaging may be helpful to confirm the diagnosis of FNH. Typical imaging characteristics are increased flow, focal uptake, and slow washout. The slow washout is due to abnormal bile ducts in the lesion that do not connect normally with the biliary system. (Note that adenomas and some hepatocellular carcinomas can also be hot on delayed HIDA imaging but will be cold on SCOL.)
- Contrast-enhanced CT or MRI demonstrates enhancement on early phases and washout on delayed phases. A central scar representing an arterial venous malformation may be seen as enhancement on delayed images.
- Angiography and Doppler US can demonstrate the “spoked wheel” arterial pattern.

✓ Pearls & ✗ Pitfalls

- ✓ More than two-thirds of FNH cases are equal or increased on SCOL compared with normal liver, and either appearance makes FNH the most likely etiology.
- ✓ A cold lesion on SCOL is nonspecific and can represent essentially anything, including FNH.
- ✓ Normal or increased SCOL uptake in a hepatic lesion makes tumor (primary or metastatic) very unlikely.
- ✓ SCOL is taken up by the reticuloendothelial system: liver, 85%; spleen, 10%; bone marrow, 5%. Colloid shift increases the splenic and marrow uptake ratios.
- ✗ A hepatic lesion needs to be large enough to be confidently characterized by SCOL (> 1.5 cm on SPECT).
- ✗ Increased regional SCOL uptake of the *quadrate* lobe can be seen with superior vena cava obstruction (with upper extremity tracer injections).
- ✗ Increased regional SCOL uptake of the *caudate* lobe can be seen with hepatic vein thrombosis (Budd–Chiari syndrome) as a consequence of separate and unaffected venous drainage from this lobe directly into the inferior vena cava.
- ✗ Artifactual cold hepatic “defects” can be caused by breast attenuation, a prominent gallbladder, and recent barium studies, particularly on planar SCOL imaging.

Case 72

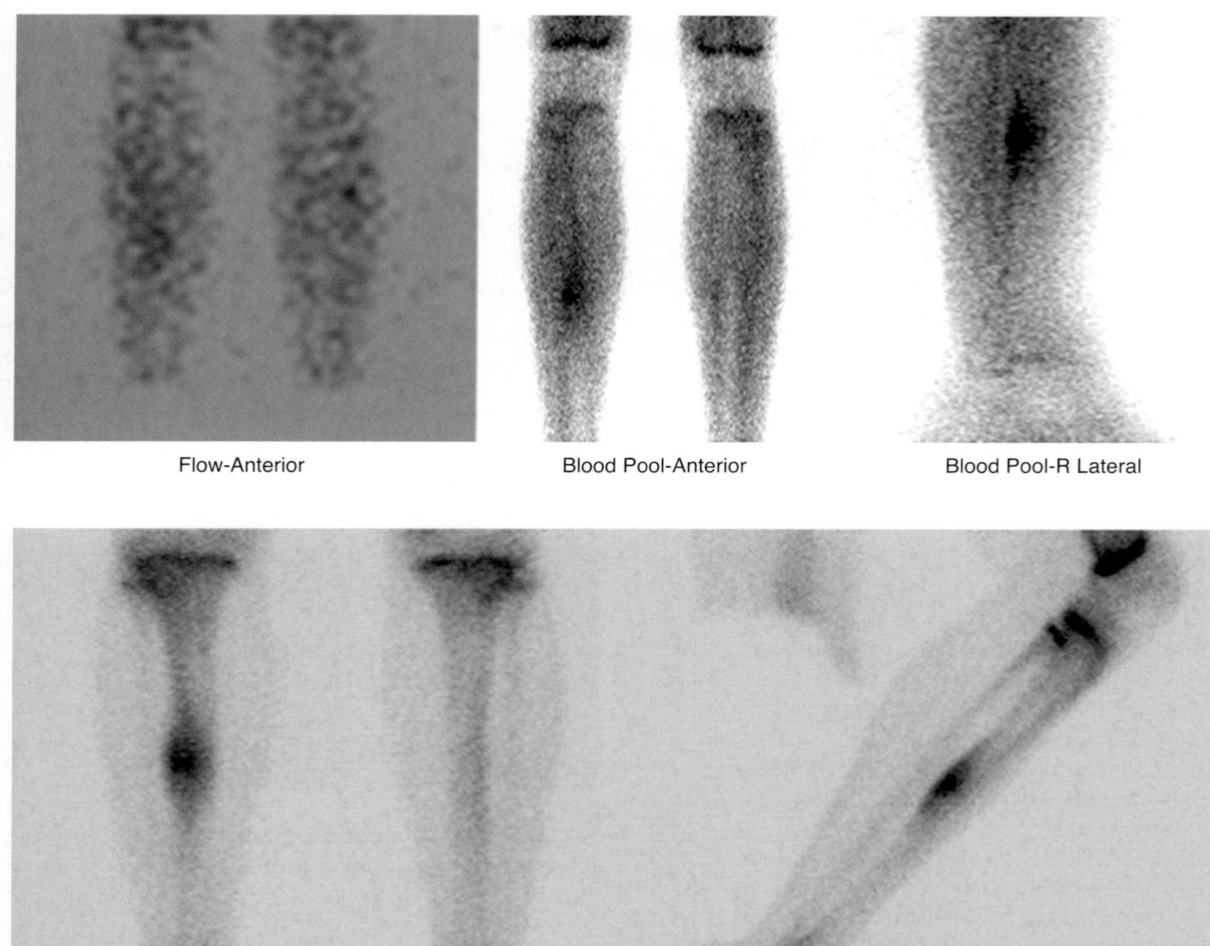

Flow-Anterior

Blood Pool-Anterior

Blood Pool-R Lateral

Delayed-Anterior

Delayed-R Lateral

Clinical Presentation

16-year-old boy with right leg pain that is most pronounced at night.

Imaging Findings

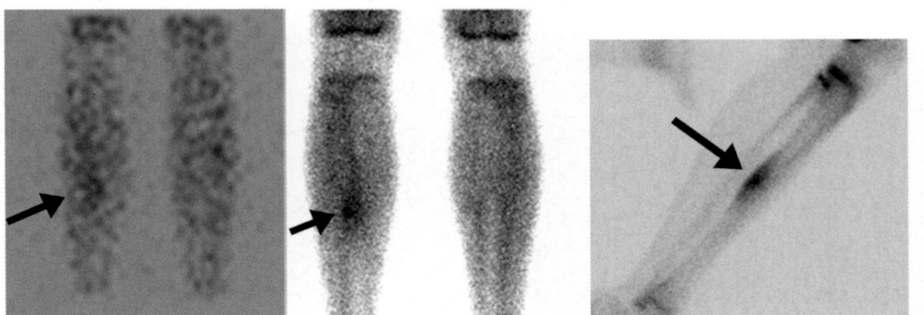

(A) Anterior and right lateral images of the lower extremities from a Tc99m-MDP three-phase bone scan demonstrate focal increase in flow and blood pool activity in the right mid tibia (*arrows*). **(B)** The delayed anterior image reveals fusiform focal uptake in the right mid tibia. The lateral view localizes this uptake to the posterior tibial *cortex*. Centrally, there is a very small focal region of more intense uptake (*arrow*). Increased uptake at multiple physes is seen, which is appropriate for the patient's age.

Differential Diagnosis

- ***Osteoid osteoma:*** Increased uptake is seen on all three phases, and a more prominent focus of cortically based uptake within a surrounding region of less intense uptake is a more specific finding indicating the nidus ("double density" sign). The history also supports this diagnosis.
- *Infection:* This is also positive on three-phase scan and may appear similar to osteoid osteoma on bone scan alone. Osteomyelitis will typically not exhibit a "double density" sign, however.
- *Stress fracture:* This is also cortically based and cannot be reliably differentiated from osteoid osteoma on bone scan alone, but the history in this case is more suggestive of osteoid osteoma.

Essential Facts

- Osteoid osteoma is a benign bone neoplasm occurring in younger patients (> 90% between 5 and 25 years).
- More common in males (4:1)
- Two-thirds of lesions are in appendicular skeleton (femur and tibia most commonly), but any bone may be involved.
- Can present with limping, painful scoliosis (lesions in spine), or growth disturbance (lesions in growth plate).
- Classically more painful at night and relieved by aspirin
- Treatment options include CT-guided percutaneous radiofrequency ablation and surgical curettage.

Other Imaging Findings

- Radiography and CT often demonstrate cortically based sclerosis/thickening. Sometimes, a lucent nidus can be found on CT scan, as in this case (*arrows;* above right). However, a clear nidus may not always be seen:

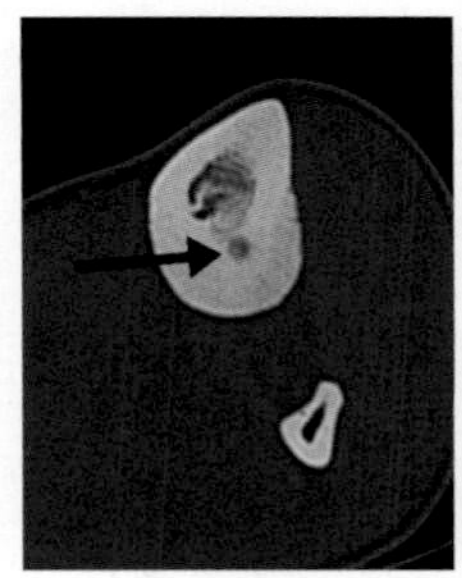

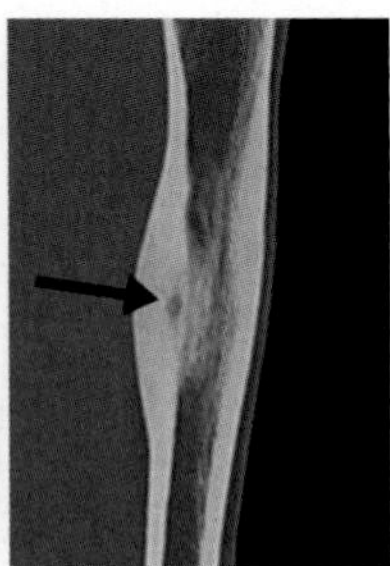

- Osteoid osteomas may be fusiform, as in this case, or demonstrate more punctate rounded uptake, as is common in the spine.

✓ Pearls & × Pitfalls

✓ As demonstrated in this case, lateral views can be very helpful to establish the lesion as based in the cortex, n the medulla, which alters the differential diagnosis.

✓ Benign bone lesions such as nonossifying fibroma and bo islands do not demonstrate increased flow or blood pool.

✓ Bone scan can be used postoperatively or intraoperatively if there is a question about complete resection of the nidu

✓ Osteoblastoma is a very similar entity, only larger (> 2 cm) and often expansile.

× Almost any benign or malignant bone tumor can have three-phase positive uptake on bone scan, including fibrous dysplasia, aneurysmal bone cyst, giant cell tumors, Ewing sarcoma, osteosarcoma, and more vascula metastases.

ase 73

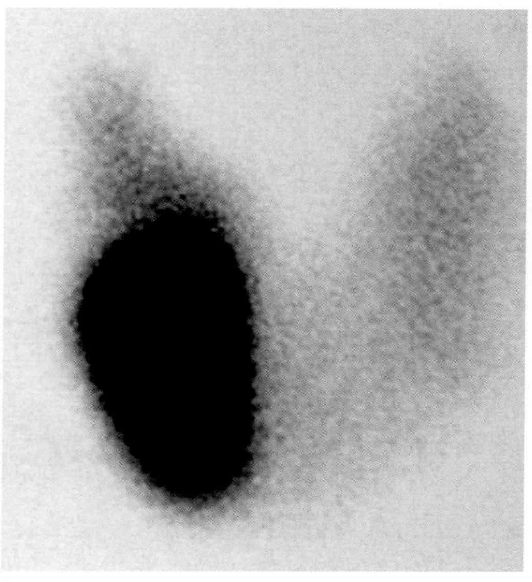

Tc04 pinhole image

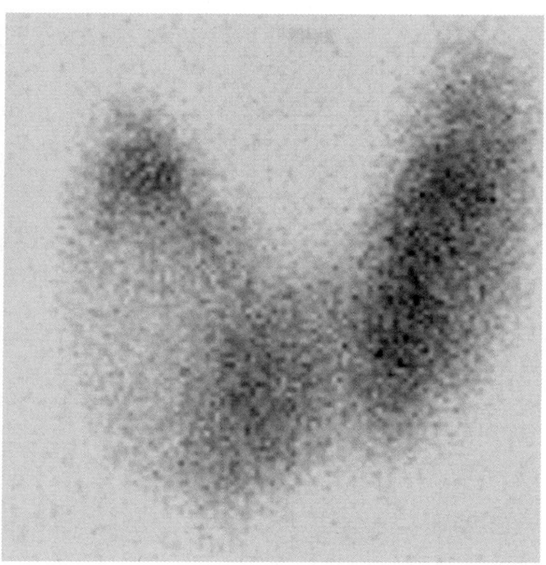

I123

B

Clinical Presentation

56-year-old woman with a palpable right thyroid nodule presents for evaluation. Pertechnetate images were acquired st. Iodine 123 and US images were obtained 2 weeks later.

rther Work-up

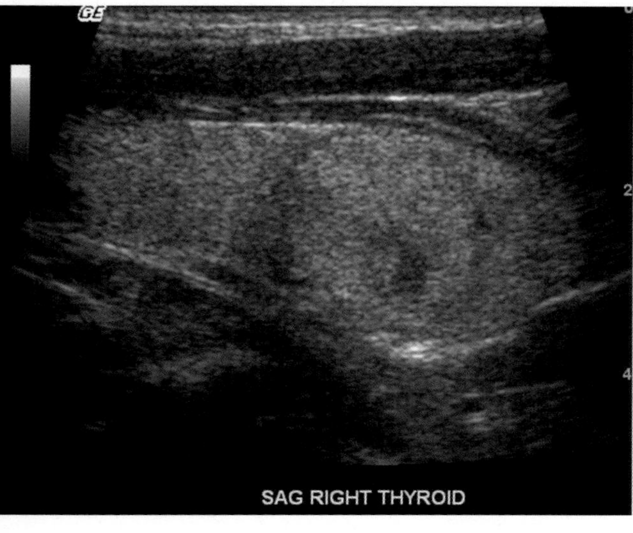

Imaging Findings

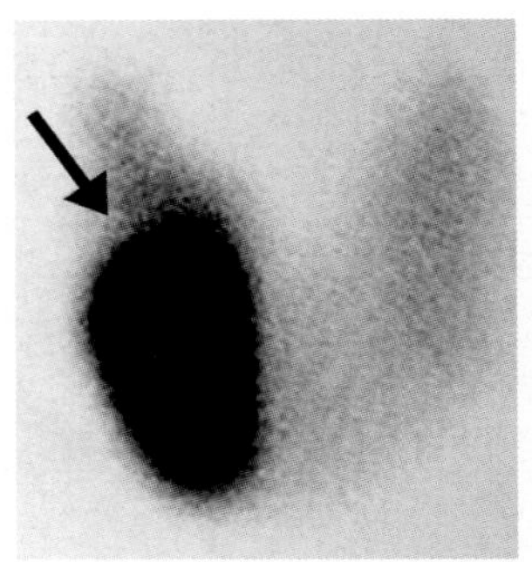

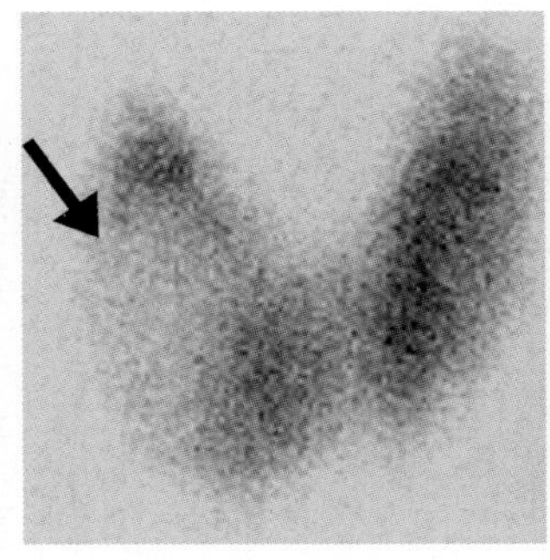

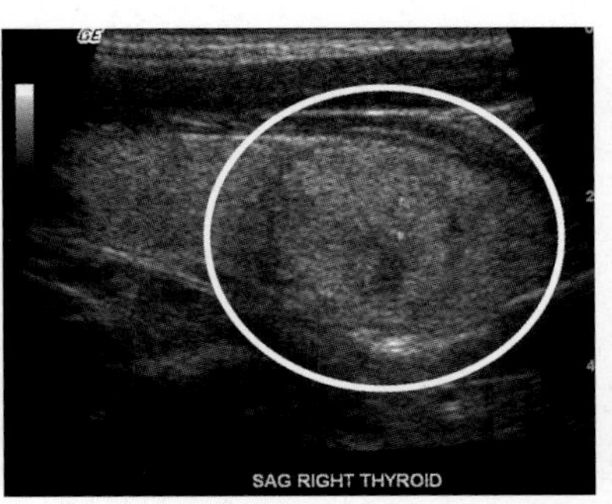

(A) Anterior pinhole image from a pertechnetate (TcO_4) thyroid scan reveals focal increase in radiotracer accumulation in a large right lower pole nodule (*arrow*). Normal homogeneous activity is seen throughout the remainder of the gland. **(B)** Anterior pinhole image from an iodine 123 thyroid scan reveals focal decrease in activity in the right lower pole nodule (*arrow*). Normal homogeneous activity is seen in the remainder of the gland. **(C)** Longitudinal thyroid US image from this patient demonstrates a medium-sized predominantly solid lesion in the right mid region and lower pole (*circle*).

Differential Diagnosis

- ***Discordant nodule indeterminate for malignancy:*** Nodules that accumulate significant TcO_4 but are cold on radioiodine are termed "discordant" and are of some concern for malignancy.
- *Benign colloid nodule:* This is one of the most common etiologies for a cold nodule on iodine scan. However, such nodules cannot be confirmed to be benign based on imaging alone.
- *Benign hyperfunctioning adenoma:* This would appear hot on TcO_4, as in this patient. However, it would also be hot on radioiodine.

Essential Facts

- TcO_4 is trapped by thyroid tissue; iodine is trapped and then organified.
- Dominant thyroid nodules that are cold on TcO_4 *or* on radioiodine scan carry a 15 to 20% risk for malignancy, and biopsy should be strongly considered.
- Nodules that are warm or hot on radioiodine are considered benign and represent (hyper)functioning adenomas.
- A nodule usually appears the same on TcO4 and iodine. However, occasionally a nodule can be warm/hot on TcO_4 but cold on iodine. These are termed "discordant" and carry the same risk for malignancy as any dominant cold nodule (15–20%), and biopsy should be considered.
- The incidence of discordant thyroid nodules is low. Fewer than 5% of nodules hot on TcO_4 are discordant on iodine.

Other Imaging Findings

- Thyroid US can confirm the presence of a nodule and determine if it is cystic, solid, or mixed. If a cold nodule i a completely simple cyst, it is benign. Otherwise, it may be malignant.

✓ Pearls & × Pitfalls

- ✓ TcO_4 is administered intravenously, radioiodine orally.
- ✓ Tracer physiology is not affected by radioactivity. I123, I131, and cold iodine have an identical biodistribution (e.g., salivary glands, thyroid, stomach).
- ✓ Although the potential for discordance exists, TcO_4 scanning is less expensive, requires less patient time, and can provide better images than I123. Different centers use different tracers.
- ✓ Thyroid cancers do not organify to a high degree but can occasionally trap significantly (and hence be discordant).
- ✓ Biopsy should be considered for any dominant nodule(s) that is cold (with either tracer) and > 1.0 cm or growing, unless it is completely cystic by US.
- × A nodule should not be characterized as warm/hot unless it is clearly seen. If a known nodule (e.g., by palpation or US) is not apparent on the scan, it should be categorized as cold and of some risk for malignancy.
- × Nodules < 1 cm are difficult to characterize with scintigraphy.

Case 74

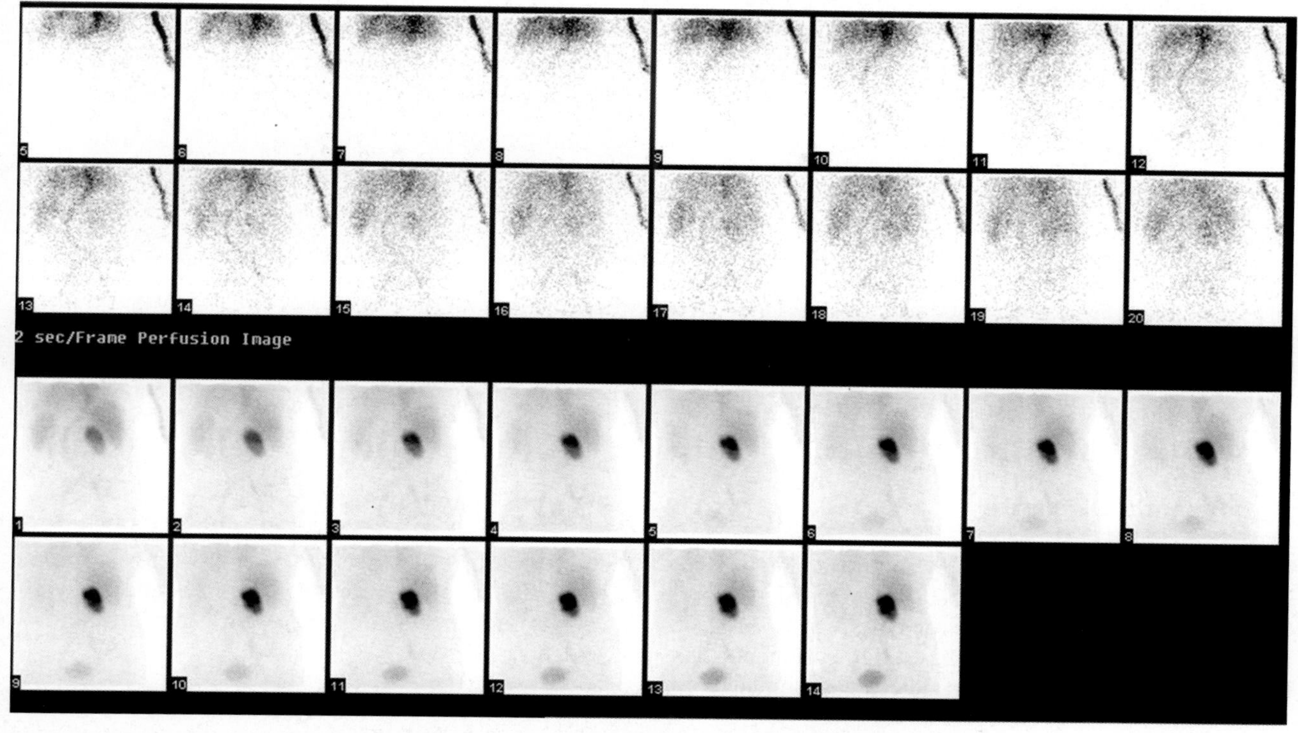

A

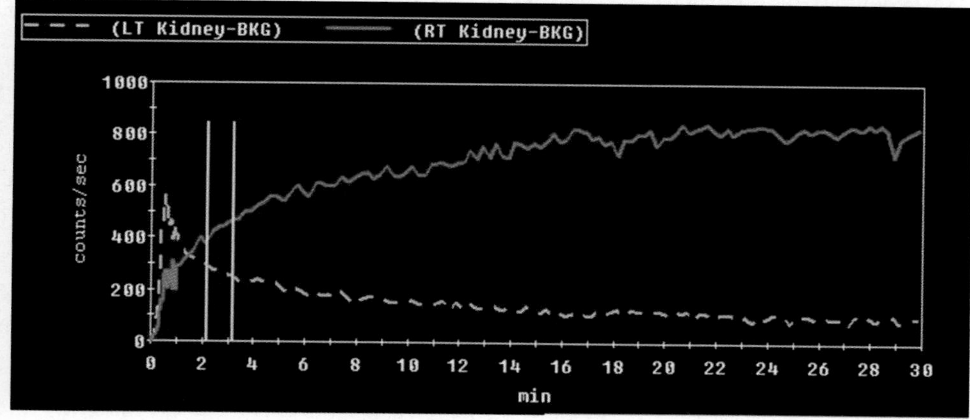

B

Clinical Presentation

A 60-year-old woman with elevated creatinine and oliguria.

Imaging Findings

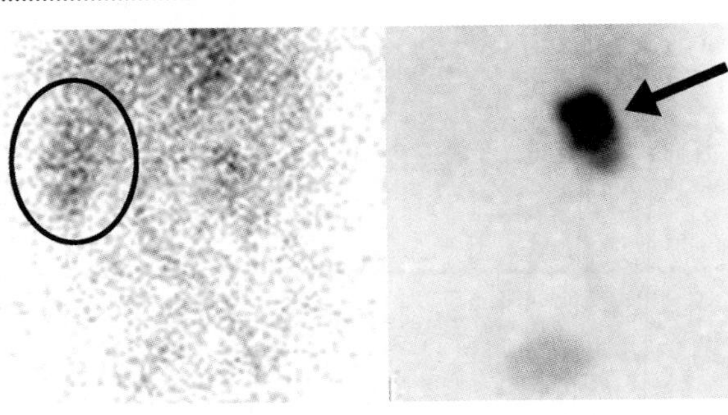

A

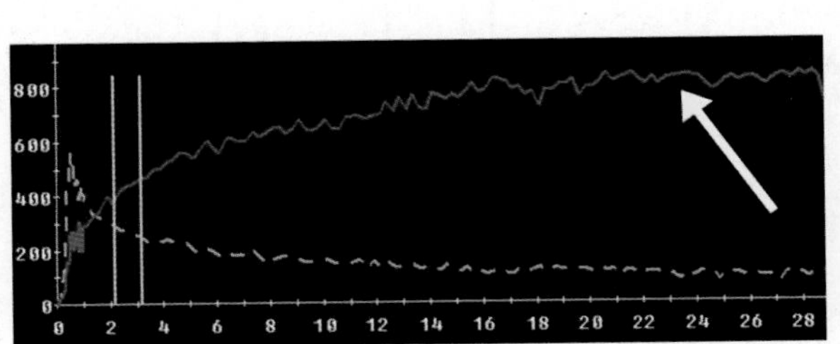

B

(A) Posterior images from a Tc99m-MAG3 renal scan. Flow images reveal decreased tracer activity in the right kidney. There is apparent flow to the left kidney; however, this represents splenic activity (*circle*). The patient had a left nephrectomy. Dynamic images reveal abnormal progressive tracer parenchymal extraction by the right kidney (*arrow*) but only minimal evidence of urinary excretion. **(B)** Curves generated from a region of interest around the entire kidney show a continually rising renogram on the right (*arrow*). The left renal curve appears to demonstrate some function because the technologist erroneously drew a region of interest around the spleen.

Differential Diagnosis

A scan demonstrating normal flow and extraction but delayed excretion indicates renal parenchymal dysfunction and can be seen with acute tubular necrosis (ATN), obstruction, and medical renal disease (glomerulonephritis, diabetic nephropathy). They can all look very similar.

- ***ATN:*** A tubular agent such as MAG3 demonstrates normal flow with normal or delayed extraction but severe cortical retention with minimal excretion into the collecting system.
- *Obstruction:* This can cause renal parenchymal dysfunction and then cannot be differentiated from other causes of renal failure. A large photopenic collecting system may indicate hydronephrosis and suggest this diagnosis.
- *Chronic medical renal disease:* This may have a similar appearance, although typically some radiotracer excretion is seen from the cortex.

Essential Facts

- Ischemia, sepsis, renal toxic drugs, and intravenous contrast are the most common causes of ATN.
- In renal transplant patients, ATN can be differentiated from acute rejection by examining the flow/extraction phase, which is normal in ATN and delayed in rejection.
- ATN will typically regress over time, so serial imaging will show improved cortical excretion.

Other Imaging Findings

- US or CT can evaluate renal size to differentiate chronic renal disease from an acute process. Evidence of hydronephrosis or polycystic disease can lead to an alternative diagnosis.

✓ Pearls & × Pitfalls

✓ The differential diagnosis for renal transplant dysfunction includes ATN, acute rejection, cyclosporine toxicity (less common now because of changes in immunosuppressive therapy), and obstruction.

✓ Renal scintigraphy can be used in differentiating ATN from renal transplant rejection. With rejection, flow will decrease, and serial exams will show worsening function.

✓ After transplant, the timing of renal dysfunction can be useful for distinguishing ATN from acute rejection. ATN typically appears earlier postoperatively.

× Poor hydration can mimic ATN on renal scintigraphy.

× Always verify that regions of interest are correctly placed to avoid errors seen in this case.

Case 75

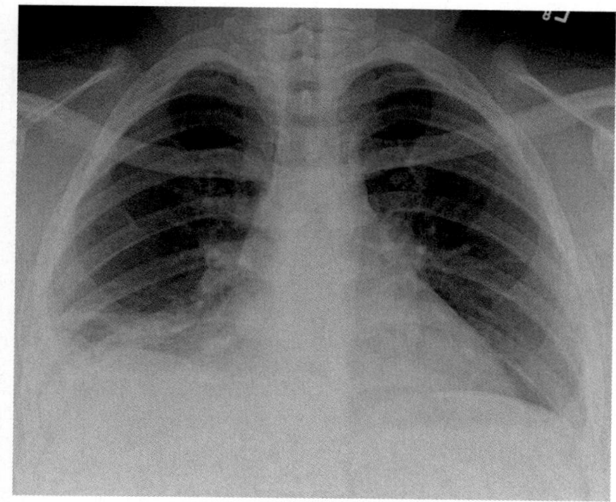

A

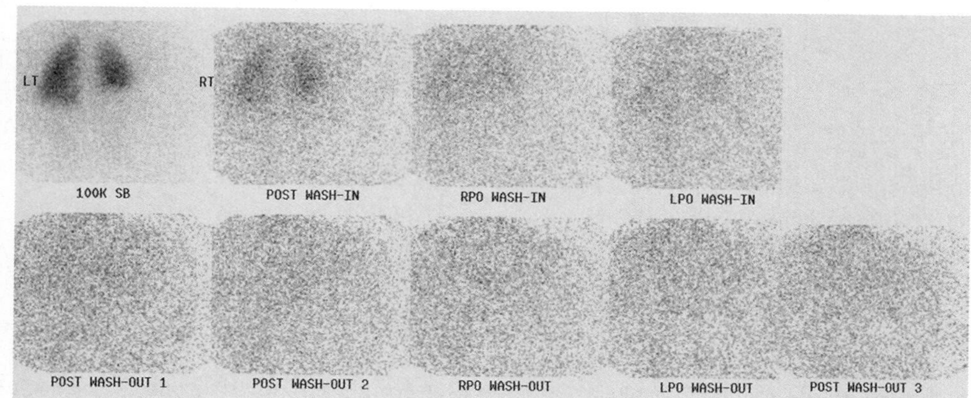

B

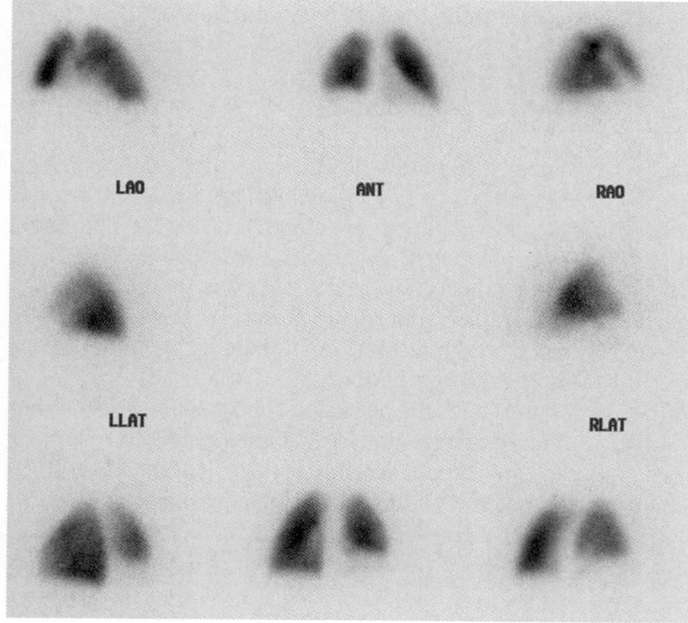

C

Clinical Presentation

A 42-year-old woman with acute shortness of breath.

Imaging Findings

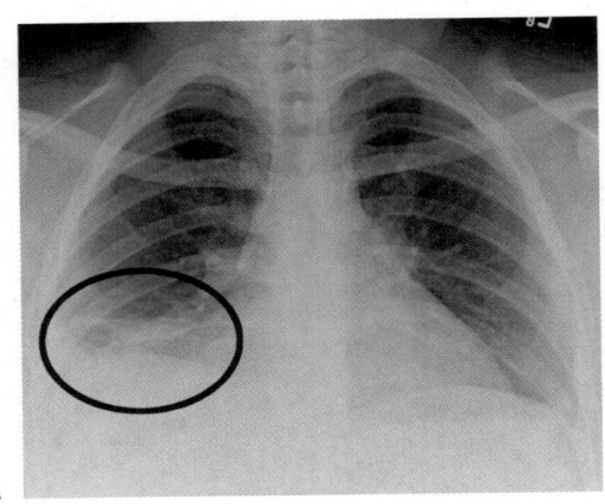

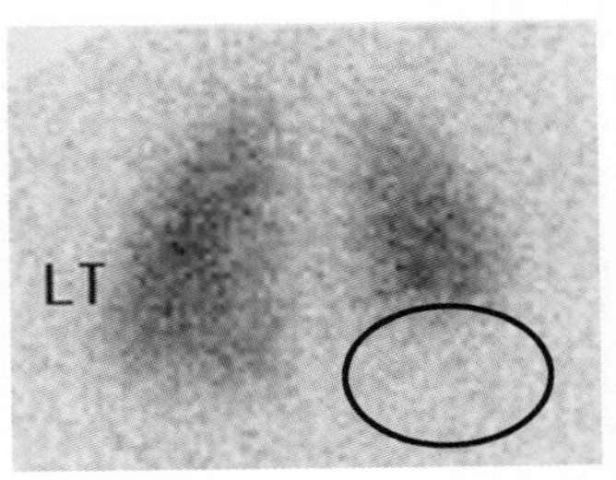

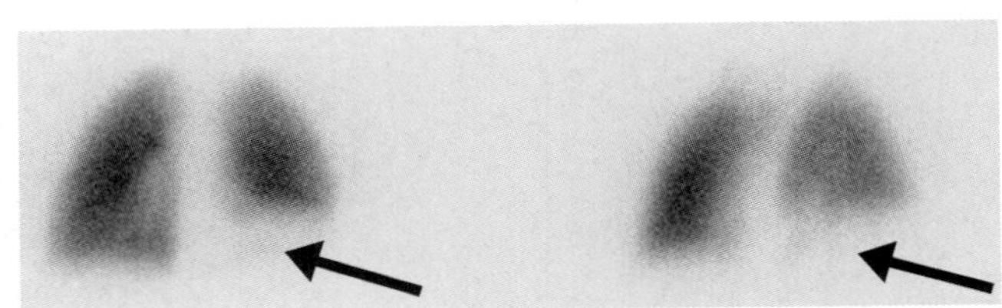

(A) Chest x-ray (CXR) demonstrates a small right pleural effusion and linear subsegmental atelectasis at the right lung base (*circle*). **(B)** Posterior and posterior oblique dynamic xenon 133 ventilation images demonstrate decreased ventilation to the right lung base on single breath (*circle*). No abnormal retention is seen on delayed imaging. **(C)** Multiple views from a Tc99m-MAA perfusion scan demonstrate a single large segmental perfusion defect in the posterior basal right lower lobe (*arrows*) that is matched to the ventilation and radiographic abnormalities (and is larger than the radiographic abnormality).

Differential Diagnosis

- ***Intermediate probability for pulmonary embolism (PE) with evidence of pulmonary infarction:*** A single moderate or large segmental perfusion defect in the lower lobe, with corresponding ventilation and CXR abnormalities, is PIOPED intermediate for PE, as it represents a "triple match" in the lower lung. The CXR findings would suggest pulmonary infarction in this setting.
- *Aspiration/pneumonia:* This would have similar findings on all three studies. However, the perfusion defect is more commonly the same size or smaller than the radiographic abnormality.
- *Lung cancer:* No mass is seen in this patient, although postobstructive effect from an occult central lesion would look similar. Cancer is less likely given the history, however.

Essential Facts

- Most PEs demonstrate perfusion defects with normal ventilation (mismatched). CXR is usually normal or nearly normal.
- Most perfusion defects are matched and due to reflex vasoconstriction from airway disease. These are usually classified as low probability (with normal CXR).
- Most PEs do not cause pulmonary infarcts, given the dual blood supply (bronchial arteries from aorta).
- Occasionally, PEs do cause pulmonary ischemia or infarction that results in effusion and air space disease (focal edema, atelectasis, or hemorrhage). This results in a "triple match" of corresponding abnormalities on CXR, ventilation (V) scan, and perfusion (Q) scan.
- By PIOPED, a single moderate or large triple match *in the lower third of the lung* is intermediate probability; in the upper two-thirds, it is very low probability.

Other Imaging Findings

- CTA, MRA, or catheter angiography can be performed to confirm PE.
- A sonographic deep vein thrombosis study can be useful in the setting of intermediate-probability VQ scans to help determine the likelihood of PE.

✓ Pearls & ✗ Pitfalls

✓ The most common intermediate-probability feature on VQ scan is 1 to 3 moderately sized (25–75% of segment) *mismatched* perfusion defects (1 large = 2 moderate).

✓ For triple match, a ventilation abnormality is actually superfluous; a lower lung perfusion defect matching a radiographic abnormality is enough to yield a "triple match" and intermediate probability, regardless of the findings on ventilation.

✗ With true PE, the perfusion abnormality should be *larger* than a corresponding CXR abnormality (the anatomic radiographic abnormality is the "tip of the iceberg" compared with the underlying physiologic perfusion defect). A defect on perfusion scan that is smaller than a CXR defect is very low probability for PE.

Case 76

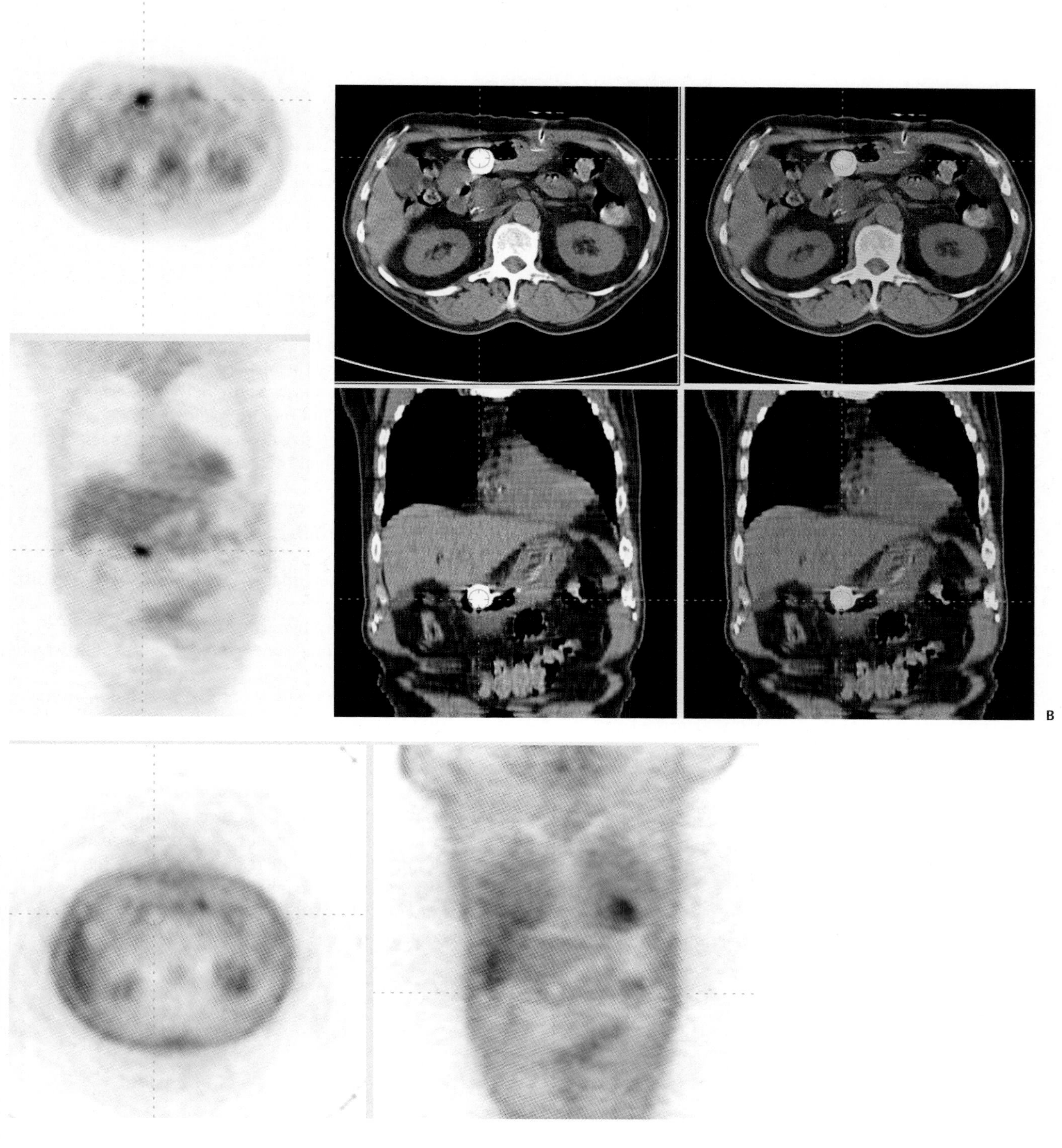

Clinical Presentation

A patient presents for head and neck carcinoma restaging.

Imaging Findings

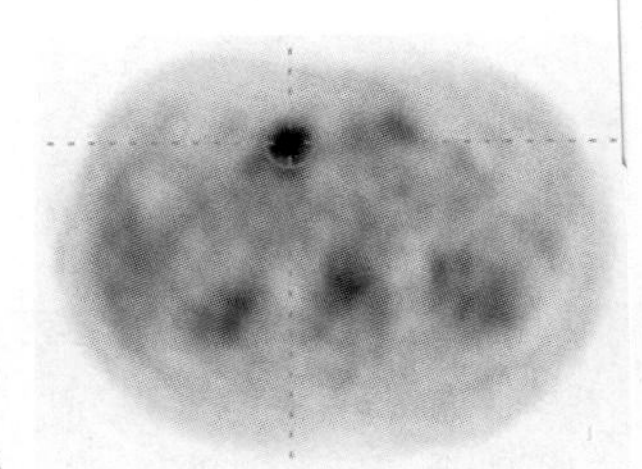

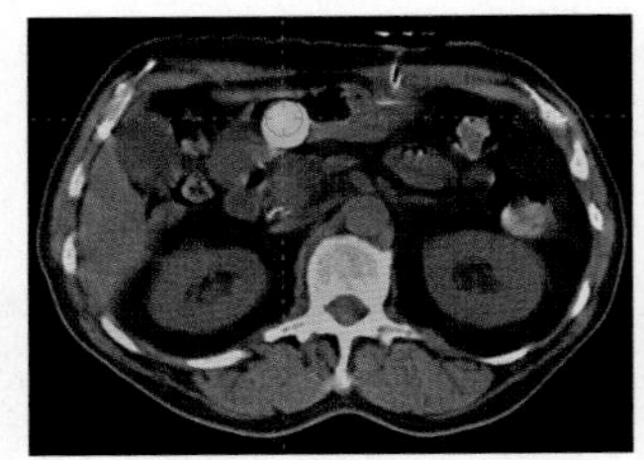

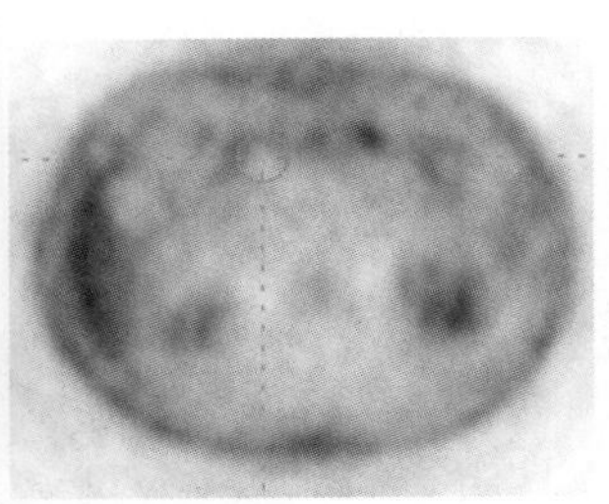

(A,B) Hybrid FDG-PET/CT imaging demonstrates a focal marked increase in radiotracer accumulation in the anterior abdomen (*crosshairs*). On CT, this corresponds to a contrast-filled gastrostomy catheter balloon. **(C)** PET emission image without attenuation correction demonstrates absent radiotracer accumulation in this same location.

Differential Diagnosis

- ***Artifact of attenuation correction (AC):*** The lack of activity on the noncorrected images proves that this is an example artifactual "pseudo-uptake" of FDG.
- *Metastasis to bowel:* This can appear similar on AC images but will have a corresponding focus of some increased uptake on the noncorrected images.
- *Inflammation of bowel:* This will also have some increased uptake on the noncorrected images (and is usually more tubular in configuration than this).

Essential Facts

- AC is required for a uniform appearance and ability to quantify (i.e., SUV calculations) the source emission (also known as noncorrected, or NAC) images.
- Transmission scans for AC can be performed on a standalone PET by using external positron decaying rods such as germanium 68 (historically) or by using CT on modern PET/CT machines.
- CT performs AC much faster than standalone PET (seconds vs. minutes) and allows much better localization of PET findings.
- However, with CT correction, the lower energies of CT (~100 keV) must be scaled to 511-keV PET to produce attenuation coefficients for correction of the emission images.
- Although these CT-based coefficients are scaled correctly for most patient densities (e.g., water, soft tissue, and bone), they are incorrect at higher densities like those of metal and higher-density contrast, causing overcorrection and creating the false appearance of increased FDG uptake on AC images.

Other Imaging Findings

- Older standalone PET units do not demonstrate this type of artifact because the energies of the transmission scan photons are the same as those of the FDG photons (both 511 keV) and do not require scaling.
- Beam hardening ("streak" artifact) can be seen on the CT portion of these high-density regions.

✓ Pearls & × Pitfalls

✓ The noncorrected images should be inspected to distinguish true hypermetabolic activity from artifact. Any true uptake from hypermetabolism will have some increased focal uptake, even if mild, on the noncorrected images.

× A change in the position of the transmission attenuation map, such as with patient motion between PET and CT or PET/CT breathing mismatches (particularly near the lung bases), can also cause artifactual uptake (increased or decreased) on the AC images.

× Intravenous and oral CT contrast agents can also create artifacts on the AC images, caused either by the inherent high density of the contrast, as discussed previously, or by the change in location of the contrast between the times of CT (transmission) and PET (emission) image acquisition.

Case 77

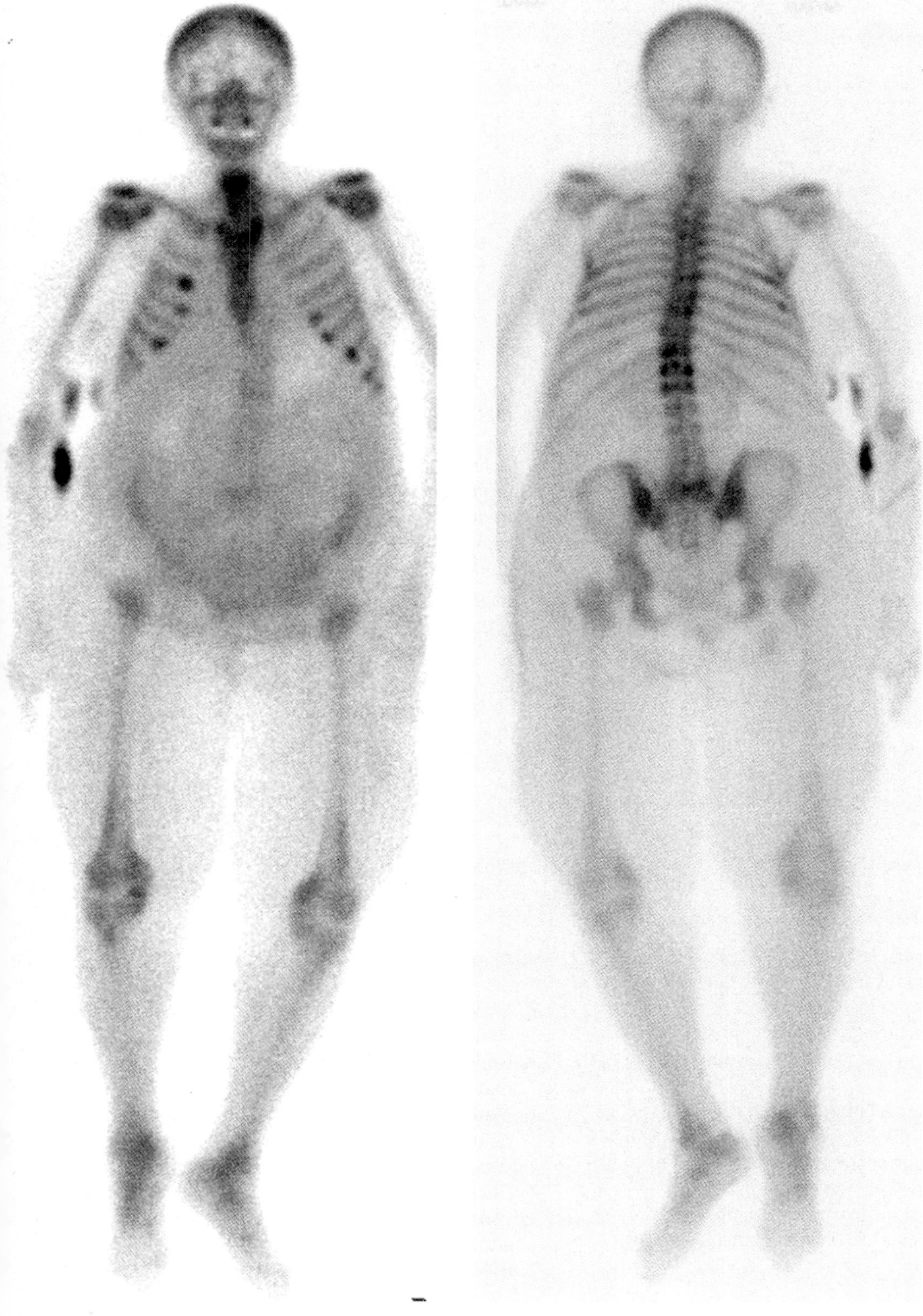

Clinical Presentation

A 51-year-old woman with a history of ovarian carcinoma now has back pain and abdominal distention.

Imaging Findings

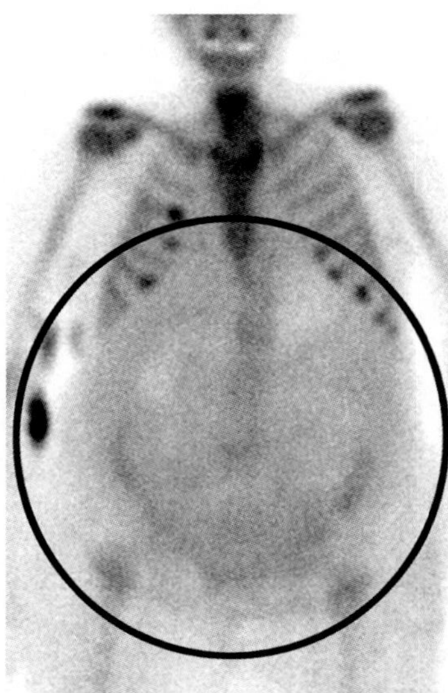

Anterior and posterior whole-body bone scan images demonstrate multiple osseous foci as well as diffuse, mildly increased abdominal soft-tissue uptake (*circle*).

Differential Diagnosis

- ***Malignant ascites (with possible bone metastases):*** A diffuse increase in soft-tissue uptake occupying the entire peritoneal cavity makes this the most likely diagnosis, given the history. And although the anterior rib lesions appear posttraumatic, the more lateral rib and the spine lesions are more suspicious.
- *Bowel necrosis:* Any soft-tissue infarction/necrosis can have increased uptake on bone scan. This would not be as diffuse as seen here, however.
- *Peritoneal mesothelioma:* Primary and metastatic soft-tissue tumors can have increased uptake on bone scan but are generally more focal than seen here.

Essential Facts

- Bone scan radiopharmaceuticals (e.g., Tc99m-HDP/Tc99m-MDP) are also taken up by soft-tissue necrosis and many primary or metastatic soft-tissue malignant processes, usually because of the avidity of abnormal calcium deposits (which may be microscopic and not visible on CT).
- Diffuse metastatic serosal implantation can result in malignant effusions (pleural, pericardial, and peritoneal), and then diffuse radiotracer uptake can be seen throughout the fluid space.
- Common primary lesions to cause this appearance include those of the ovaries, bladder, pancreas, colon, stomach, and breast.
- Tapping the fluid space can be performed to assess for tumor cells and markers.
- The fluid volumes are often large and symptomatic, so tapping can also be therapeutic.

Other Imaging Findings

- US can detect pleural or peritoneal fluid but cannot assess for malignant effusion. It can help guide pleural or abdominal paracentesis.
- CT can also detect fluid and can identify enhancing pleural or peritoneal soft-tissue thickening, which would be suggestive of a malignant etiology.
- FDG-PET can demonstrate increased uptake of peritoneal lesions, but the volume of tumor may be below the resolution of PET.

✓ Pearls & × Pitfalls

- ✓ Most ascites is not malignant but rather caused by cirrhosis.
- ✓ Nonmalignant fluid is not increased on bone scan. It may actually be seen as a region of decreased activity.
- × Malignant effusions are typically found incidentally on bone scan performed for osseous metastatic surveillance.
- × Do not confuse increased uptake in all the patient's soft tissues (including those in the extremities) for a malignant effusion, which should be confined to a single space. Diffuse soft-tissue uptake can be caused by renal failure.

Case 78

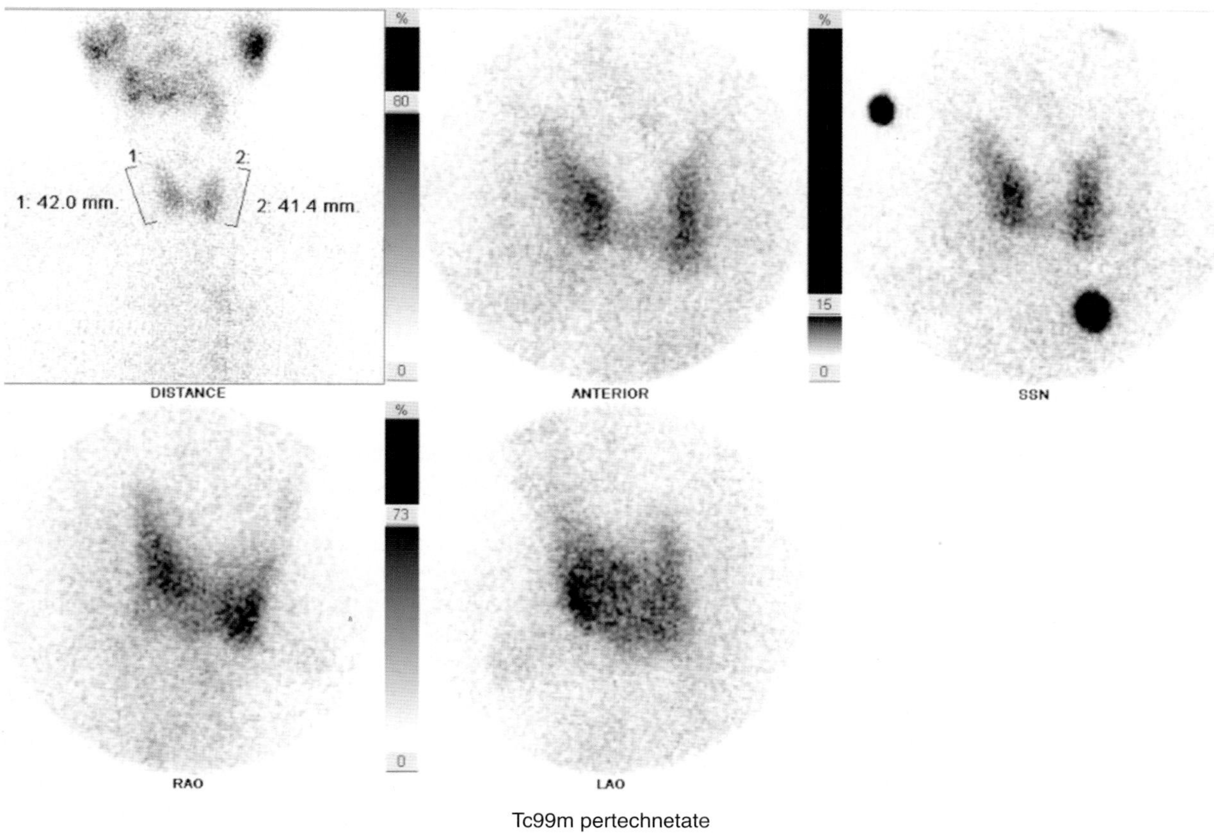

A

Tc99m pertechnetate

I123

Planar

B

24-hr thyroid radioiodine uptake = 1.5%

Clinical Presentation

A 9-year-old girl with hypothyroidism and goiter.

Imaging Findings

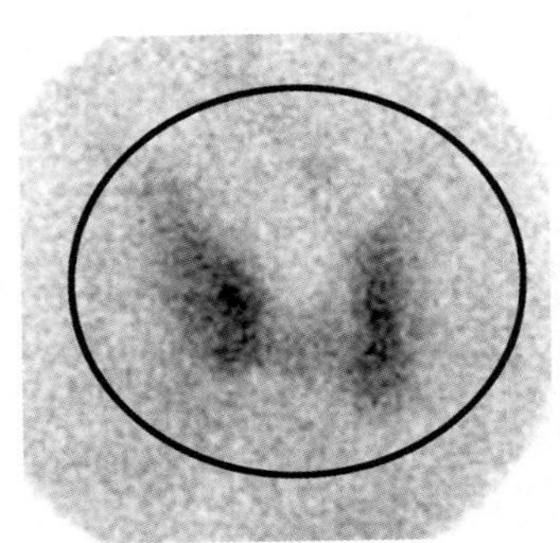

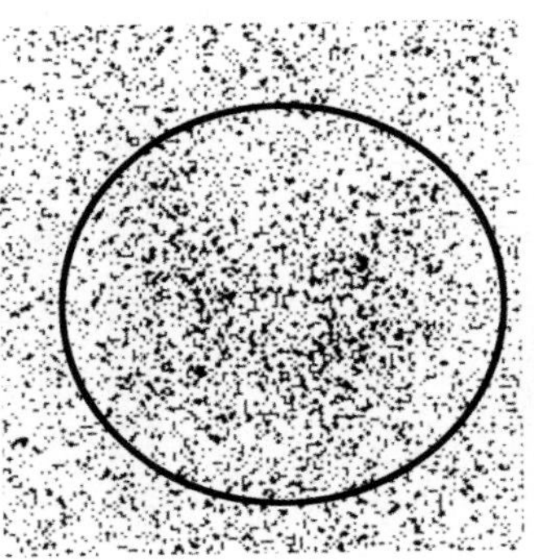

(A) Anterior planar and pinhole images from a pertechnetate thyroid scan reveal normal uniform activity throughout the thyroid gland (*circle*). **(B)** However, the 24-hour radioiodine uptake and scan are markedly uniformly decreased (*circle*) at 1.5% (normal, 10–30% at 24 hours).

Differential Diagnosis

- ***Organification defect:*** The pertechnetate scan (which is performed shortly after injection) will show normal uniform tracer uptake given that the ability of the thyroid gland to trap is normal. A defect in the process of organifying iodine allows washout of iodine, as seen on the 24-hour–delayed uptake and scan.
- *Antithyroid medications:* Medications such as propylthiouracil (PTU) and methimazole will look similar, as they block the organification of iodine but do not interfere with trapping. However, no such history is provided.
- *Subacute thyroiditis:* The typical finding is one of diminished pertechnetate and diminished iodine uptake.

Essential Facts

- Thyroid hormone synthesis requires iodide trapping followed by oxidation and incorporation into tyrosine (organification).
- An organification defect can be congenital (such as with a genetic peroxidase deficiency) or acquired (as in chronic thyroiditis) and results in hypothyroidism.
- Treatment is with thyroid hormone replacement.

Other Imaging Findings

- A related scintigraphic exam, the perchlorate washout test, can also be used to confirm an organification defect. Oral perchlorate will displace any iodine in the gland that is not organified. This causes a decrease in the iodine uptake measurement when compared with a baseline measurement on serial uptakes obtained over 2 hours. An uptake drop of $>$ 10% from peak is considered diagnostic for an organification defect.

✓ Pearls & × Pitfalls

✓ Pertechnetate is trapped by the thyroid gland but is not organified. Drugs such as perchlorate and nitroprusside interfere with trapping.

✓ Iodine (cold or radioactive) is trapped and organified by the thyroid gland. Drugs that interfere with organification (but not trapping) include methimazole, PTU, and sulfonamides.

✓ The normal 24-hour thyroid uptake of radioiodine is approximately 10 to 30% of ingested activity. The normal 24-hour uptake of (injected) pertechnetate is zero (it washes out by then).

× The recovery phase of thyroiditis, during which trapping may return to normal while organification remains inhibited, could look similar to this case (normal pertechnetate and decreased radioiodine uptake).

Case 79

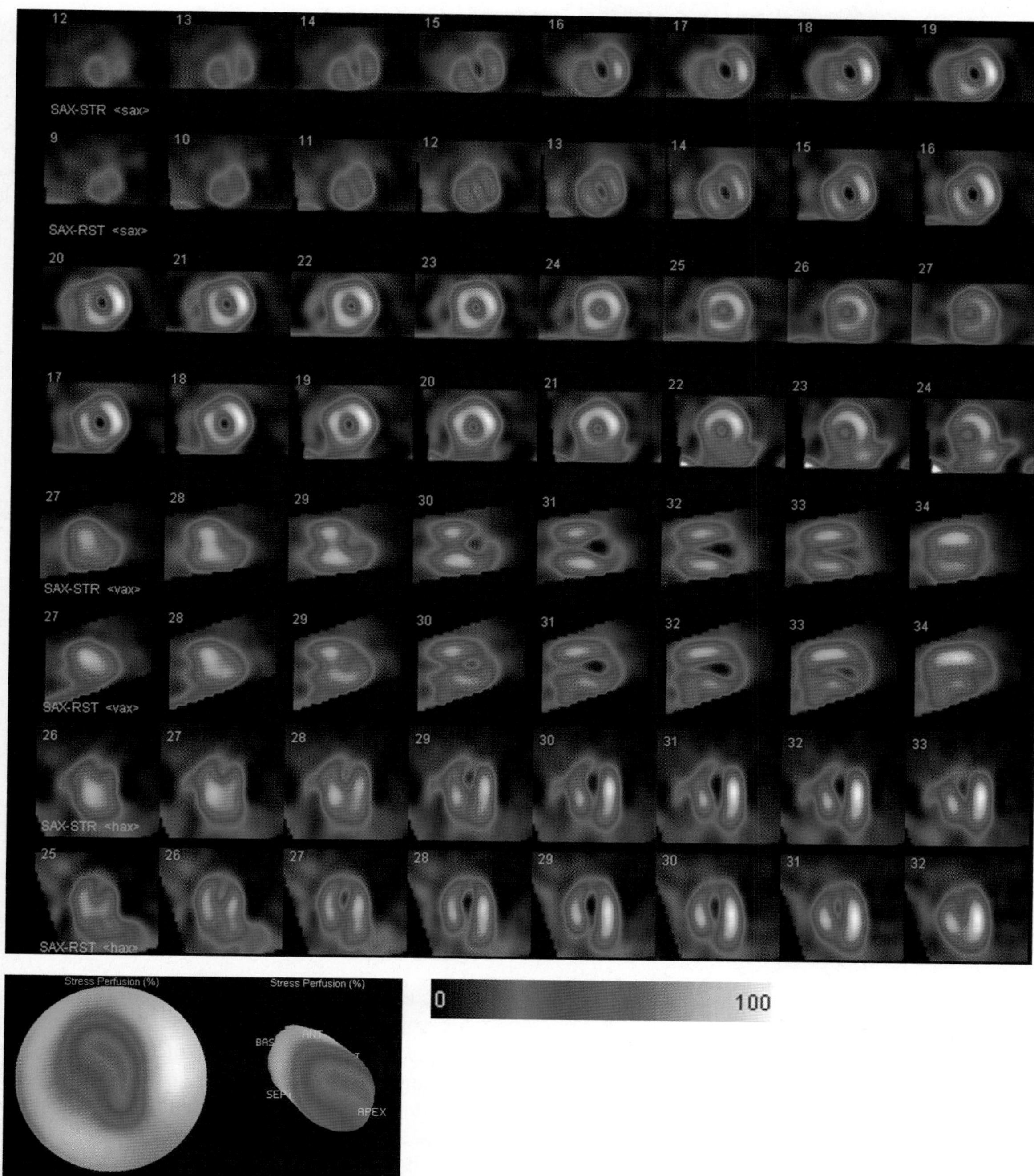

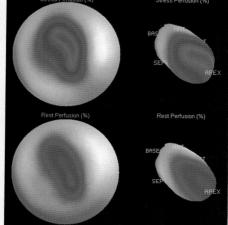

Clinical Presentation

68-year-old woman presents with chest pain and undergoes myocardial perfusion scintigraphy at rest and then at stress. he gated images (not shown) demonstrated an apical wall motion abnormality.

Imaging Findings

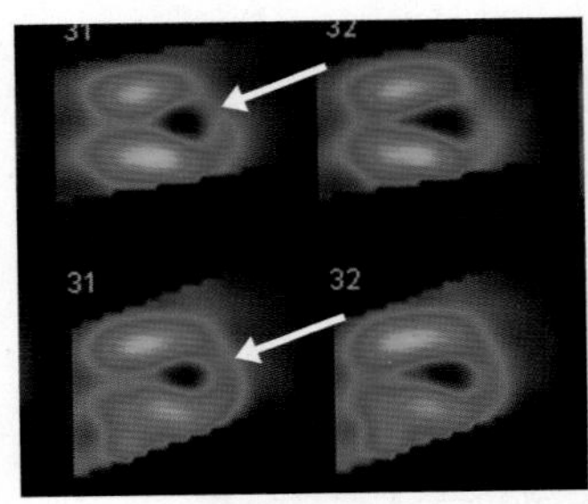

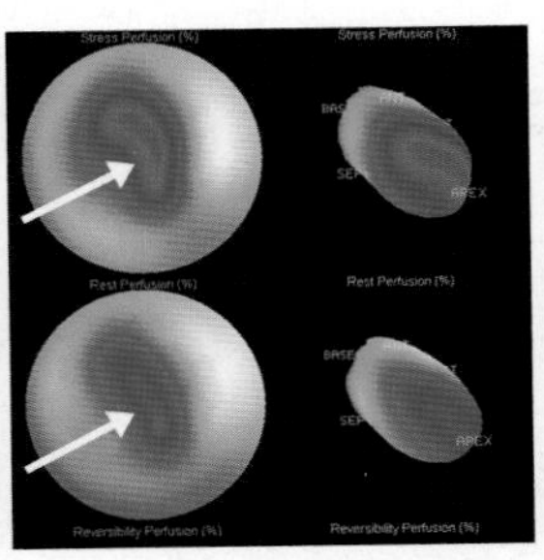

(A) Myocardial perfusion SPECT images demonstrate a medium-sized defect of marked severity in the anterior apex at stress that improves mildly at rest (*arrows*). Mild aneurysmal dilatation of the apex is also seen. **(B)** Stress and resting polar maps again demonstrate the severe, slightly reversible defects (*arrows*).

Differential Diagnosis

All three diagnoses can demonstrate defects on the rest and stress scans. However, attenuation artifacts should not have regional wall motion abnormalities, and hibernating myocardium requires additional imaging to document.

- ***Left anterior descending territory myocardial infarction with mild peri-infarct ischemia:*** This is the most likely diagnosis to account for a resting defect that worsens on stress and has a regional wall motion abnormality.
- *Hibernating myocardium:* This can appear similar, with fixed or partially reversible perfusion defects at rest and stress, and would also have a wall motion abnormality. However, redistribution on a 24-hour–delayed thallium 201 image or good uptake on a cardiac FDG-PET would be needed to make this diagnosis.
- *Breast attenuation artifact:* This can demonstrate a largely fixed defect in this location but should not worsen at stress and should not have an associated wall motion abnormality.

Essential Facts

- Myocardial perfusion scintigraphy is more sensitive than stress ECG or stress echocardiography in detecting reversible myocardial ischemia.
- Any combination of perfusion agents—Tl201, Tc99m-MIBI, and Tc99m-TETRO—can be used at rest and stress, but the two most common protocols are same-day Tl201 at rest and a Tc99m agent at stress or a low-dose/high-dose Tc99m agent at rest and stress.
- Gated SPECT images are required to assess for regional wall motion abnormalities, determine the left ventricular ejection fraction, and to problem-solve potential attenuation artifacts.
- Any method of stress—exercise or pharmacologic—can yield images equally sensitive for detecting reversible ischemia.
- Both infarcts and hibernating tissue have "fixed" perfusion defects at rest and stress. They both have resting wall motion abnormalities. (Gated images are acquired with the heart *at rest* before and/or after stress injections.)
- Reversible ischemia is a perfusion defect at stress that improves at rest and generally has normal resting wall motion.

Other Imaging Findings

- Resting echocardiography can demonstrate a regional wall motion abnormality in infarct or hibernating tissue.
- Stress echocardiography can demonstrate a regional wall motion abnormality *during stress* with reversible ischemia.
- Rest and stress myocardial perfusion imaging can also be performed with cardiac PET using rubidium 82 or N13-ammonia to reveal *perfusion* findings similar to those demonstrated by SPECT, but with improved accuracy due to better spatial resolution and attenuation correction.
- Cardiac *viability* PET can be performed with FDG to distinguish infarct from hibernating tissue, similar to delayed redistribution of Tl201 (again with improved accuracy on FDG-PET vs. thallium SPECT).
- Contrast-enhanced CT and MRI are rapidly evolving in the field of cardiac imaging and will play an increasing role.

✓ Pearls & ✗ Pitfalls

✓ Regional wall motion is the key to distinguishing a true resting perfusion defect (seen in both hibernating myocardium and infarct) from attenuation artifacts in myocardial perfusion imaging.

✗ Thallium is a potassium analogue (marker of cell membrane integrity) and the only clinical SPECT agent that can be used to assess for redistribution/viability (FDG can be used with PET). MIBI and TETRO (mitochondrial binding) do *not* redistribute to viable tissue. The disadvantages of thallium, however, are higher patient radiation dose and poorer overall image quality.

✗ Moderate or severe reversible defects may require coronary angiography for further evaluation and possible angioplasty or coronary artery bypass graft. Milder defects can often be managed medically.

Case 80

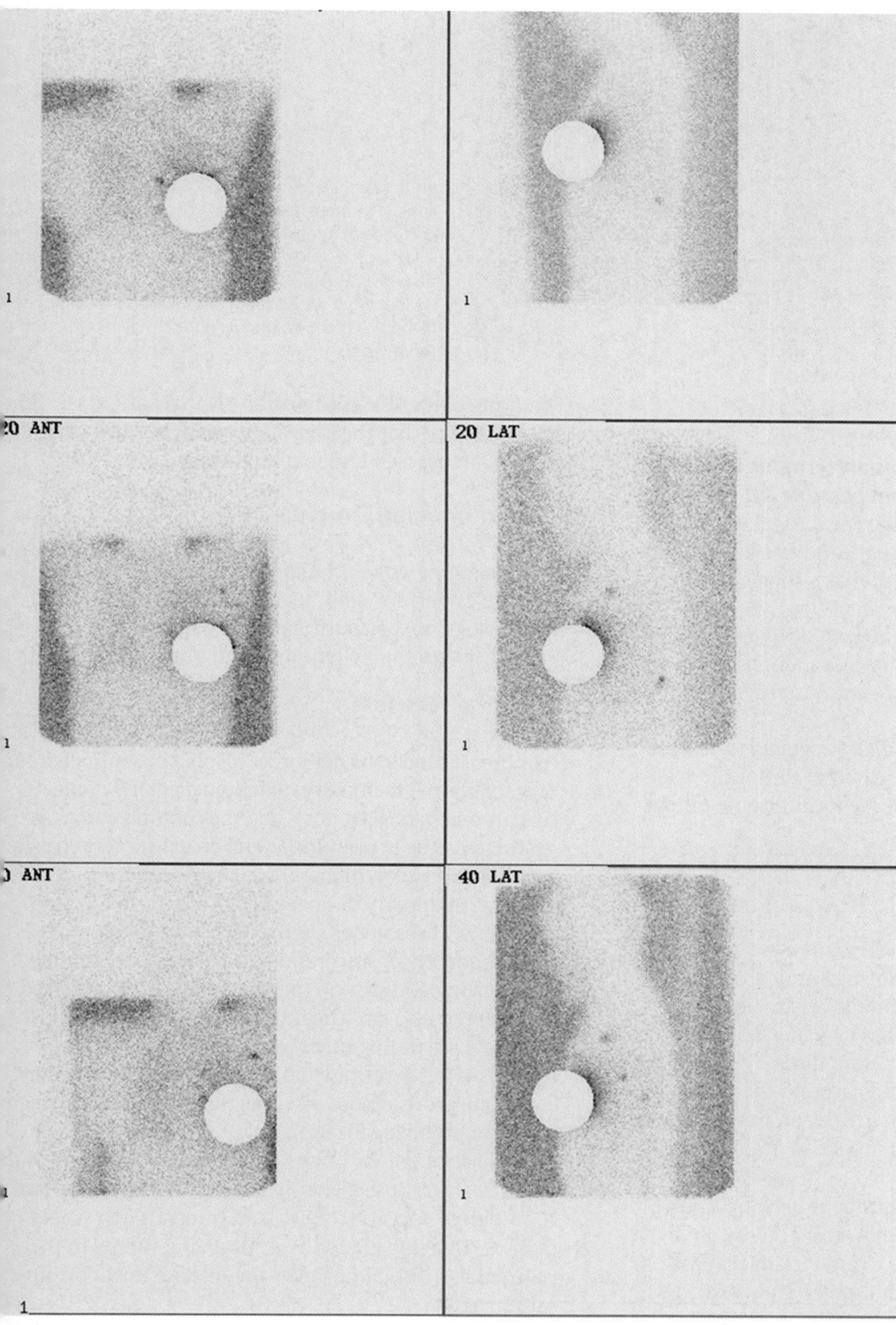

Clinical Presentation

65-year-old woman with a new diagnosis of breast carcinoma.

Imaging Findings

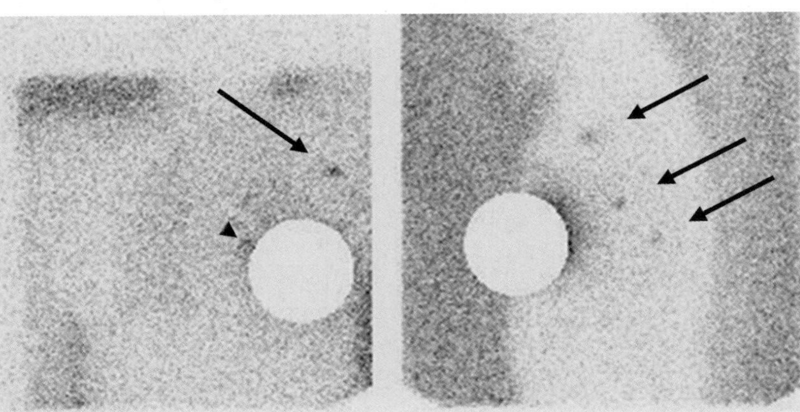

Immediate, 20-minute, and 40-minute anterior and left lateral lymphoscintigraphy images with Tc99m-SCOL reveal three separate lymph nodes (LNs) in the left axillary region, with the lowest-positioned LN identified first. The superior LN is identified second and the mid LN identified last (*arrows*). There is also the suggestion of subtle LN activity in the left internal mammary chain (*arrowhead*).

Differential Diagnosis

- ***Emission/transmission lymphoscintigraphic images demonstrating left axillary (and possible left internal mammary) sentinel nodes (SNs):*** Focal uptakes in the left thorax indicate the SNs. Visualization of the patient's body contour and lungs indicates that a cobalt transmission source was also used.
- *SNs on emission-only lymphoscintigraphic images:* Visualization of the patient's body contour and lungs indicates that a cobalt transmission source was also used (not just emission).
- *Lymphoscintigraphy showing axillary regional metastases:* Nodal uptake does *not* indicate whether or not there is tumor involvement, only that these locations are where regional drainage first occurs.

Essential Facts

- Lymphoscintigraphy is performed to improve accuracy and reduce patient morbidity during surgical regional (N) staging of tumor in breast carcinoma and melanoma.
- Lymphoscintigraphy is performed by using 0.5 to 1.0 mCi of Tc99m-SCOL filtered with a 22-µm filter.
- Subcutaneous injections are made around the tumor site (for melanoma and occasionally breast) or areola (breast), and imaging is performed until uptake in draining LN(s) is visualized.
- At surgery, a handheld gamma probe is used to remove any node(s) with significant radiotracer activity. Blue dye is also often injected at surgery to aid visual localization. The blue dye–identified and radiotracer-identified LNs are usually, but not always, concordant.
- As opposed to complete lymphadenectomy of the basin in question, selective sentinel LN resection results in less patient morbidity (i.e., lymphedema) and a higher sensitivity for detecting micrometastases because a more detailed pathologic assessment can be performed on fewer nodes.
- If the SN contains tumor, a complete lymphatic dissection may be performed for staging. If the SN is free of tumor, it is assumed there are no regional metastases.
- The probability of identifying an SN in a patient is ~85 to 90%. Accuracy that the identified nodes are truly SNs is $>$ 95% (rare missed regional metastasis).

Other Imaging Findings

- US is emerging as an SN mapping tool. At some institutions, US is performed first, and LNs with abnormal morphology or vascularity are sampled. If the result is positive for tumor, no lymphoscintigraphy is required.

✓ Pearls & ✗ Pitfalls

✓ For breast cancer, do not forget to look for sentinel drainage to internal mammary nodes (particularly if injecting around medial tumors) and the *contralateral* axilla (if there has been prior ipsilateral breast surgery that can disrupt and alter lymphatic drainage). However, identified internal mammary drainage can present a dilemma to surgeons. These nodes are much more difficult to access, less frequently positive, and so not commonly sampled.

✓ SN imaging and/or skin marking may *not* be required following injection. The intraoperative probe is most accurate, assuming that the correct lymphatic basin is known (as determined on the images). Accordingly, some surgeons do not use imaging but inject the tracer and use probe localization only.

✓ Lymphoscintigraphy can be performed on the day of or day before surgery (use higher Tc99m-SCOL dose for the latter).

✓ Combined emission (of SN) and transmission (sheet source) imaging is useful for localizing the SN in the patient. Lead shielding over the intense injection sites is also useful.

✗ The rate of sentinel LN detection declines as the tumor involvement of the SN increases. Failure to identify a sentinel LN raises the question of the existence of a completely tumor-filled SN (which can no longer take up the SCOL). Alternatively, this can lead to false identification of a secondary (benign) node as the SN.

✗ Focal skin contamination by radiotracer can simulate lymph node uptake.

✗ Liver/spleen visualization can occur if some injected SCOL enters a vein.

Case 81

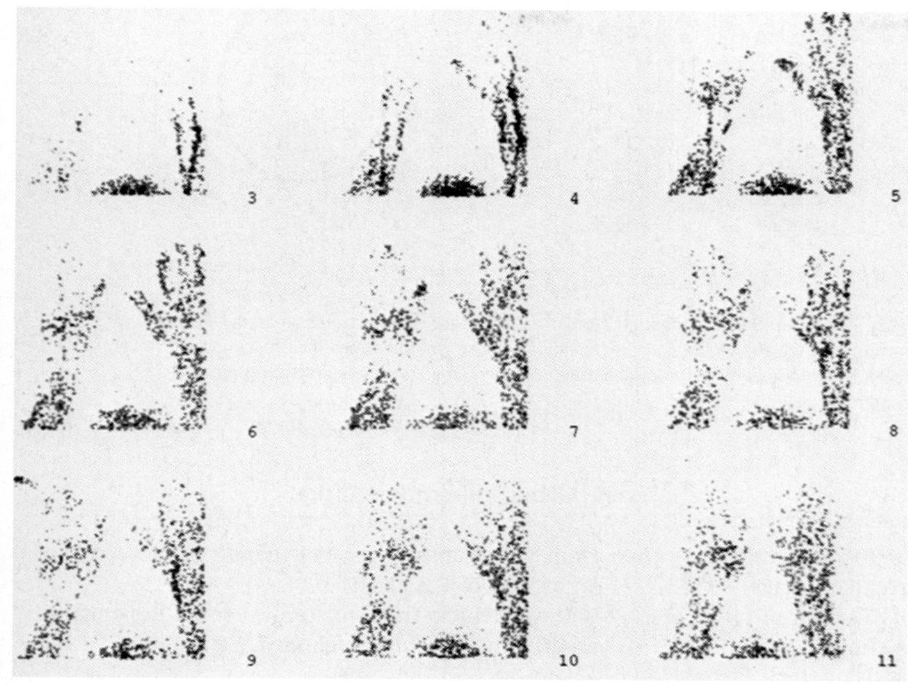

A

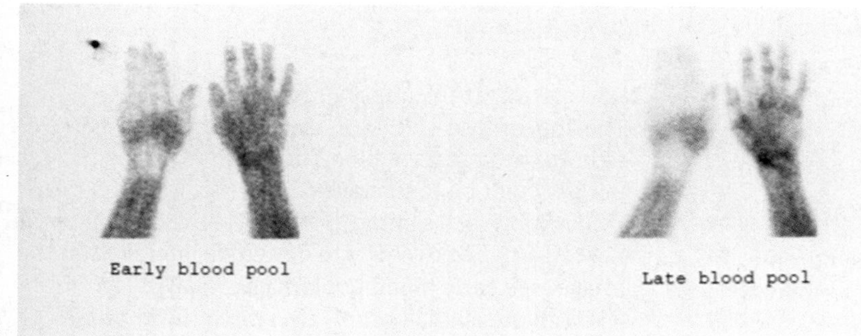

B

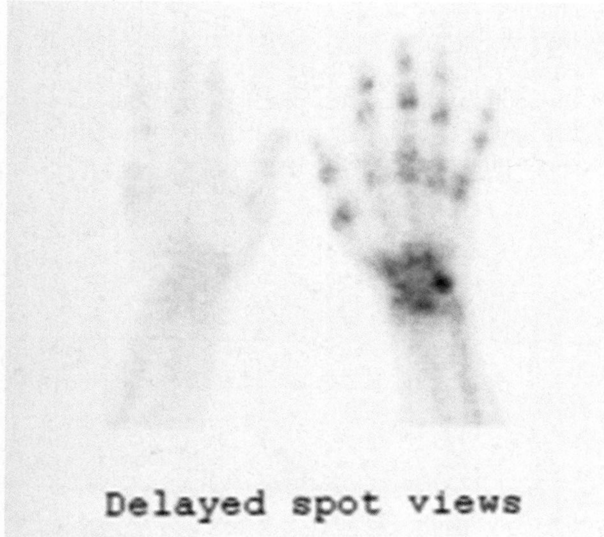

Clinical Presentation

patient with left hand pain and swelling.

Imaging Findings

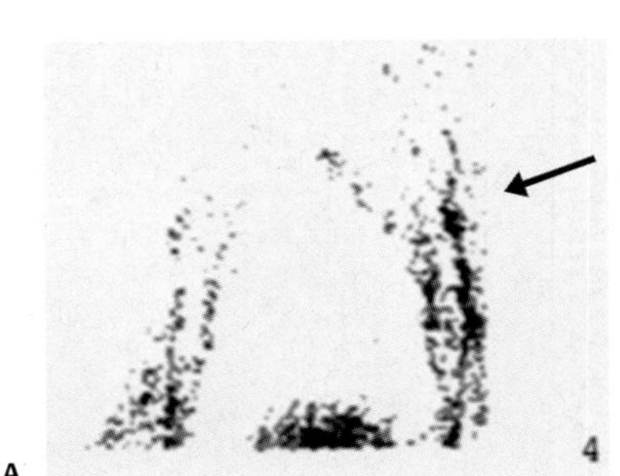

A

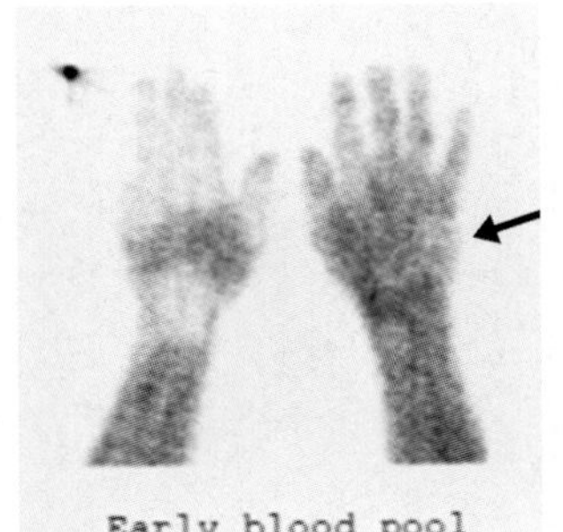

B

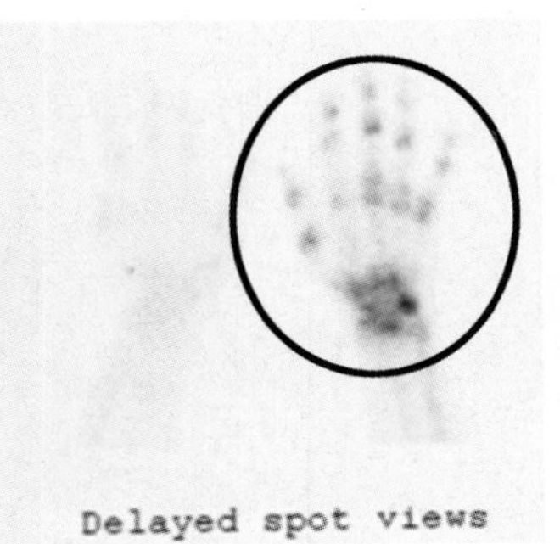

C

(A) Three-phase bone scintigraphy of the distal upper extremities was acquired. Angiographic phase demonstrates an asymmetric increase in blood flow to the left upper extremity (*arrow*). **(B)** Blood pool (extracellular) phase demonstrates increased uptake throughout the left hand and wrist (*arrow*). **(C)** Delayed phase demonstrates increased left-sided osseous uptake, most pronounced at the wrist and all periarticular sites of the left hand (*circle*).

Differential Diagnosis

- ***Reflex sympathetic dystrophy (RSD):*** Increased blood flow, blood pool, and delayed periarticular uptake diffusely is the classic appearance of this entity.
- *Inflammatory arthritis:* This can also show increased blood flow, blood pool, and delayed activity but will not involve all joints uniformly.
- *Osteomyelitis:* This can also be positive on three-phase scan but will involve only limited osseous sites and is not necessarily periarticular.

Essential Facts

- RSD is also known as complex regional pain syndrome, Sudeck atrophy, causalgia, algodystrophy, or peripheral trophoneurosis
- Pathogenesis is poorly understood, so diagnosis and treatment are challenging. RSD is thought to be related to inflammation and central nervous system hypersensitization, often following injury/surgery or a vascular event.
- Symptoms include severe pain, burning, hypersensitivity, and swelling of an affected limb. Increased sweating and skin changes can also be seen, with an eventual decrease in range of motion and osteopenia. Symptoms can be unilateral or bilateral.
- More common in adults, women > men, although can also be seen in children
- Treatment options include physical therapy and systemic or injected analgesics (e.g., sympathetic nerve blocks)/ anti-inflammatory agents. Electrical nerve stimulators and surgical sympathectomy are less common options for more severe refractory cases.
- Early diagnosis and treatment are important to shorten the course of the disease. Following successful therapy, blood flow will normalize first and periarticular uptake last on three-phase bone scan.

Other Imaging Findings

- Plain radiography is insensitive but can show periarticular osteopenia, as can CT.
- MRI can demonstrate soft-tissue edema and enhancement, skin thickening, and muscle atrophy.

✓ Pearls & × Pitfalls

✓ RSD can affect the upper or lower extremities.

✓ The appearance of RSD on the bone scan is likely related to both the increased blood flow *and* resulting increased periarticular bone turnover.

✓ By convention, a scintigraphic marker is usually placed next to a *right* extremity to designate laterality on the image (see early blood pool image, Fig. B).

× RSD can occasionally show *decreased* three-phase activity to the affected side. This is more common in children.

× Decreased three-phase activity can also be seen in chronic “burned-out” RSD.

× Immobilization or disuse of a limb from another cause can appear similar to chronic RSD on bone scan (i.e., three-phase decreased).

Case 82

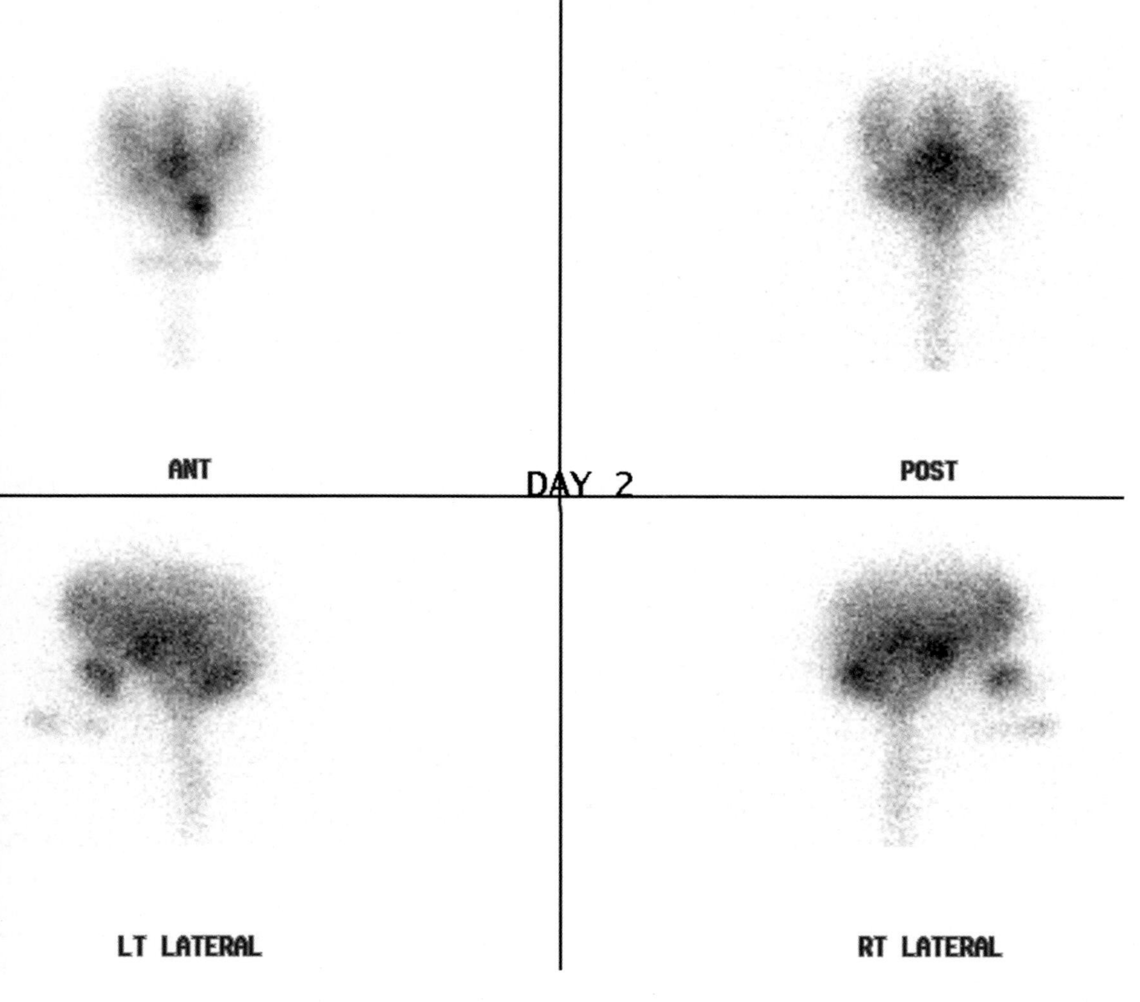

Clinical Presentation

History withheld.

Imaging Findings

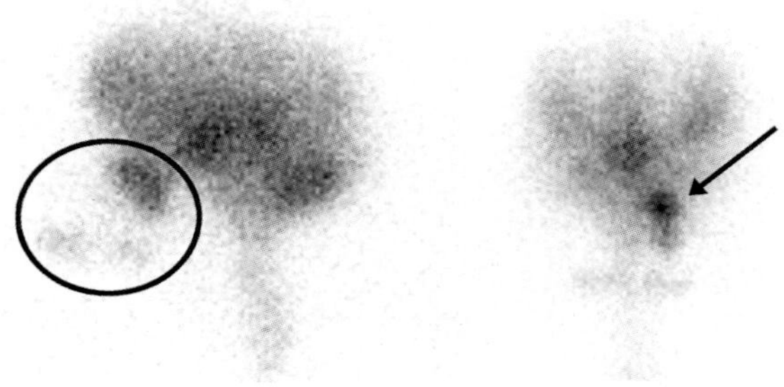

Anterior, posterior, and lateral head and neck images are obtained 48 hou after the intrathecal administration of indium 111-DTPA (cerebrospinal flu [CSF] cisternography). Abnormal extracranial nasal activity is noted bilatera (*circle*), most intensely in the left upper portion (*arrow*).

Differential Diagnosis

- ***Anterior CSF leak:*** Extracranial passage of CSF is abnormal and makes this the correct diagnosis.
- *Arachnoid cyst:* This can also appear as an abnormally increased collection of CSF if it communicates with the remainder of the CSF space. However, it should appear intracranial.
- *Normal pressure hydrocephalus:* Although this is the other common indication for radionuclide cisternography, no reflux into the third or lateral ventricles is present.

Essential Facts

- CSF leaks can take the form of rhinorrhea or rarely otorrhea.
- Leaks are commonly posttraumatic (including postsurgical) but can also result from high pressure hydrocephalus or congenital defects.
- Radionuclide cisternography can ascertain that leaked fluid is indeed CSF and can localize the leak.
- The exam is usually performed in conjunction with the placement of pledgets by the otolaryngologist in the upper and lower nasal regions bilaterally.
- Pledgets improve images by keeping leaked radiotracer in location; also, their activity can be measured individually (i.e., left, right, upper, lower) to confirm and localize a leak (to the region of the hottest pledget measured individually in a well counter).
- Because CSF is eventually absorbed into the circulation, the patient's blood is also measured; only a pledget-to-blood count ratio of $>$ 3:1 is considered positive (because body secretions are now slightly radioactive even without a leak).
- CSF rhinorrhea usually resolves spontaneously. Persistent leaks warrant surgical intervention because of patient discomfort and infection risk.

Other Imaging Findings

- High-resolution sinus CT following intrathecal iodinated contrast can also detect the presence and location of a CSF leak.
- In111-DTPA SPECT/CT can often localize the site of the leak better than SPECT or CT alone.

✓ Pearls & × Pitfalls

- ✓ The cribriform plate is the region most likely to fractur
- ✓ CSF leaks are often positional. Before imaging, place th patient in the position that replicates the leak.
- ✓ Temporal bone fractures can lead to otorrhea, which can also be detected by cisternography. Leaks into the nasal region are more commonly encountered, howeve
- × DTPA for CSF imaging can be labeled to In111 or Tc99n For leak studies (and normal pressure hydrocephalus evaluation), In111 is recommended as the long physical half-life allows for delayed imaging (as opposed to ventriculoperitoneal shunt studies, which are complet quickly, so that a Tc99m label can be used with less expense, less radiation, and better image quality than an In111 label).
- × Some authors argue that because pledget counts are more sensitive, actual imaging is not necessary for lea studies.

Case 83

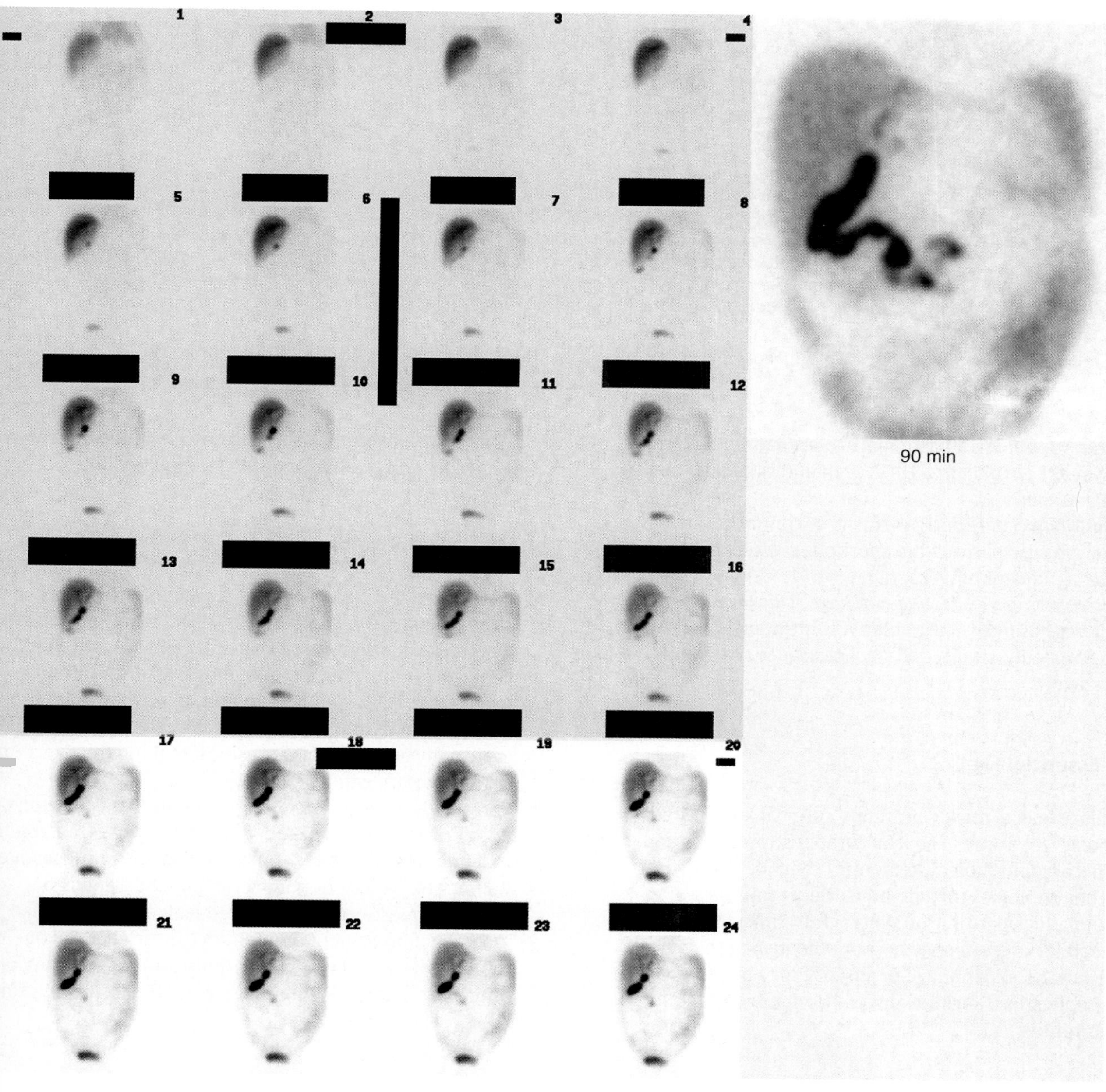

3 min/frame

Clinical Presentation

ising bilirubin following left hepatic resection and hepaticojejunostomy for cholangiocarcinoma.

Imaging Findings

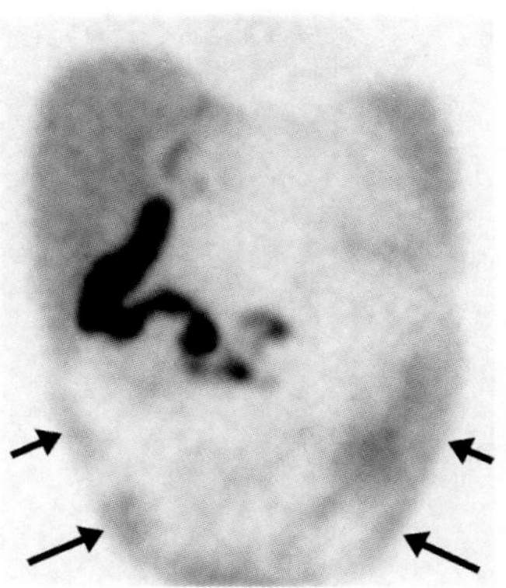

Sequential anterior imaging of the abdomen immediately following injection of Tc99m-mebrofenin demo strates prompt clearance of radiotracer from the blood pool and homogeneous distribution throughout the rig liver (left liver was removed). Prompt formation and extrahepatic passage of biliary activity is seen. Passage some bile into bowel is noted, as well as a more focal collection below the right liver. Over time, tracer is seen t appear throughout the periphery of the abdomen (*arrows*).

Differential Diagnosis

- ***Biliary leak:*** Intraperitoneal accumulation of tracer is always abnormal on a HIDA scan and is usually due to biliary leak.
- *Small-bowel perforation:* This is uncommon and less likely, particularly as intraperitoneal tracer appears before significant bowel activity.
- *Active intraperitoneal hemorrhage:* This is conceivable but very unlikely, particularly as intraperitoneal tracer appears only after blood pool clearance of tracer has occurred.

Essential Facts

- Biliary leak is most commonly surgical and secondary to cholecystectomy. The leak complication rate is higher for laparoscopic cholecystectomies than for open ones.
- Other etiologies include nonsurgical trauma and gallbladder perforation with acute cholecystitis.
- Small leaks often resolve spontaneously; otherwise, percutaneous drainage or surgery may be required.
- Complications include abscess formation and peritonitis.

Other Imaging Findings

- CT and US can demonstrate intraperitoneal fluid but are nonspecific. Only HIDA can prove the fluid is bilious.

✓ Pearls & × Pitfalls

✓ Intraperitoneal HIDA tracer is always abnormal and almost always indicates a biliary leak, whether or not a discrete leak origin or abnormal loculus is visualized.

✓ Look for outlining of bowel and/or the "disappearing liver" sign; as liver activity decreases with excretion and abnormal diffuse peritoneal activity increases, the eventually are of equal intensities, making the liver seem to disappear.

✓ Conversely, if a leak is contained, no free intraperitonea accumulation may be seen. But in these cases, an abno mal migration or collection of labeled bile is suggestive

✓ Rolling the patient or having the patient stand can resolve a questionable contained leak.

× Tracer in a prominent duodenum can simulate a contained leak. If in the bowel, activity will move and wax and wane over time. A lateral view may also be helpful

Case 84

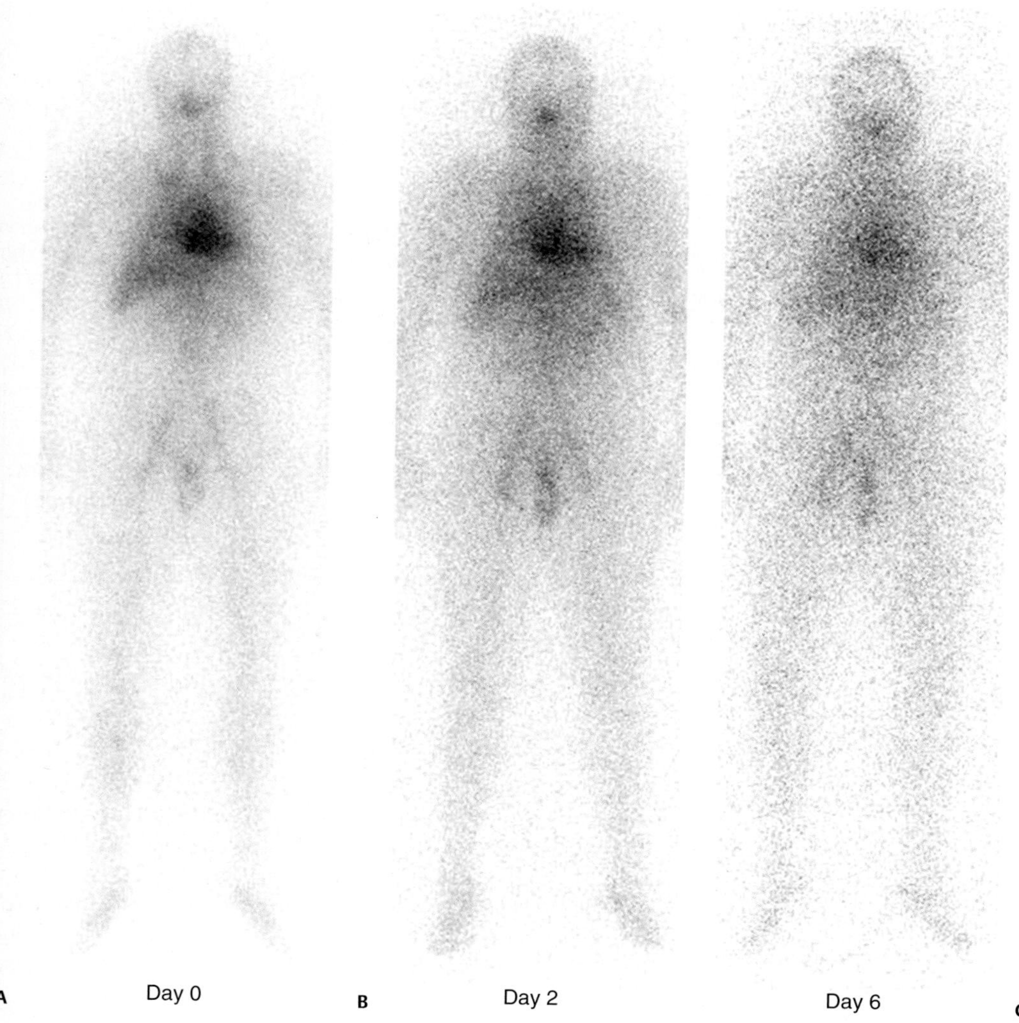

A B C

Clinical Presentation

A 54-year-old woman with a relapsed low-grade lymphoma presents for therapy. Which therapy did the patient receive? Is the biodistribution normal?

Imaging Findings

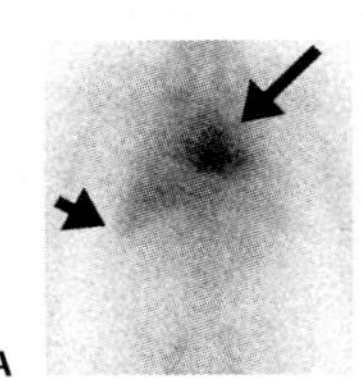
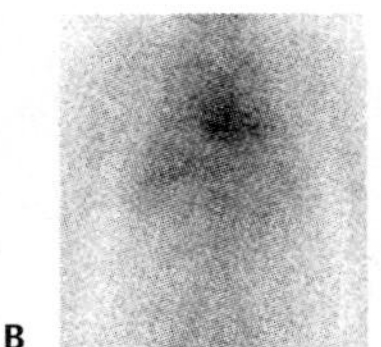
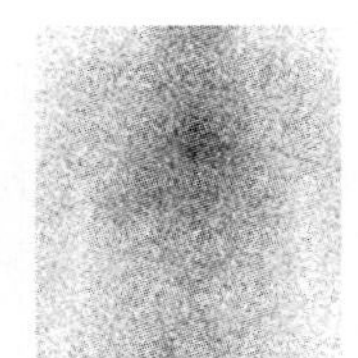

(A–C) The three anterior whole-body images are low count and are further degraded over time. Liver and blood pool activity is seen throughout the entire exam (*arrows*).

Differential Diagnosis

- ***Bexxar therapy:*** Given the low-count and low-resolution images (I131 label) and given the prolonged imaging delay, this is consistent with Bexxar therapy. There is no evidence of altered biodistribution.
- *Zevalin therapy:* Zevalin therapy has superior image quality, given the larger In111 dose (and better photon energies) used for pretreatment imaging (but with a similar biodistribution; see image at the bottom).
- *ProstaScint scan:* Like Bexxar and Zevalin, ProstaScint is a radiolabeled antibody and hence has a similar normal biodistribution (largely blood pool and liver). However, it is not a therapeutic agent.

Essential Facts

- There are two radionuclide therapy agents available for treating relapsed, follicular, or transformed low-grade non-Hodgkin lymphoma: Bexxar and Zevalin.
- They are both monoclonal antibodies that target CD20 receptors expressed on > 90% of B cells.
- Iodine 131-Bexxar is a γ- and β-emitter; hence, the same agent can be used for imaging and subsequent therapy (low dose, then high dose). However, the γ-emissions necessitate more extensive dose calculations and radiation safety precautions. Thyroid blocking is also needed (because of free I131).
- Yttrium 90-Zevalin is a pure β-emitter, so the γ-emitting In111-Zevalin must be first given for imaging, but then no special precautions are required for therapy.
- Both therapies yield very good response rates, even for patients who have failed conventional chemotherapy. A lower response rate is seen in patients whose disease has proved refractory to (nonradioactive) rituximab.
- Myelotoxicity is the primary adverse event, causing thrombocytopenia and leukopenia. Patients with lower platelet counts can receive a lower therapy dose. If their platelet count is too low, they will be untreatable, however.
- For both therapies, cold rituximab is given before the radiolabeled antibodies. The therapeutic effect is from both naked antibody and β-emission destructive "crossfire" effects.

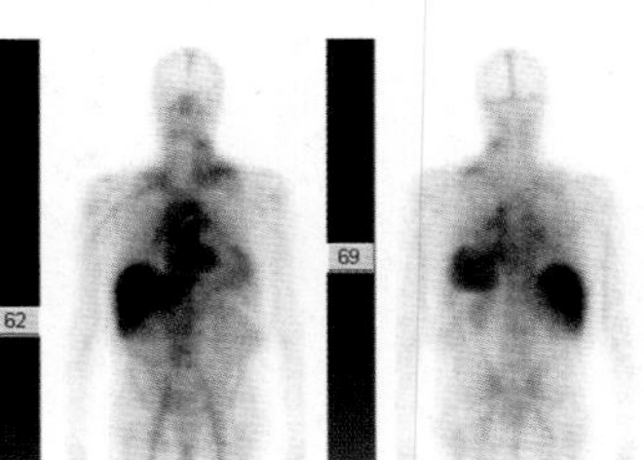

- An indium 111-Zevalin image for comparison (similar biodistribution, better image quality than I131-Bexxar) is at the bottom left.
- Comparison of the radiopharmaceuticals:

	I131	Y90
Emission	γ and β	β only
Imaging	Yes	No
Path length of β-particle	Maximum, 2.9 mm (average, 0.4 mm)	Maximum, 11 mm (average, 2.5 mm)
Radiation to others	Yes	No (even at high doses)
Cost	Low	High
Thyroid protection	Yes	No

Other Imaging Findings

- With both therapies, imaging is performed to assess for rare *altered biodistributions* (e.g., increased lung or liver uptake) that would preclude therapy. Patients may be treated whether or not the tumor is seen on the imaging portion of the study.
- CT or PET/CT can be used to stage or restage disease.

✓ Pearls & × Pitfalls

✓ A plastic syringe shield should be used with Zevalin. With a lead shield, the lead–β-particle interaction would increase the radiation dose to the injecting individual.

✓ Both therapies can be performed on an outpatient basis.

× Carefully monitor the patient for 10 to 15 minutes after slow injection for immediate adverse anaphylactoid reactions (rare).

× Contraindications to therapy include > 25% bone marrow involvement by tumor, platelet count < 100,000/mm^3, neutrophil count < 1500/mm^3, and known hypersensitivity to rituximab/murine proteins.

× Myelosuppression can occur in any patient. The nadir for platelets and WBCs is approximately 8 weeks, with levels normalizing by 12 weeks. (This suppression therefore occurs later than that seen with traditional chemotherapies.)

Case 85

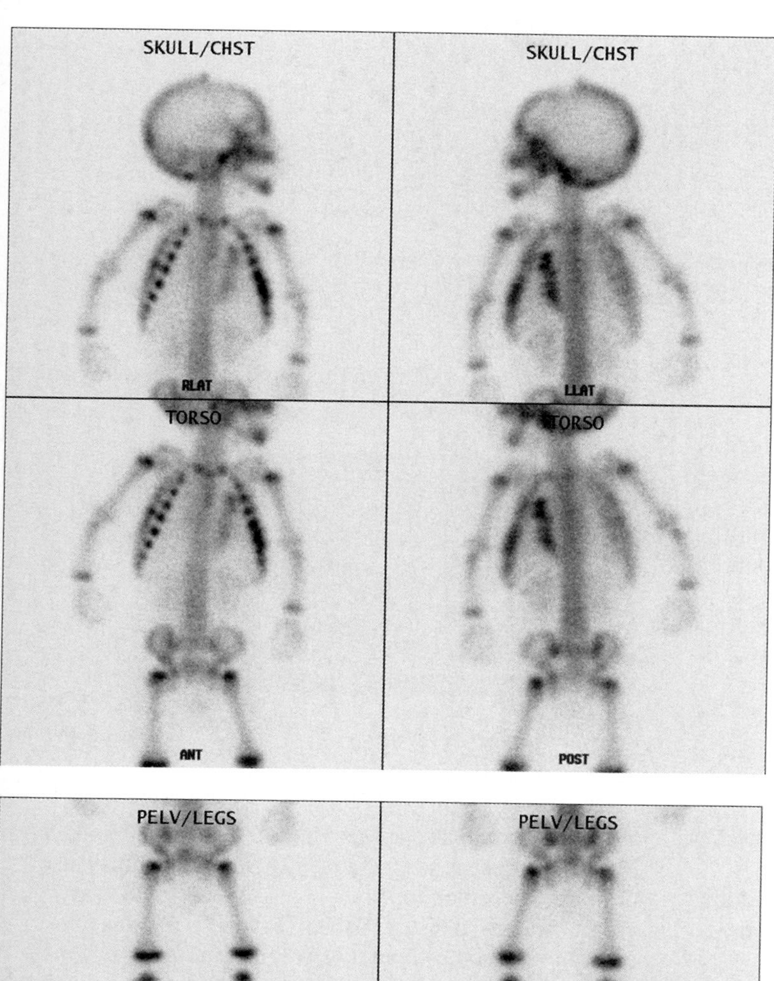

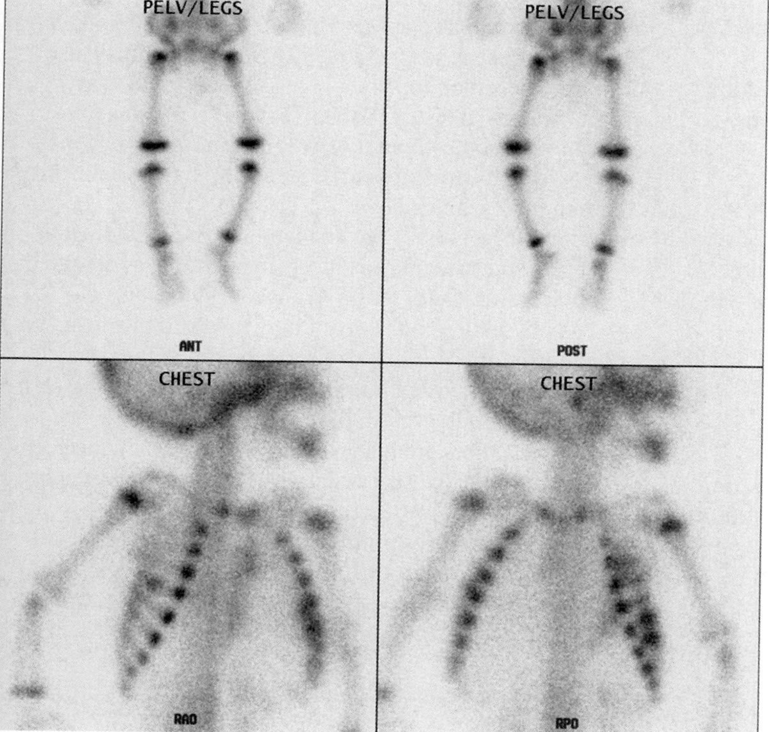

Clinical Presentation

A 6-month-old infant with failure to thrive.

Imaging Findings

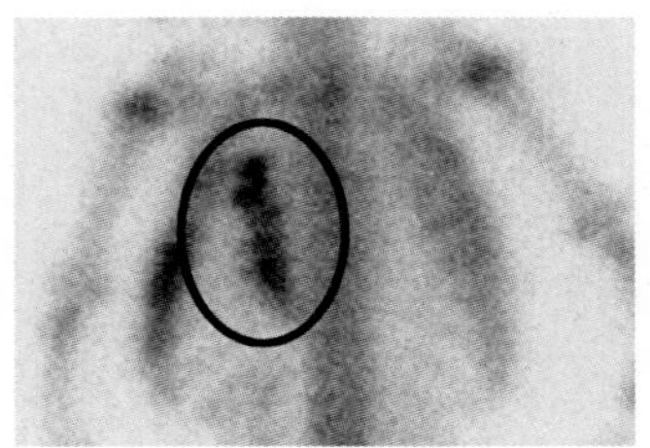
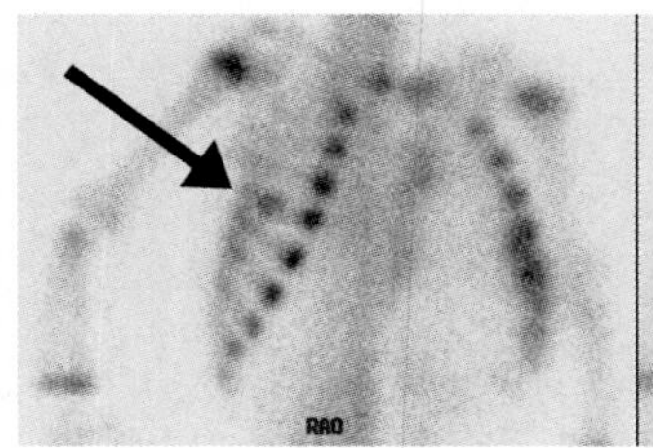

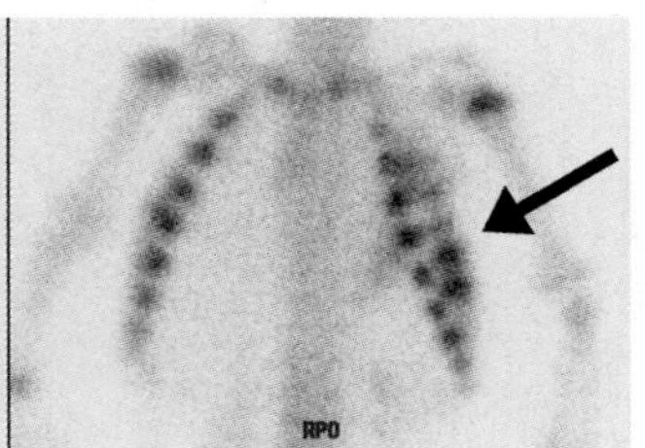

Spot images from a whole-body bone scan demonstrate multiple intense adjacent left posterior rib foci grouped in a linear fashion (*circle*) as well as milder anterolateral rib foci bilaterally (*arrows*).

Differential Diagnosis

- ***Nonaccidental trauma:*** Multiple focal, adjacent, linearly arranged rib lesions suggest fractures. Multiple fractures of different ages/intensities strongly suggest abuse.
- *Bone metastases:* These can commonly appear as multiple rib lesions. However, they are more segmental and more randomly distributed than the ones seen here.
- *Polyostotic osteomyelitis:* This can also appear as multiple bone lesions and is more common in children. Again, however, such lesions are not adjacent, as seen here.

Essential Facts

- Unexplained fractures in children should raise suspicion of nonaccidental trauma.
- Multiple fractures of various ages are the typical findings.
- The ribs are most commonly involved. Skull and long-bone (especially metaphyseal, "corner," or spiral) fractures are also common.
- A plain radiographic skeletal survey is performed first at most institutions. Bone scan can follow if results are negative/equivocal but clinical suspicion still remains.
- When abuse is suspected, alerting the proper social service is mandatory.

Other Imaging Findings

- Brain and other soft-tissue injuries, including lacerations and hemorrhage, are also frequently present and best imaged on CT.
- Brain MRI can demonstrate additional abnormalities, such as diffuse axonal injuries with "shaken baby syndrome."
- Here is the chest CT from this same infant showing one of the rib fractures (*circle*):

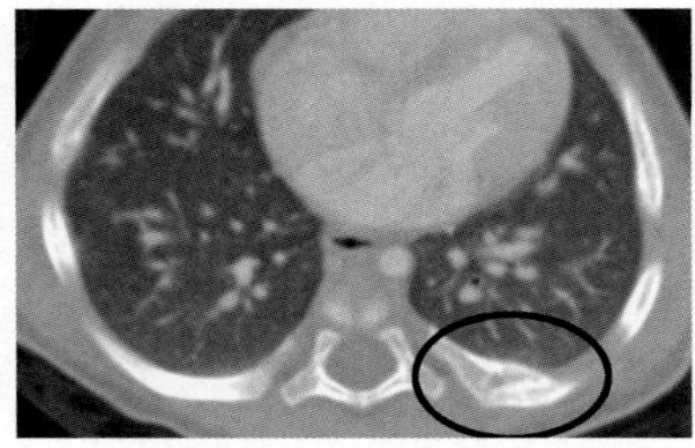

✓ Pearls & × Pitfalls

✓ Make sure to also survey the soft tissues on bone scan when abuse is suspected. Soft-tissue injury may also have abnormal uptake.

✓ In children, fractures usually have initial uptake on bone scan by 24 hours. After 3 to 4 months, they may return to normal uptake (but can still have a deformity seen radiographically).

✓ Do not forget about the analogous possibility of elder abuse. Fractures in the elderly may not have increased bone scan activity for up to a week, however.

× The physeal region is commonly involved in abuse, but abnormalities in this region can be difficult to detect given the intense uptake normal in children. Look carefully for subtle growth plate asymmetry.

× Skull fractures are insensitively detected on bone scan owing to normal suture activity. Skull radiography or CT is better.

× Multiple fractures mimicking abuse may have a valid underlying cause. Consider bone abnormalities such as osteogenesis imperfecta or Caffey disease, as well as trauma from cardiopulmonary resuscitation.

Case 86

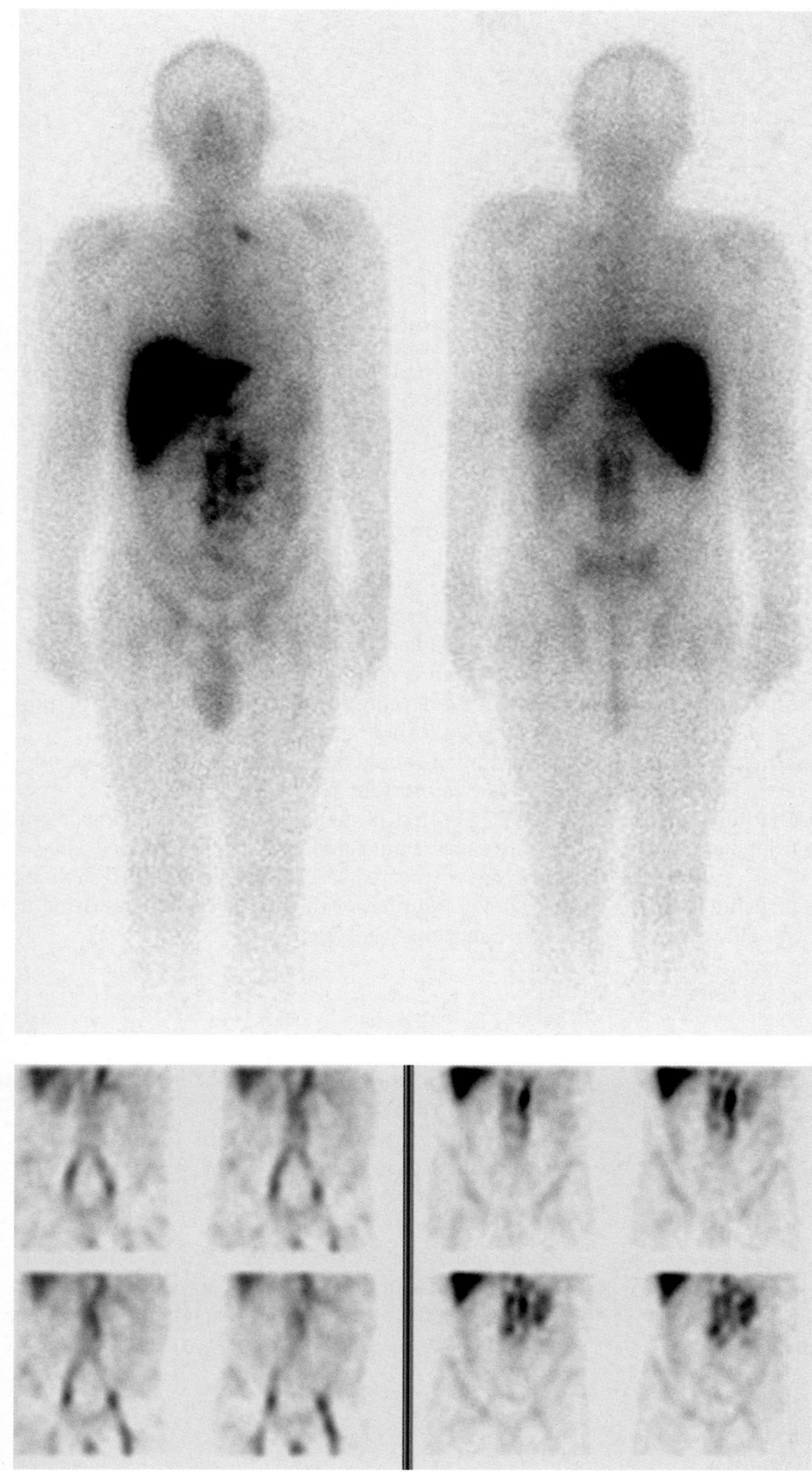

Clinical Presentation

A 54-year-old man presents for cancer restaging.

Imaging Findings

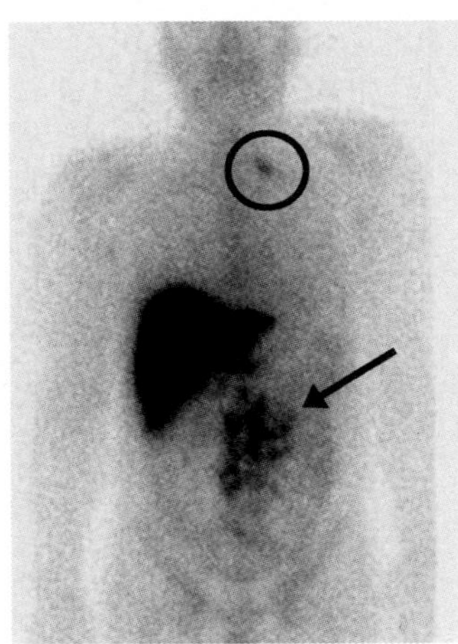

A

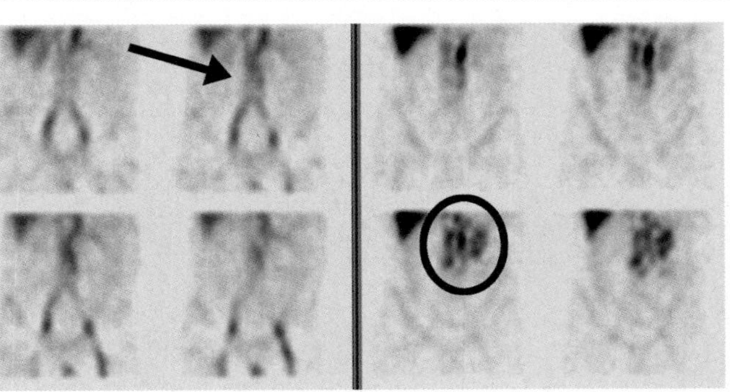

B

(A) Anterior and posterior whole-body imaging demonstrates intense physiologic uptake in the liver diffusely as well as milder blood pool, marrow, and bowel activity. Multifocal abnormal radiopharmaceutical uptake in the mid abdominal region (*arrow*), as well as focal uptake in the left supraclavicular region (*circle*), is seen. **(B)** Dual coronal SPECT imaging with Tc99m-RBCs (left images) at the same time as acquisition from the original tracer in A (right images) demonstrates abnormal accumulation in retroperitoneal aortocaval lymph nodes (*circle*), separate from the physiologic blood pool distribution mapped simultaneously on RBC scan (*arrow*).

Differential Diagnosis

- ***ProstaScint scan with metastasis within the mid abdomen and left supraclavicular region:*** Distribution of the radiopharmaceutical is consistent with an antibody study (blood pool, intense liver, bone marrow, and bowel). Focally abnormal uptake that is separate from blood pool is specific for prostate cancer metastases.
- *ProstaScint scan showing tortuous abdominal vessels:* Although physiologic antibody activity in blood pool can mimic tumor, the tagged RBC study shows that the focal uptake on the ProstaScint scan is separate from blood vessels.
- *Gallium scan showing lymphoma:* Ga67 biodistribution does include liver, spleen, marrow, and bowel. However, salivary and lacrimal uptake should also be seen; liver is not as intense, and blood pool is not visible (see "Interpreting Whole-Body Scans").

Essential Facts

- ProstaScint is indium 111-labeled capromab pendetide, which is an antibody targeted to prostate-specific membrane antigen (PSMA).
- Although PSMA is expressed in all forms of prostate tissue, it is overexpressed in prostate carcinoma.
- ProstaScint scanning is indicated for detecting recurrent/metastatic *soft-tissue* tumor in the prostate bed or more distally in at-risk patients.
- Imaging is performed 4 to 6 days following injection of the (In111-labeled) ProstaScint tracer. Typically, dual-energy imaging of Tc99m-RBCs (injected on the day of imaging) can allow mapping of the blood pool and decrease false-positives (antibodies normally persist in the blood pool, which can be adjacent to lymph nodes and simulate lymph node tumor involvement).
- ProstaScint imaging can be used to guide radiotherapy.

Other Imaging Findings

- Prostate/pelvic MRI can identify the initial prostate cancer and detect local recurrence.
- Abdominal/pelvic CT can detect regional lymph node metastases but is not sensitive or specific.
- SPECT/CT is emerging as the modality of choice to most accurately perform ProstaScint imaging.
- Bone scanning should be performed to detect *skeletal* metastases in prostate cancer.
- With PET, FDG has limited avidity for typical lower-grade prostate cancers but can detect more aggressive subtypes. Newer tracers like C11-acetate and C11-choline have shown promise for the more accurate assessment of prostate cancer with PET/CT.

✓ Pearls & ✗ Pitfalls

✓ If the Gleason score is < 6, it is unlikely that patient has distant metastases.

✗ Human antimouse antibody (HAMA) limits repetitive ProstaScint injections. Up to 40% of patients can have some level of side effects from the whole antibody injection.

✗ Rarely, other tumor types may be ProstaScint-avid. If the lesion distribution appears atypical for prostate cancer, consider other entities, like lymphoma. Tumor neovascularity has been associated with several PSMA markers.

Case 87

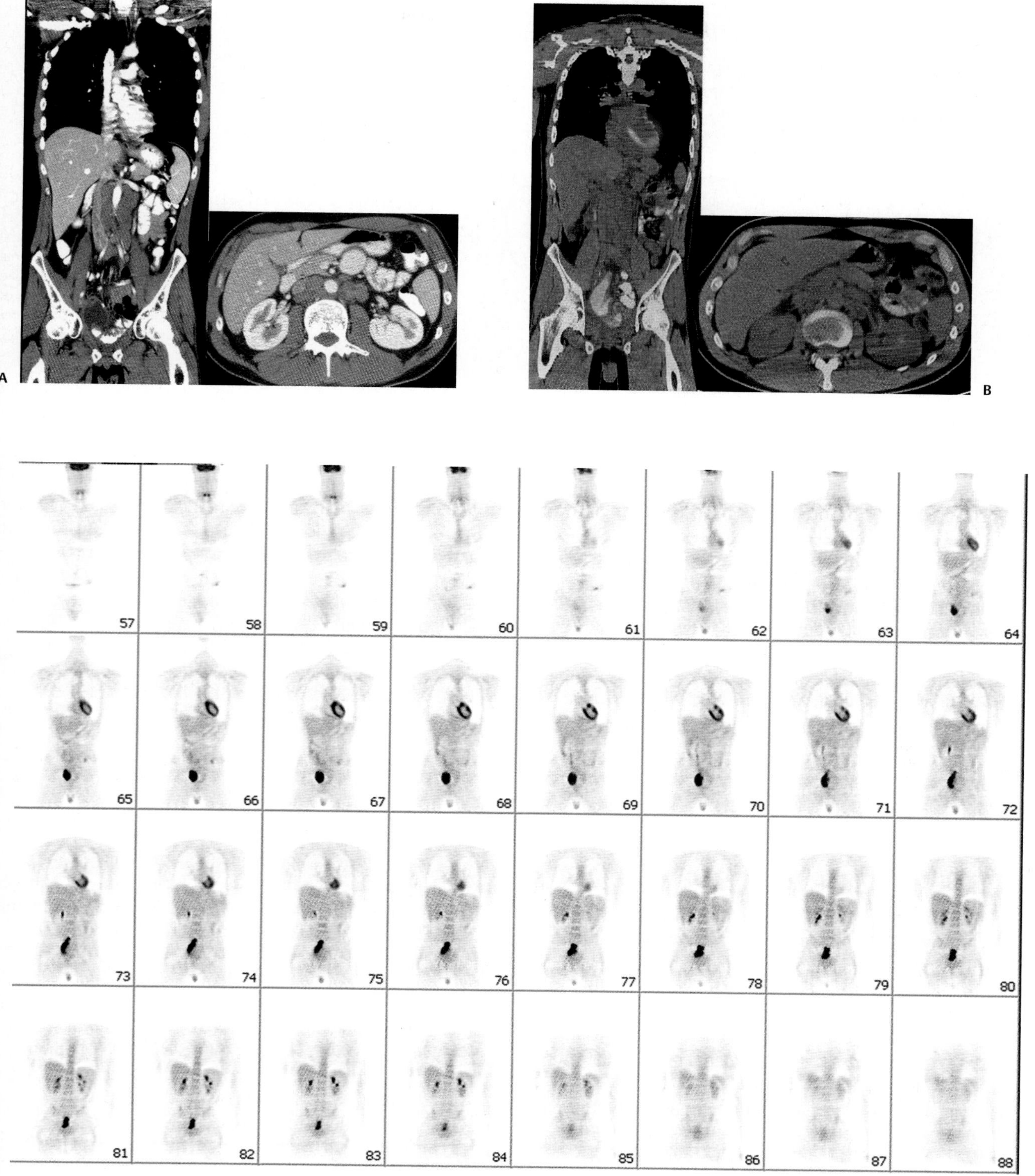

A B C

Clinical Presentation

A 30-year-old man with colorectal cancer (mucinous type) status post resection and chemotherapy presents for restaging. He is also status post bladder reconstruction. Baseline CT (not shown) was normal. No presurgical FDG-PET was performed.

Imaging Findings

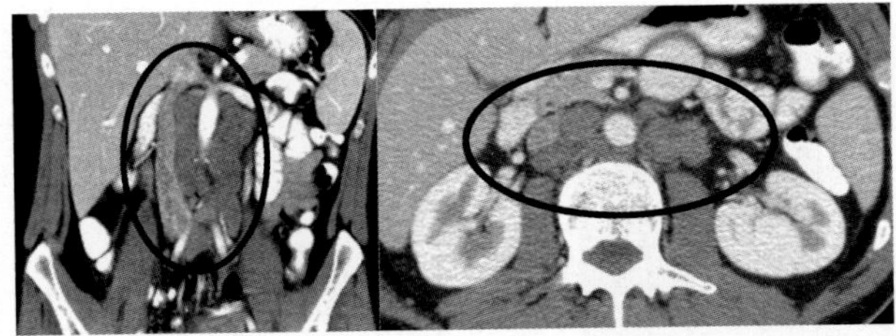

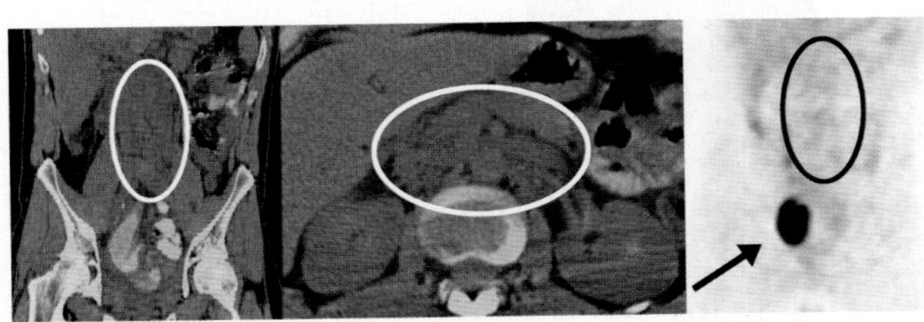

(A) Selected coronal and axial slices from contrast-enhanced CT demonstrate multiple enlarged retroperitoneal lymph nodes (*circles*), which are new from the previous scans. **(B,C)** Coronal whole-body FDG-PET images and selected axial and coronal hybrid PET/CT images demonstrate no abnormal FDG uptake to correspond to the enlarged retroperitoneal lymph nodes or elsewhere (*circles*). Physiologic excretion is noted in the reconstructed bladder in the right pelvis (*arrow*).

Differential Diagnosis

- ***Progression of non–FDG-avid colorectal metastases:*** Abnormal enlarging lymph nodes on CT in a patient with a known cancer are highly suspicious for metastatic disease, even without FDG uptake. Mucinous cancers are often non–FDG-avid, so this is the diagnosis of exclusion.
- *Development of secondary lymphoproliferative neoplasm:* This is a consideration because neoplasms such as low-grade lymphomas or leukemias can also appear as enlarging non–FDG-avid lymph nodes. Patients with prior chemotherapy are at an increased risk for the development of these secondary tumors.
- *Benign reactive adenopathy:* Systemic illness and other diffuse inflammatory diseases can also appear as abnormally large, non–FDG-avid lymph nodes. This is less likely given the history, however.

Essential Facts

- Although the vast majority of malignancies are moderately or markedly FDG-avid, a minority will demonstrate little or no uptake on PET.
- In general, these include lower-grade or low-cellularity (e.g., mucinous) tumors.
- Common examples include bronchoalveolar lung, papillary thyroid, mucosa-associated lymphoid tissue (MALT) and other low-grade lymphomas, renal cell cancers, lower-grade prostate cancers, hepatomas, neuroendocrine tumors, and mucinous colorectal and ovarian tumors.
- For some of these tumor types, FDG-PET may be attempted for staging, but if the tumor proves to be nonavid, restaging PET exams are generally not performed unless there is reason to believe the tumor has transformed to a more aggressive form.
- These non–FDG-avid tumors are then followed with diagnostic CT only.

Other Imaging Findings

- Anatomic imaging with CT or MRI is used in conjunction with PET for staging and restaging.
- Bone scan can assess for bone metastatic disease even for non–FDG-avid tumors like prostate cancer (assesses bone remodeling even from non–FDG-avid metastases).
- ProstaScint can be used to assess for prostate cancer soft-tissue lesions, which are often not FDG-avid.
- Other PET tracers are in development that measure factors like tumor cellular proliferation (as opposed to glucose hypermetabolism) and can detect non–FDG-avid lesions (e.g., F18-fluorothymidine [FLT]).

✓ Pearls & × Pitfalls

✓ Any enlarging lesion on CT (e.g., lymph node, hepatic lesion, lung nodule) should be viewed with suspicion for tumor/progression even if negative on FDG-PET.

✓ Despite the nonavidity for FDG of some tumors, the vast majority are FDG-avid, and adding PET to CT for staging and restaging increases accuracy by approximately one-third.

✓ Edema/fluid overload can also lead to enlarged, non–FDG-avid lymph nodes.

× Just as not all malignancies are FDG-avid, not all FDG-avid neoplasms are malignant. As examples, benign adenomas of adrenal, colonic, or hepatic origin can occasionally be markedly FDG-avid.

× Benign granulomatous diseases such as sarcoidosis typically appear as enlarged lymph nodes that *are* significantly FDG-avid.

× Baseline FDG-PET should be performed *before* implementation of any therapy to determine if the tumor is FDG-avid and can be followed with PET.

Case 88

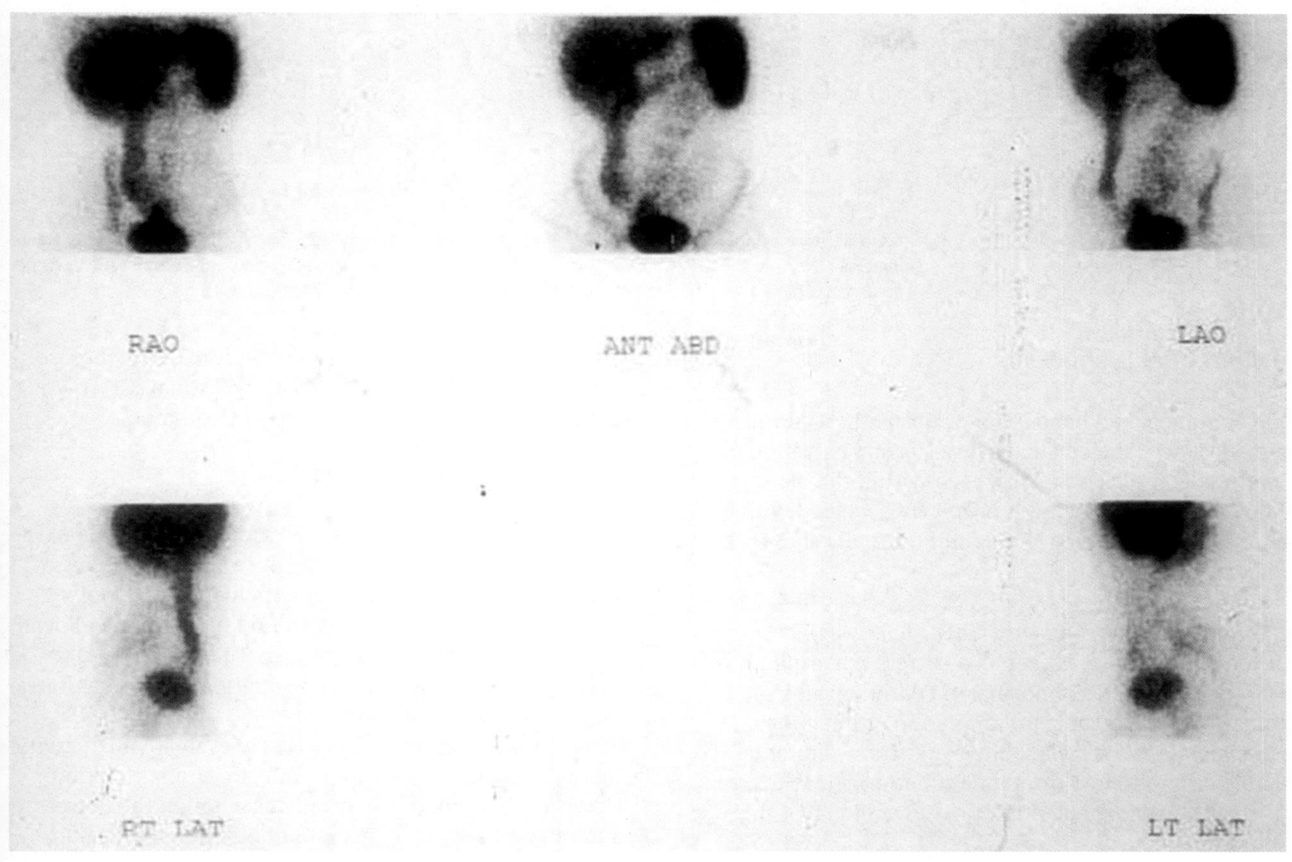

Clinical Presentation

A 32-year-old woman with abdominal pain, fever, and diarrhea.

Imaging Findings

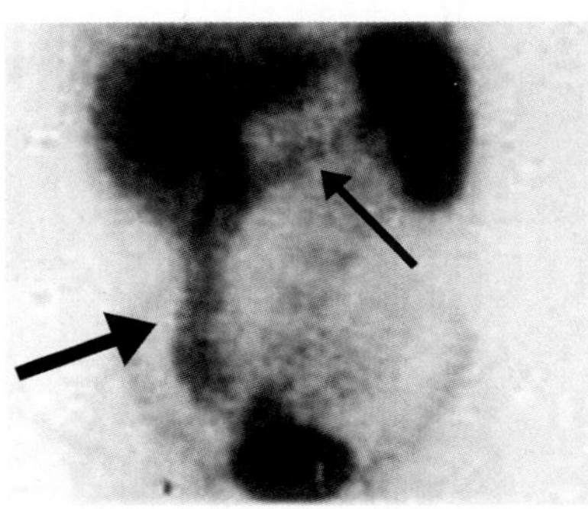

Multiple static images from a Tc99m-HMPAO (Ceretec) WBC study were obtained 30 minutes after tracer injection. Normal activity is seen within spleen, liver, bone marrow, and bladder. Abnormal WBC accumulation is seen to involve a long segment of the right and transverse colon (*arrows*).

Differential Diagnosis

The liver, spleen, and bone marrow normally accumulate Tc99m-HMPAO–labeled leukocytes. Normal excretion of technetium complexes are also seen within the bladder and bowel on *later* imaging (unlike WBCs labeled with indium 111-oxine, which should not normally show bladder/bowel excretion).

- ***Inflammatory bowel disease (IBD):*** Tc99m-HMPAO–labeled WBC activity is seen in a pattern corresponding to large bowel that is abnormal (on early imaging) and compatible with colonic inflammation or infection.
- *Pseudomembranous colitis:* Bowel infection cannot be reliably differentiated from inflammation on WBC scan. A history of prolonged antibiotic use would favor this diagnosis.
- *Gastrointestinal bleeding:* This can look similar to IBD if active. Tracer will move over time if sequential images are obtained.

Essential Facts

- Tc99m-HMPAO and In111-oxine–labeled leukocytes are both acceptable for evaluating IBD.
- Tc99m-HMPAO has the advantage of earlier imaging (can begin by 20 minutes), shorter imaging times due to the higher dose used, and a lower patient radiation exposure than In111 (due to shorter physical half-life).
- Physiologic Tc99m-HMPAO excretion into the bowel can be seen by as early as 1 hour in children and by 4 hours in adults, which is a disadvantage compared with In111.
- In111-labeled leukocytes are not normally excreted into the bowel or bladder, which is an advantage over Tc99m-HMPAO.
- With In111, imaging is usually performed 24 hours after injection, although imaging as early as 4 hours may be performed in an acute setting (e.g., abdominal abscess) or to determine the location of IBD (before the inflamed mucosal cells with labeled WBCs slough off and move distally).
- The intensity and extent of WBC uptake correlate with findings seen on histology and endoscopy.
- Both ulcerative colitis (UC) and Crohn disease can be evaluated. UC involvement begins at the rectum and proceeds proximally without skip lesion. Crohn disease can affect any portion of the gastrointestinal (GI) tract, with terminal ileal involvement most common.

Other Imaging Findings

- Endoscopy (capsule or direct) provides visualization of the GI tract but may not be possible in severely ill patients. WBC scan can guide endoscopic evaluation and biopsy.
- CT and MRI can detect IBD with findings including bowel thickening, enhancement, stenosis, "creeping fat," and fistulae. However, WBC scan is superior for demonstrating current disease activity.
- FDG-PET is also emerging as a tool to evaluate IBD activity.
- Gallium can also detect active infection/inflammation. However, as gallium is normally excreted in the bowel and imaging may take up to 48 hours, it is not ideal for evaluating IBD.
- US can also be used to evaluate for bowel thickening with IBD, especially in the pediatric population.

✓ Pearls & × Pitfalls

✓ Normal biodistribution showing spleen > liver and bone marrow activity makes a WBC scan likely (see "Interpreting Whole-Body Scans").

✓ Uptake can be contiguous or multifocal with IBD. Scintigraphy can be used to evaluate the response to anti-inflammatory therapy.

✓ Bowel preparation is not required, and the study can be performed in very ill patients.

× Swallowed WBCs from an upper respiratory infection can cause a false-positive exam for GI disease.

× Accessory splenic tissue can simulate bowel uptake.

× Infectious diseases such as pseudomembranous colitis as well as bowel infarction cannot be differentiated from IBD on WBC imaging.

× Neutropenia can decrease the sensitivity of the exam. A granulocyte count of $> 2 \times 10^6$ cell/mL is recommended for adequate labeling.

× Excreted bladder activity seen with Tc99m-HMPAO labeling can obscure rectal disease. Postvoid, posterior, or lateral imaging may be useful.

× Rarely, some tumors (e.g., melanoma) will also accumulate labeled leukocytes.

Case 89

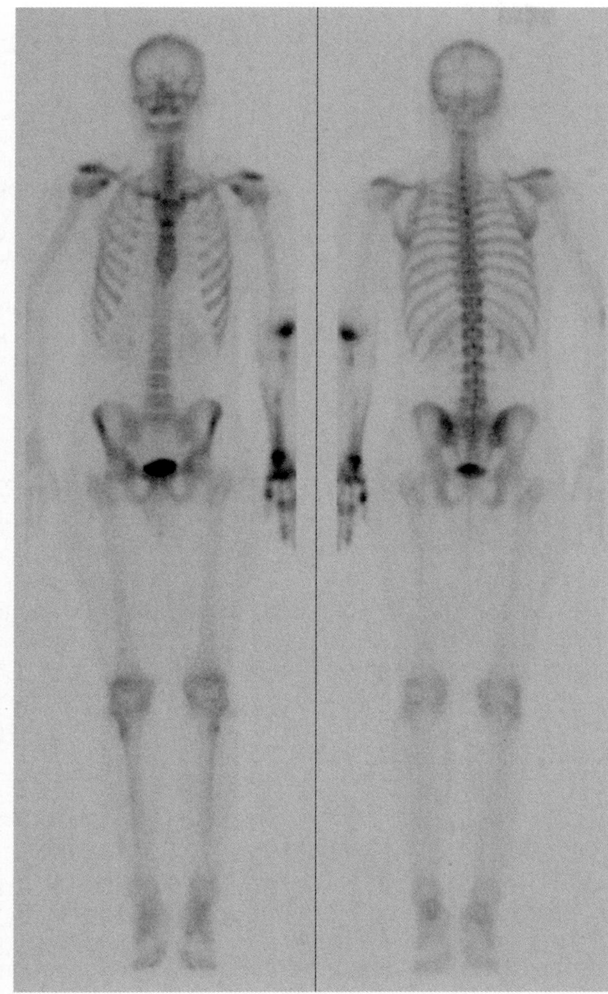

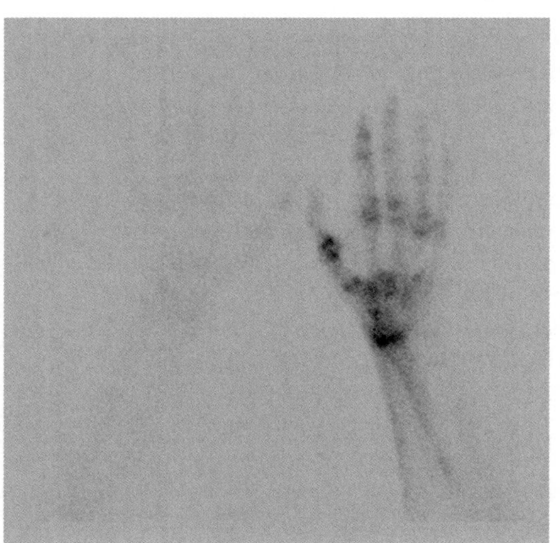

B

Clinical Presentation

A 20-year-old man with a history of left tibial plateau stress fracture to confirm healing.

Imaging Findings

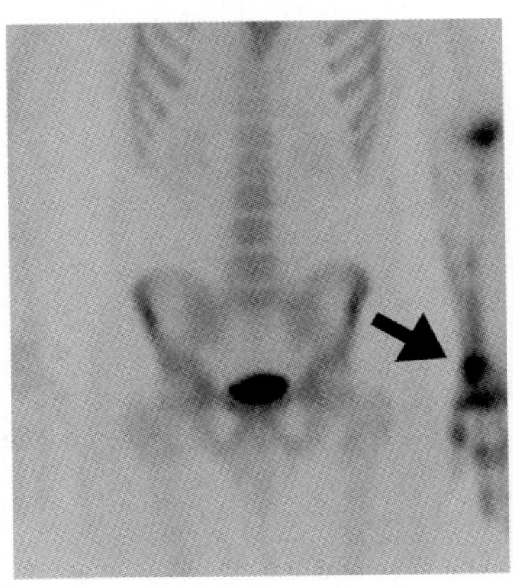

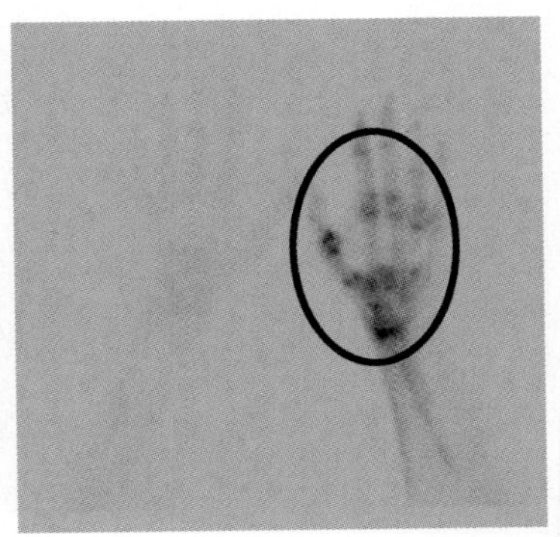

(A) Three-hour–delayed anterior and posterior whole-body bone scan image demonstrates focal uptake involving the left distal radius, wrist, and hand (*arrow*). Uptake is also noted in the left antecubital region, as well as possible skin uptake on the left arm. No tibial plateau uptake is evident, suggesting completion of fracture healing. **(B)** Spot views of both hands demonstrate increased radiopharmaceutical uptake in the distal radius as well as multiple bones diffusely in the left hand and wrist, most pronounced along the radial aspect (*circle*).

Differential Diagnosis

- ***Inadvertent radial artery injection of the radiopharmaceutical:*** Distribution of the radiopharmaceutical is most consistent with radial artery injection, which involves the radial side of the forearm, wrist, and thumb through fourth finger.
- *Reflex sympathetic dystrophy:* This is less likely, given that the radiopharmaceutical does not involve the fifth digit or the ulnar aspect of the palm and wrist. Also, the skin uptake does not support it.
- *Arthritic changes:* This is unlikely for an inflammatory or osteoarthritis as the distribution in this case is both proximal and distal and not confined to the joints.

Essential Facts

- Radial artery injection is a technical error by the nuclear medicine technologist. Typically, this error is made by technology students, as in this case, or other inexperienced individuals.
- It most likely occurs in the radial artery distribution, given the typical attempted injection into the adjacent cephalic vein along the radial side of the wrist.
- Tracer distribution on a bone scan is determined by both regional tracer delivery (regional blood flow or tracer concentration) and osteoblastic activity.
- The significant first-pass osseous extraction of the highly concentrated tracer gives this characteristic appearance on bone scan.
- The patient may feel warmth and tingling during the injection and bright arterial blood may be encountered, but there is otherwise no associated patient morbidity (injection site compression is recommended to avoid a hematoma).

Other Imaging Findings

- Similar findings can occur at the ankle and foot if an inadvertent arterial injection is made in the lower extremity.
- The remainder of the bone scan is usually diagnostic, and unless the symptoms involve the affected extremity, no repeat bone scan is typically necessary.

✓ Pearls & ✗ Pitfalls

✓ If the radiopharmaceutical distribution is not classic for arterial injection (i.e., most pronounced on the radial side of the hand), consider other etiologies, such as reflex sympathetic dystrophy, which has more diffuse periarticular involvement.

✓ Interviewing the technologist and patient for symptoms experienced during the injection can often help confirm the suspicion of arterial injection.

✗ If the clinical problem involves the extremity where an arterial injection was made, a repeat study (venous injection and imaging) should be performed after 48 hours. Here is a repeat scan (normal venous injection) from this same patient 1 week later, confirming no osteoblastic abnormality of the hands:

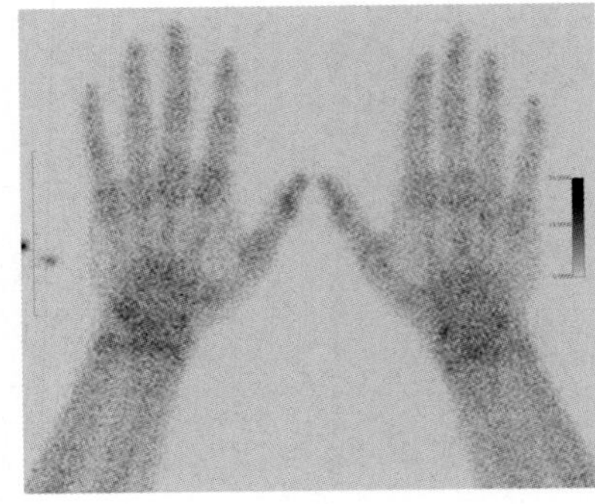

Case 90

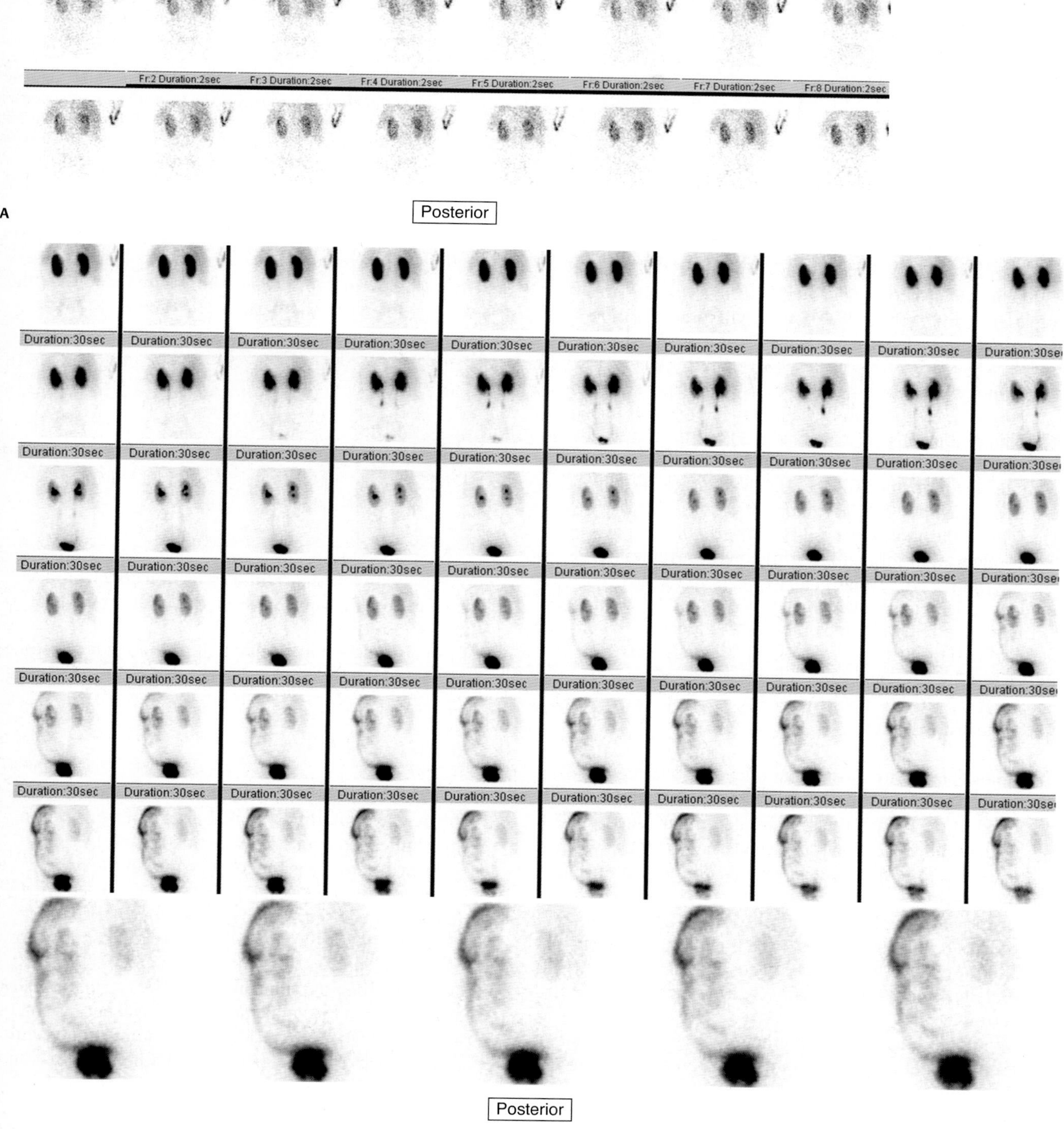

Clinical Presentation

32-year-old woman with left flank pain persisting after a hysterectomy. CT of the abdomen revealed ascites.

Imaging Findings

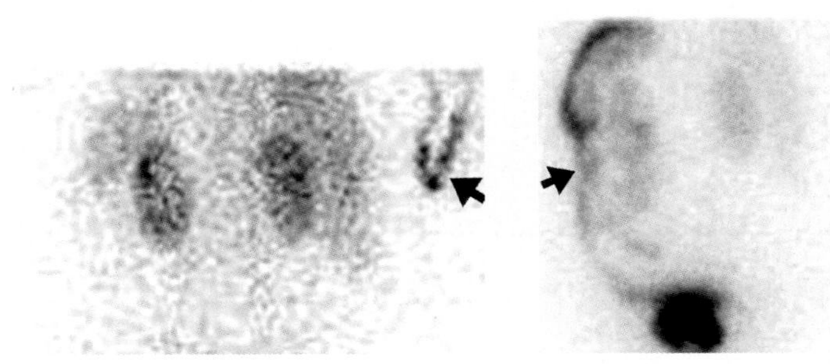

(A) Posterior dynamic Tc99m-MAG3 images reveal normal symmetric radiotracer flow and parenchymal extraction by both kidneys. Activity seen along the right side of the body is due to some persistent radiotracer at the injection site (*arrow*). **(B)** Dynamic images reveal normal radiotracer excretion and clearance from both kidneys, indicating normal function. However, abnormal radiotracer activity is seen outside the urinary tract, extending from the left side of the bladder along the left abdomen (*arrow*). This activity progresses along the left paracolic gutter and terminates superior to the spleen.

Differential Diagnosis

Tc99m-MAG3 activity outside the urinary system in a patient with a recent history of pelvic surgery is most compatible with a urinary leak.

- ***Urinary leak:*** Review of the dynamic images show abnormal activity extending along the left side of the abdomen that begins near the bladder. Locating the site of the leak may be difficult scintigraphically, but in this case the site was confirmed to be at the distal ureter.
- *Urinary enteric fistula:* Abnormal activity will also be seen in the abdominal cavity. However, it will have a configuration compatible with bowel (intraluminal).
- *Alternative physiologic biliary excretion of MAG3:* This can be seen on delayed images but should be within the biliary system only (including gallbladder) and eventually within bowel.

Essential Facts

- Ureteral leaks are most commonly due to iatrogenic injury. Trauma and obstruction are other etiologies.
- Leaks at the renal level are most commonly due to trauma; however, they can also be seen after transplant or be due to obstruction. Iatrogenic injury is an uncommon cause.
- Urinary bladder leaks are most commonly seen after trauma or pelvic fractures. Most are extraperitoneal.
- Aspiration of a fluid collection suspicious for urinary leak will demonstrate an elevated creatinine compared with serum levels.
- Minor leaks may resolve on their own or with the placement of stents. More severe leaks may require surgical intervention.

Other Imaging Findings

- On scintigraphy, a renal leak will typically appear as a photopenic region around the kidney, which fills in with radiotracer over time.
- Intravenous pyelography has a sensitivity of only 30% in detecting renal leaks.
- Retrograde pyelography can demonstrate the level of the leak, as seen in this same patient (*arrow*):

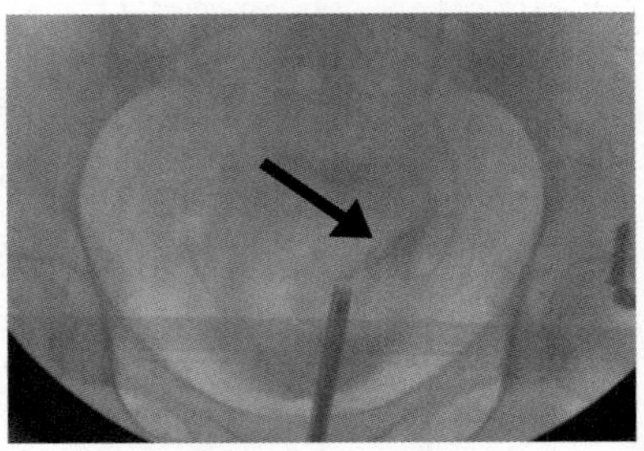

- US is useful in locating a fluid collection and may raise the concern for a leak. However, it cannot prove that the fluid represents leaked urine.
- CT can also show nonspecific fluid, although it can sometimes show the precise level of the leak.

✓ Pearls & × Pitfalls

✓ Contrast-enhanced CT is the most sensitive test for the diagnosis of urinary leak. Delayed imaging out to 20 minutes after contrast injection is useful.

✓ Renal scintigraphy is the test of choice if the patient cannot receive contrast. DTPA or MAG3 labeled with Tc99m can be used. MAG3 is superior, particularly if renal function is diminished, but is significantly more expensive.

× On delayed scintigraphic imaging, MAG3 can normally appear within the gallbladder and bowel because of alternative biliary excretion, which should not be confused with a urinary leak or other pathology. This is *not* seen with DTPA.

× Abnormal tracer seen before 2.5 minutes cannot represent a urinary leak given that radiolabeled urine is not yet formed.

Case 91

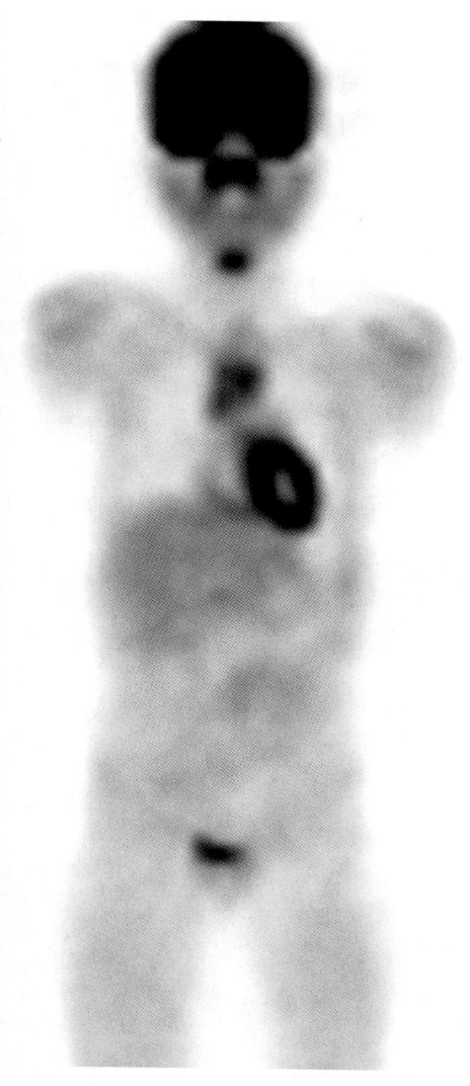

A

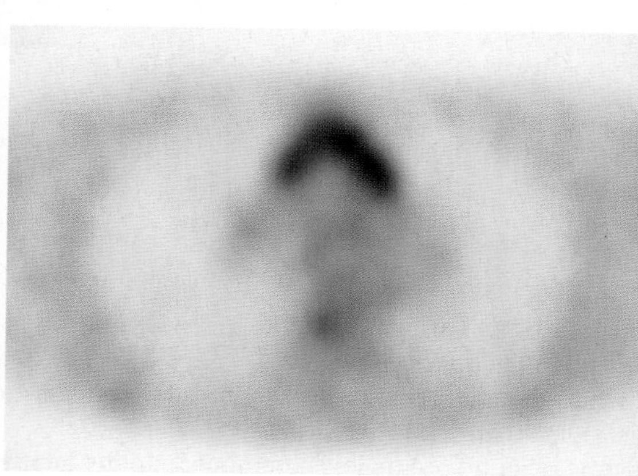

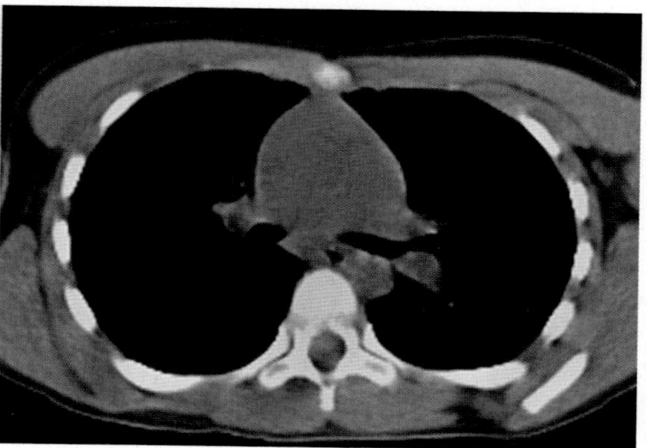

B

Clinical Presentation

A 9-year-old girl with lymphoma presents for restaging 6 months after chemotherapy.

Imaging Findings

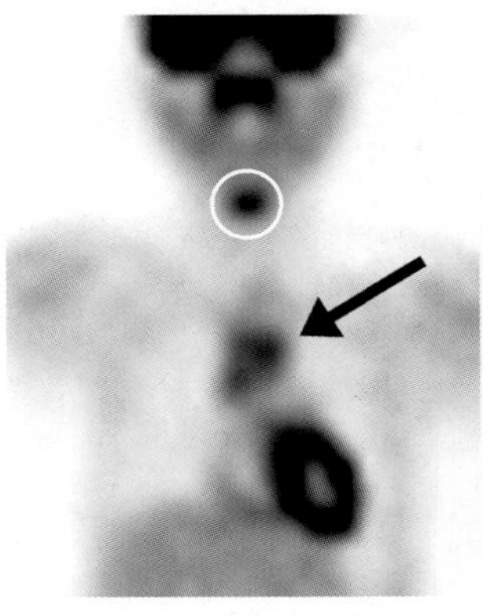

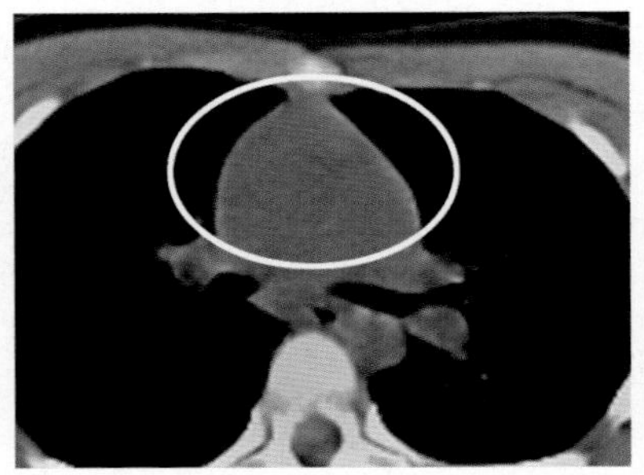

(A) A whole-body FDG-PET coronal image demonstrates hypermetabolic focus in the superior mediastinum (*arrow*). Physiologic laryngeal activity is noted in the midline nec (*circle*). **(B)** Axial registered PET/CT images demonstrat a sail-shaped focus of uniformly increased uptake in th anterior superior mediastinum in the location of the thymu (*circle*).

Differential Diagnosis

- ***Benign thymic hyperplasia:*** Uniformly increased thymic uptake in a child following chemotherapy makes "thymic rebound" the most likely diagnosis.
- *Recurrent lymphoma:* This should also be considered but is typically more nodular and masslike.
- *Germ cell tumor:* This is also a consideration but is also usually more irregular and may have varying density like calcification on CT.

Essential Facts

- Benign thymic hyperplasia is caused when the thymus "rebounds" in size following atrophy from severe illness, steroids, or most commonly chemotherapy.
- It is seen in children and young adults, with the hyperplasia usually occurring within 1 year following chemotherapy.
- During this time, the thymus increases in size and becomes avid for FDG (and gallium).
- Although some studies have shown that a higher thymic SUV on PET increases the likelihood a thymic lesion is malignant, there is considerable overlap with benign hyperplasia. Anatomic features on CT (see subsequent images) are likely more reliable.
- Thymic rebound is asymptomatic, and no therapy is necessary.

Other Imaging Findings

- Chest radiography does not usually demonstrate the enlarged thymus, except in very young children if the thymus becomes very large.
- Gallium scan will show similar thymic uptake with hyperplasia following chemotherapy, steroids, or illness.
- CT may be useful to further characterize and will show regular, straight, or slightly convex thymic margins for hyperplasia and irregular, densely enhancing, or asymmetric margins for tumor.
- Here is the PET/CT in another patient with anterior mediastinal lymphoma. Note the more nodular appearance on both the PET and CT portions:

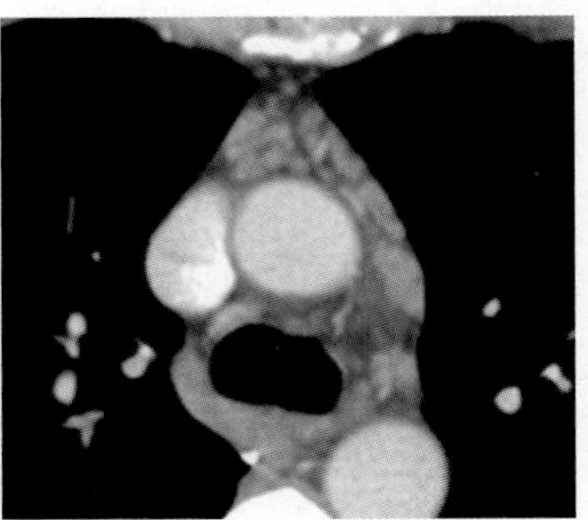

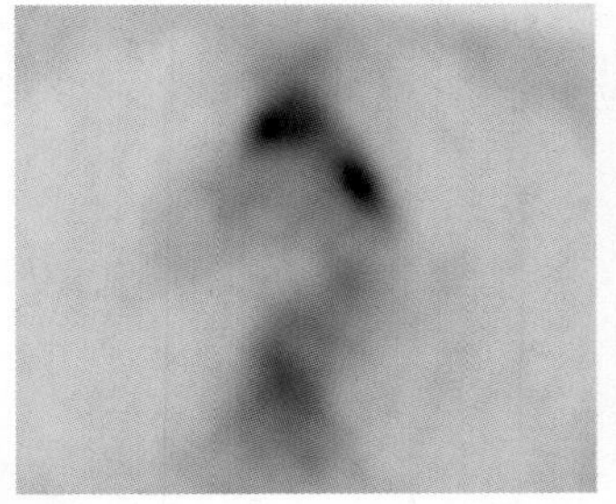

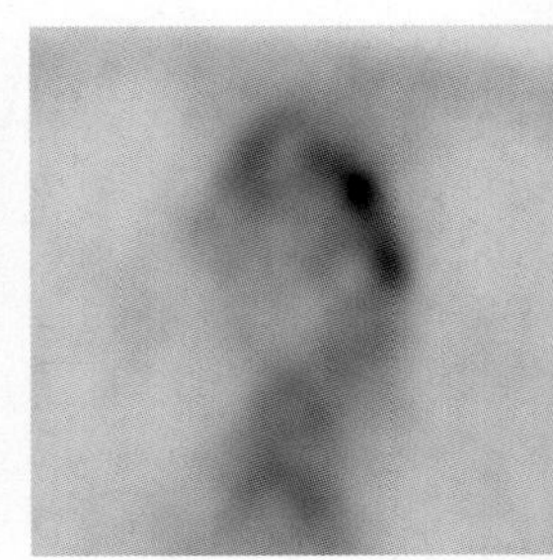

- MRI can demonstrate chemical shift in benign thymic hyperplasia (which is fat-containing).

✓ Pearls & ✗ Pitfalls

✓ The thymus will often rebound to a size significantly larger than its original size.

✓ Thymic rebound occurs more rapidly following cessatio of steroids than with chemotherapy.

✗ Thymic rebound occurs less commonly in older adults. If the patient is older than 30 years, suspicion should b higher for tumor.

Case 92

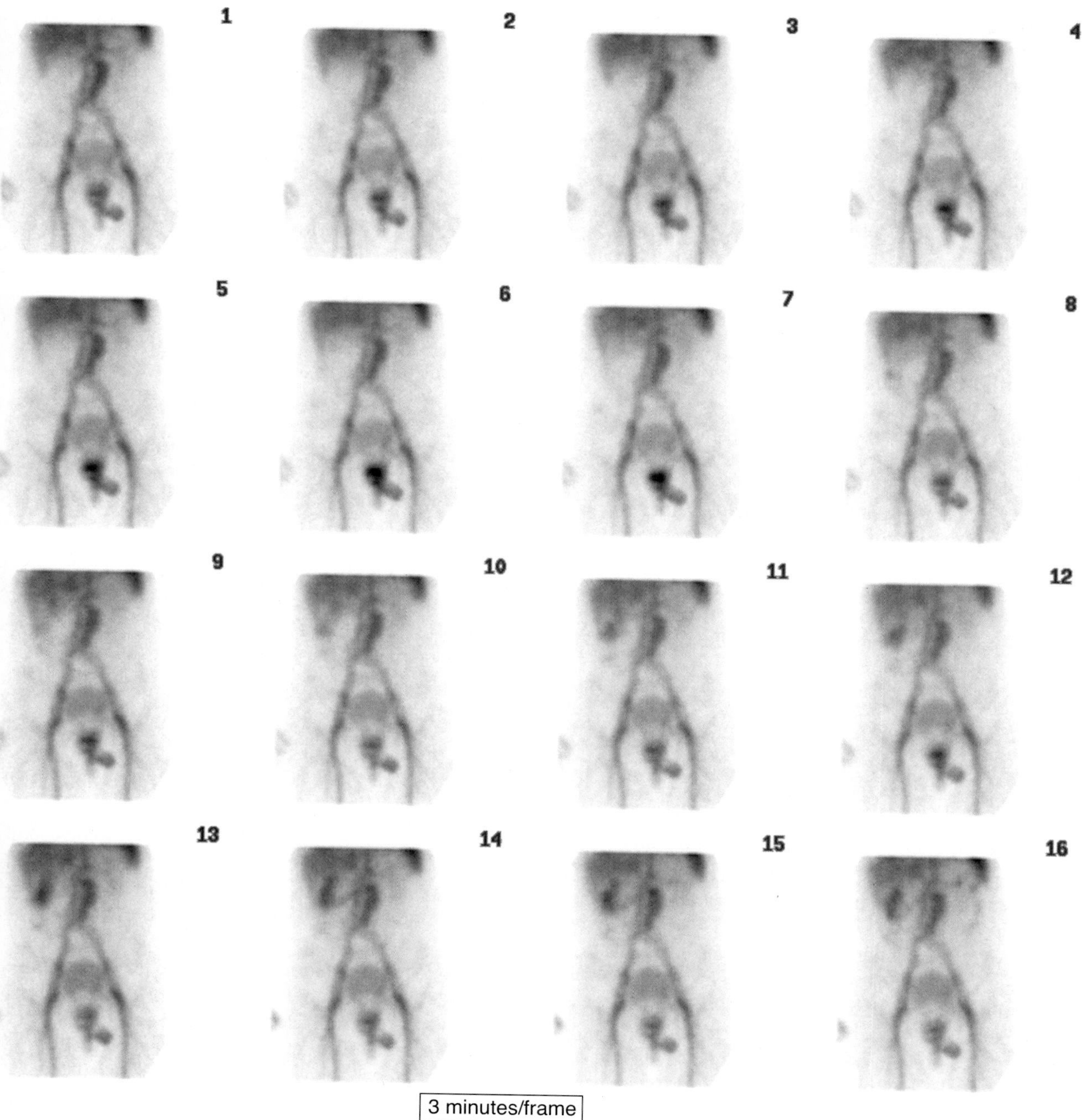

Clinical Presentation

History withheld.

Imaging Findings

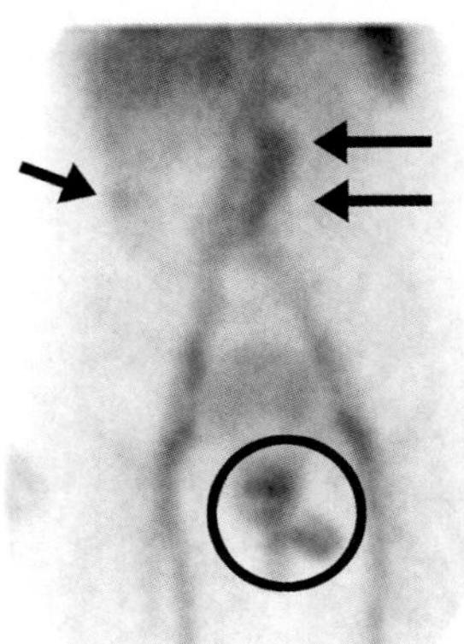

Sequential images acquired immediately following injection of Tc99m-labeled RBCs demonstrate an abnormal focus appearing in the right mid abdomen (*single arrow*). Over time, this becomes tubular, moving to the right upper quadrant and across to the left abdomen. Also noted is aneurysmal dilatation of the distal abdominal aorta (*double arrows*) as well as physiologic tubular activity in the corpora cavernosa of the penis (*circle*).

Differential Diagnosis

- ***Active colonic hemorrhage:*** Given the peripheral location and large caliber, this is the most likely etiology for the abnormal tubular activity.
- *Small-bowel bleed:* This is usually of smaller caliber and located more centrally in the abdomen. It typically migrates from the left upper to the right lower quadrant.
- *Vascular intraperitoneal tumor:* Vascular (even nonhemorrhagic) lesions can appear as an abnormal focus on RBC scan because of increased circulating RBCs. However, they do not move over time.

Essential Facts

- Etiologies for lower gastrointestinal (GI) hemorrhage include angiodysplasia, diverticula, polyps, and neoplasm.
- Colonoscopy can identify many lower GI bleeds. However, bleeding can be occult in small bowel and even in colon. Bleeding can also be difficult to assess via colonoscopy if briskly active.
- Labeled RBC imaging can identify and localize an active GI bleed, with an imaging window of several hours.
- Normal intense RBC accumulation on an RBC scan includes "blood pool" spaces: larger vessels, cardiac chambers, diffuse spleen (red pulp), and penis (corpora cavernosa) activity. Additionally, some urinary excretion of free radiotracer often yields bladder activity.
- Criteria for calling a GI bleed are (1) abnormal activity in (2) a tubular configuration that (3) moves over time.

Other Imaging Findings

- Catheter angiography can be used to confirm and better localize bleeding as well as provide embolization therapy. However, sensitivity for detecting an active bleed is lower (need 1–2 mL/min as opposed to 0.2 mL/min for RBC scan), and the timing window for bleed activity is only seconds (vs. hours for RBC scan).
- CTA is also emerging as a sensitive noninvasive tool and unlike RBC scintigraphy may not require the bleed to be active to localize.
- Tc99m-SCOL has also been used, but clearance of tracer from the blood pool in 15 to 20 minutes makes the imaging window small for detecting active hemorrhage.

✓ Pearls & ✗ Pitfalls

- ✓ When possible, always look at the dynamic cine images instead of static captures. This improves sensitivity and specificity.
- ✓ Angiographic images (within the first 60 seconds) from an RBC scan can be useful to localize a very rapid bleed or detect the *source* of a bleed (e.g., identify the perfusion "blush" of a colonic tumor), even if it is not actively bleeding.
- ✓ If initially negative, delayed RBC imaging can be useful to document interval, intermittent bleeding. However, as GI blood can move forward and backward, accurate localization is usually not possible on these more delayed images.
- ✓ A lateral and/or posterior view can be useful to differentiate rectal bleed from normal bladder or penis (rectal bleed is posterior on lateral view and becomes hotter on posterior view—opposite for penile activity).
- ✗ Variceal and collateral vessels can be abnormal and tubular but will not continuously move over time.
- ✗ Arteriovenous malformations and vascular tumors can be visualized as an abnormal hot focus even if not actively bleeding but also will not move over time.
- ✗ Hepatic hemangiomas can be seen as a focal lesion on more delayed RBC imaging. Accessory spleens can also be seen, typically in the left upper quadrant.

Case 93

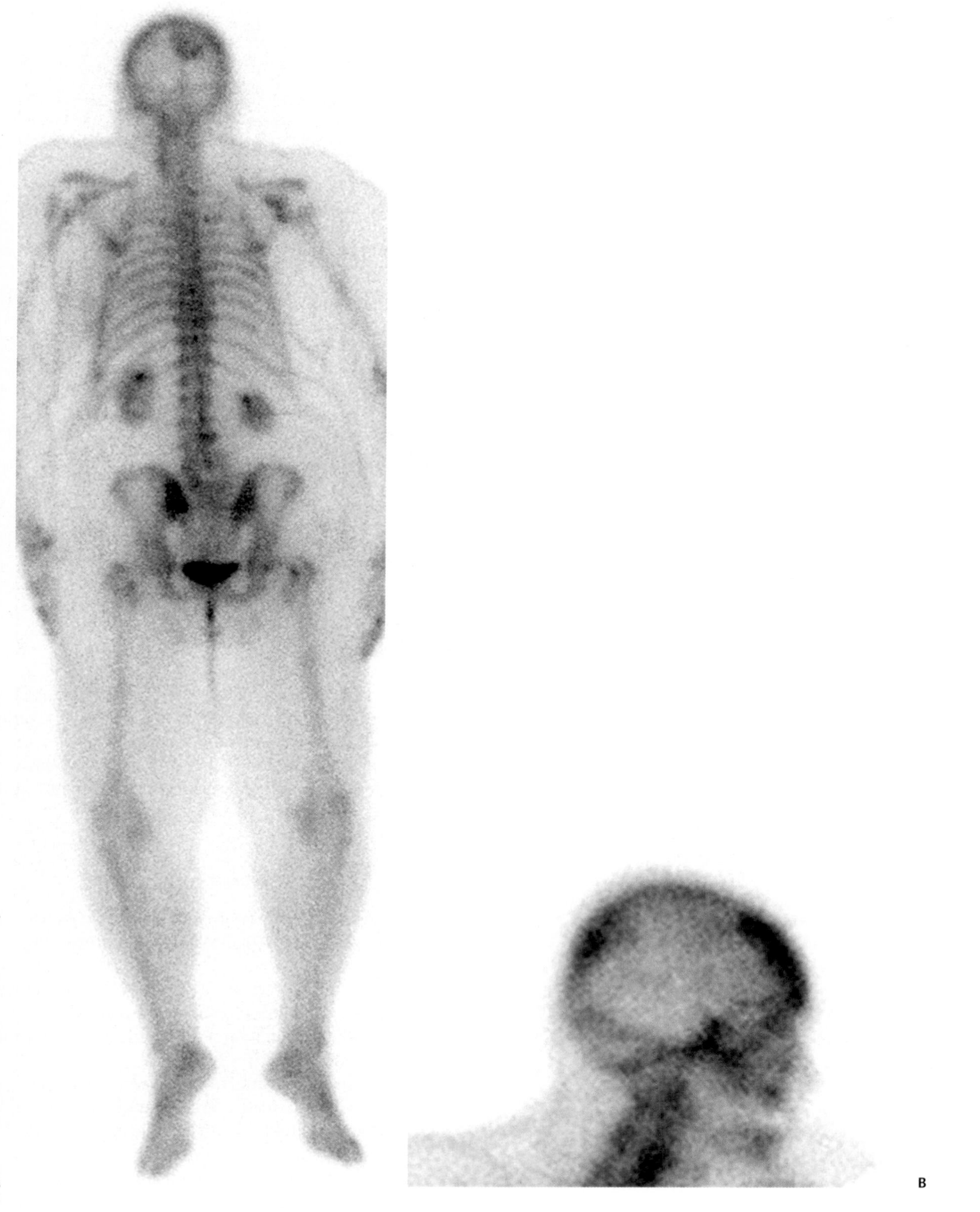

Clinical Presentation

A 74-year-old woman with newly diagnosed breast cancer. What is the most likely etiology for the appearance of the skull?

Imaging Findings

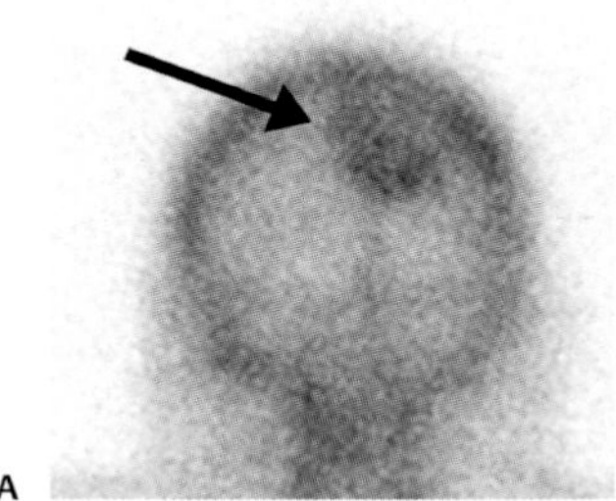
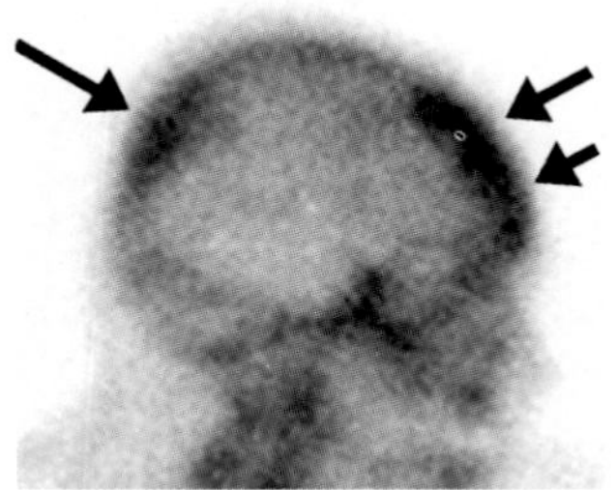

(A,B) Posterior image from a Tc99m-MDP whole-body bone scan reveals a large, round focus of increased tracer uptake in the right posterior parietal region (*long arrow*, A). This can be seen posteriorly on the right lateral spot view as well (*short arrow*, B). Tracer uptake in the frontal skull is typical for benign hyperostosis (*double arrows*, B). Degenerative uptake is seen in the right shoulder, lower lumbar spine, and hips.

Differential Diagnosis

Tracer uptake in the region of the skull is difficult to evaluate on planar imaging because such uptake cannot always be differentiated from soft-tissue uptake in the adjacent brain.

- ***Intracranial soft-tissue uptake:*** This can be difficult to differentiate from bone uptake on planar images without SPECT. However, solitary skull region uptake is not uncommonly due to intracranial pathology (benign or malignant), which should be considered before the lesion is called a skull metastasis.
- *Skull metastasis:* This could have an identical appearance on planar imaging. SPECT could be used to assess if the lesion is osseous or involves the intracranial soft tissues.
- *Craniotomy defects:* These will also appear as round skull foci but are most commonly increased only at the periphery (ring).

Essential Facts

- Solitary "skull" uptake on bone scan is not uncommonly due to intracranial soft-tissue pathology, including benign and malignant tumors and prior brain infarcts.
- Soft-tissue uptake of bone tracer is due to calcium deposition within the tissues. Disruption of the blood–brain barrier is required for intracranial soft-tissue uptake of bone agents.
- Meningiomas are one of the most common of such lesions and are usually encountered incidentally on bone scan.
- Meningiomas are the most common primary intracranial tumor in adults (15% of tumors). More than 90% are supratentorial.
- Most are asymptomatic (> 90%) and benign. Malignant meningiomas are less common.
- They are typically seen in middle age, somewhat more commonly in women and African Americans.
- Treatment is surveillance for the typical asymptomatic lesion. Symptomatic or malignant lesions can be resected.

Other Imaging Findings

- Bone scan SPECT imaging can differentiate osseous skull uptake from intracranial soft-tissue uptake.
- With meningiomas, CT and MRI will demonstrate a densely enhancing extra-axial lesion. Here is this same patient's MRI demonstrating the meningioma (*arrow*):

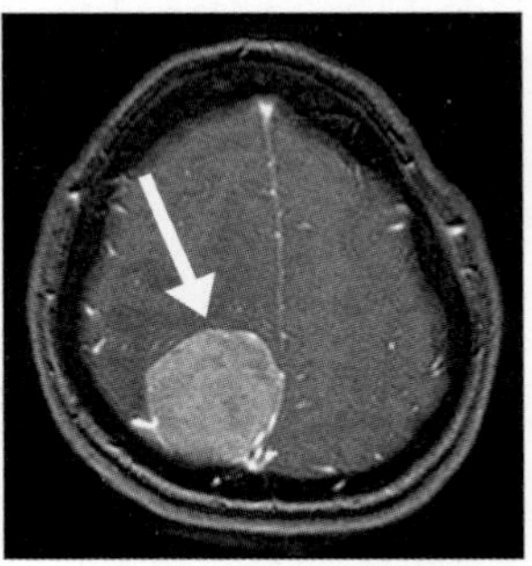

- FDG-PET demonstrates absent or only mildly increased uptake with benign meningiomas but can show markedly increased uptake with malignant meningiomas.
- Octreotide imaging can be used to evaluate and follow up meningiomas because nearly all express somatostatin receptors.

✓ Pearls & × Pitfalls

✓ A solitary skull focus in a patient with known cancer has an approximately 50% likelihood of representing a bone metastasis.

✓ Other causes of intracranial soft-tissue focal uptake that can simulate a skull lesion on bone scan include brain metastases, prior brain infarct, calcified aneurysms, and dural calcifications.

✓ Soft-tissue uptake in tumors can be seen elsewhere on whole-body bone scan (e.g., primary breast tumor, neuroblastoma in children, testicular seminoma, and liver metastases).

× Paget disease can commonly mimic bone metastases anywhere. In the skull, Paget disease can appear similar to the uptake on this patient's image, with a large round region of uptake (osteoporosis circumscripta).

Case 94

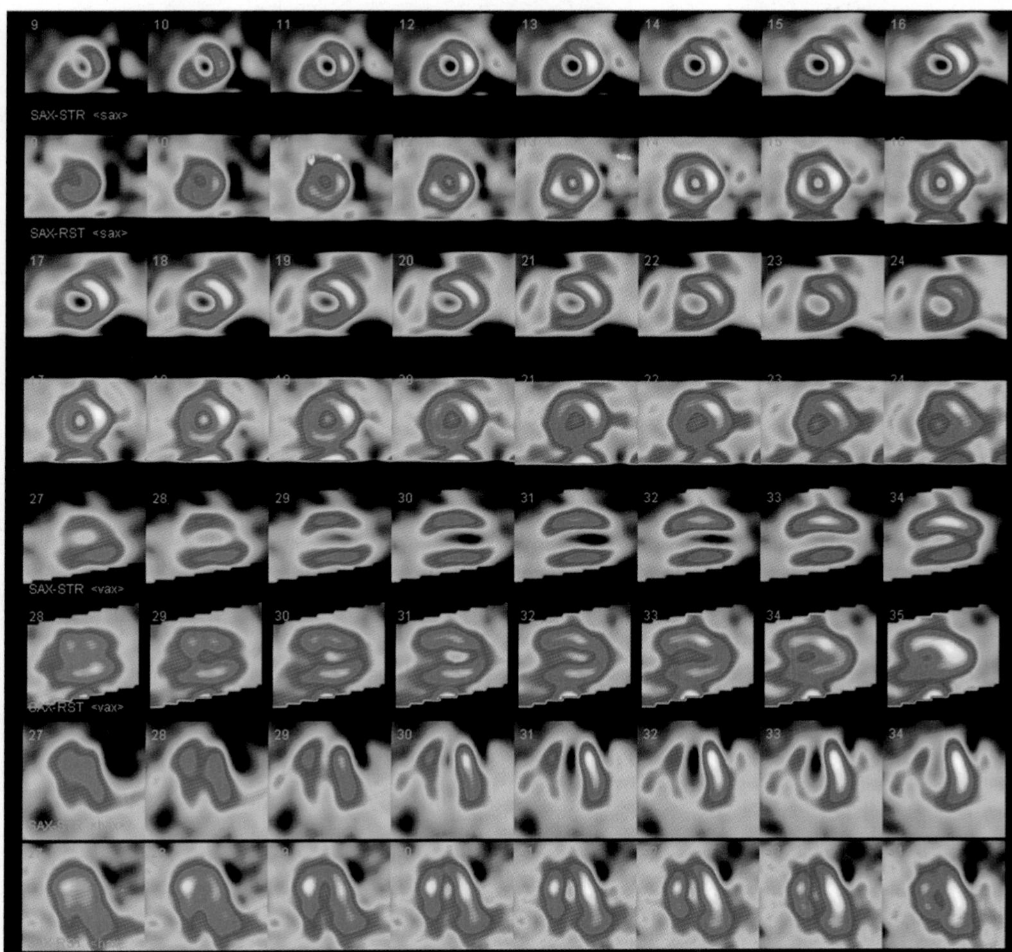

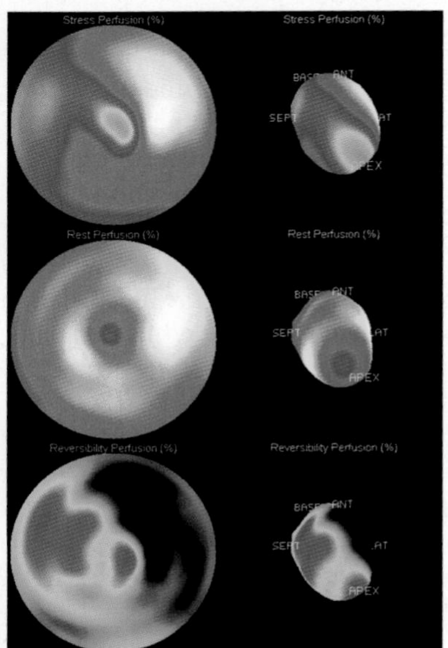

Clinical Presentation

A 64-year-old woman with chest pain on exertion.

Imaging Findings

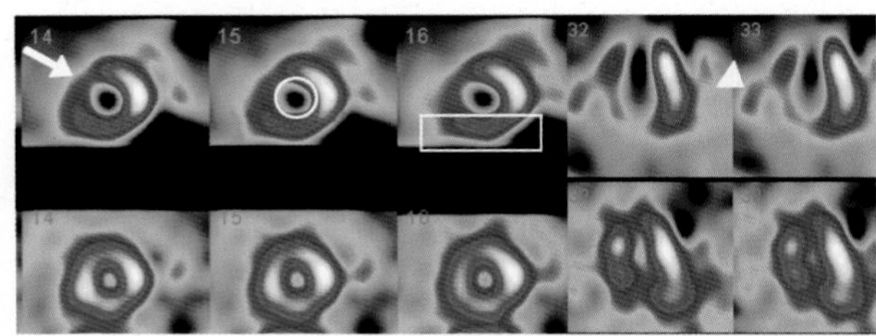

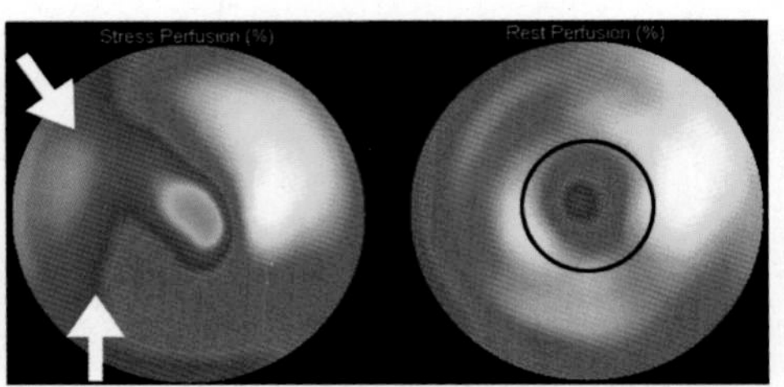

A B

(A) Rest and stress myocardial perfusion scintigraphy demonstrates a large, severe, almost completely reversible perfusion defect in the anteroseptal and apical segments (left anterior descending territory; *arrow*) with a moderate, completely reversible defect in the inferior wall (right coronary territory; *rectangle*). Additionally, increased right ventricular (RV) uptake (*arrowhead*) and an increase in left ventricular (LV) chamber size ("transient ischemic dilation"; *circle*) are seen at stress. **(B)** Rest and stress polar maps and surface renderings display the same nearly completely reversible abnormalities (*arrows*). A small apical perfusion defect persists at rest (*circle*).

Differential Diagnosis

- ***Reversible ischemia in the left anterior descending (LAD) artery and right coronary artery (RCA) territories:*** Reversible perfusion defects indicate that this is the most likely diagnosis. (The small fixed apical component may represent a small superimposed infarct.)
- *Shifting breast artifact:* This can occasionally simulate reversible LAD artery disease. However, it would not affect the inferior wall.
- *Diaphragmatic creep artifact:* This can simulate reversible RCA disease. However, it would not affect the anterior wall. It is rarely encountered with current imaging protocols.

Essential Facts

- Myocardial perfusion–gated SPECT imaging (myocardial perfusion imaging [MPI] or myocardial perfusion SPECT) has emerged as a reliable noninvasive method for detecting patients with significant coronary artery disease (CAD).
- Such disease may be symptomatic and indicate myocardial tissue at risk for infarct. MPI indentifies patients for whom angiography and possible intervention may be warranted.
- Patients are imaged at rest and then post stress with one of several perfusion tracers (thallium 201 and/or Tc99m-labeled MIBI or TETRO).
- Stress can be exercise (with a target heart rate [HR] > 85% of 220 minus patient's age) or chemical with dobutamine (same target HR) or adenosine/regadenoson (no target HR because they are direct vasodilators). Dipyridamole has a similar effect to that of adenosine/regadenoson but has been largely replaced by these agents.
- A reversible perfusion defect (defect on stress only) indicates ischemia (narrowed coronaries), whereas a persistent defect at stress and rest indicates infarct.
- Gated imaging is also typically performed with MPI to assess for regional wall motion (WM) abnormalities and global left ventricular ejection fraction (LVEF); reversible ischemia has normal WM on MPI; infarct has abnormal regional WM; normal LVEF > 50%.

Other Imaging Findings

- Stress electrocardiography (which can be performed alone or in conjunction with MPI) can identify ST-segment depression during stress-induced ischemia but is less sensitive than MPI.
- Stress cardiac echo identifies abnormal WM at peak stress in patients with reversible ischemia but is also less sensitive than MPI.
- Cardiac *perfusion* PET (with rubidium 82 or N13-ammonia can be performed at rest and during pharmacologic stress to identify infarct and ischemia with more accuracy (PET routinely utilizes attenuation correction and has better image spatial resolution than SPECT).
- CTA and catheter coronary angiography can confirm significant coronary disease; angioplasty/stenting can be performed during catheter studies for therapy.

✓ Pearls & × Pitfalls

- ✓ Most centers use MIBI or TETRO at stress and Tl201 or MIBI/TETRO at rest. Tl201 has significantly higher patient radiation and poorer image quality but can be used for redistribution imaging if there is a resting perfusion defect to assess for possible viability (see Case 5).
- ✓ Exercise and chemical stress provide equivalent exam sensitivity for CAD. Adenosine is contraindicated with active bronchospasm and heart block, and its vasodilator effects are inhibited by caffeine or similar drugs, which can result in false-negative studies. Regadenoson is a newer, similar agent causing less bronchospasm.
- ✓ Aminophylline can be given to reverse unwanted effects of dipyridamole/regadenoson (e.g., heart block, patient symptoms). It is generally not needed with adenosine, given the very short biologic half-life of adenosine (can just stop giving adenosine).
- × Like any SPECT, MPI demonstrates *relative* perfusion, so balanced triple-vessel disease may appear normal at rest and stress. Transient ischemic dilation and/or increased RV uptake at stress are clues that this may be present (or that there is more severe underlying disease), as seen in this case. These ancillary findings are more specific with exercise stress than with adenosine/regadenoson, however.
- × Increased pulmonary tracer uptake at rest and stress indicates resting LV dysfunction (or pulmonary inflammation). Increased pulmonary uptake only at stress suggests stress-induced LV dysfunction and likely significant underlying CAD.

Case 95

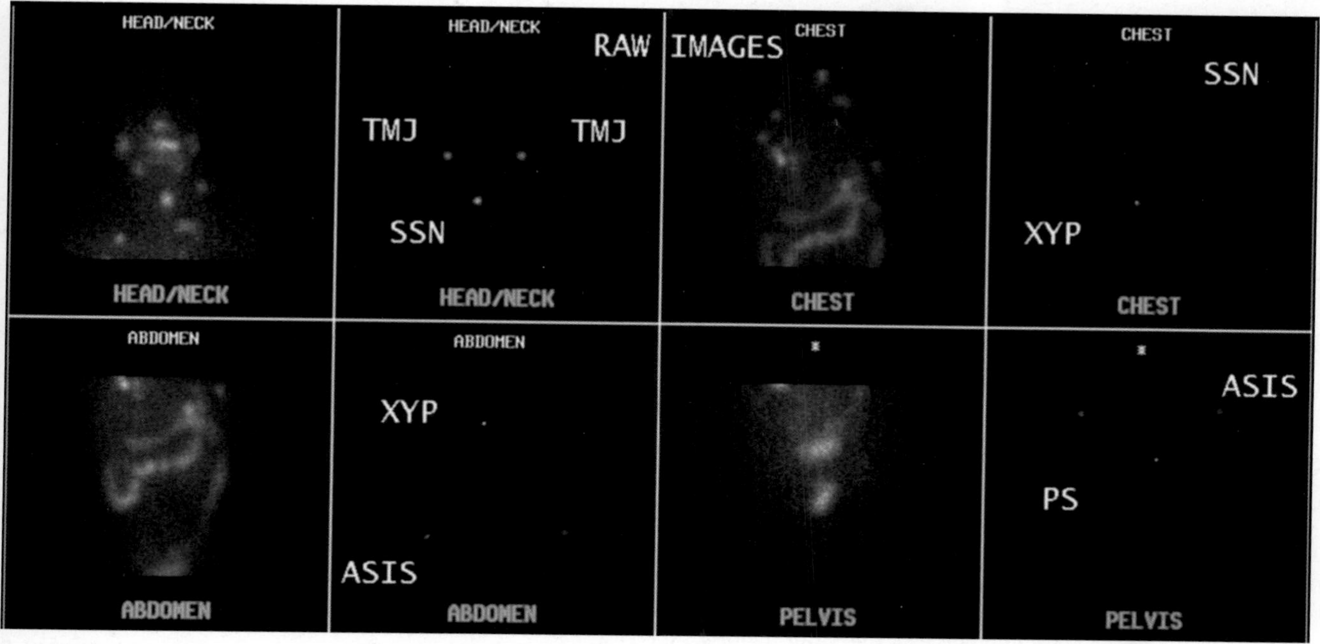

Clinical Presentation

A 38-year-old woman with a history of malignancy presents for restaging.

Imaging Findings

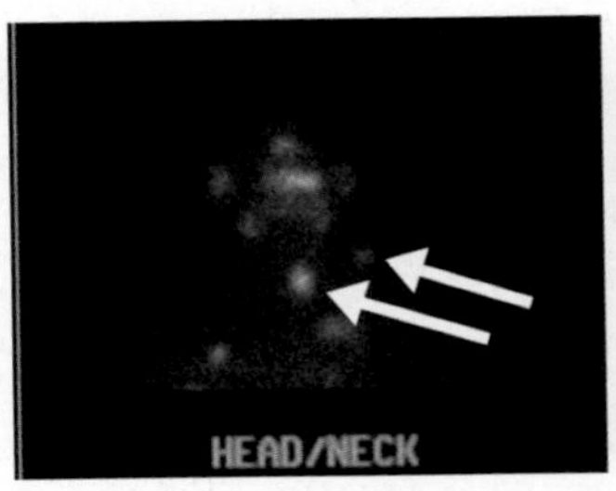

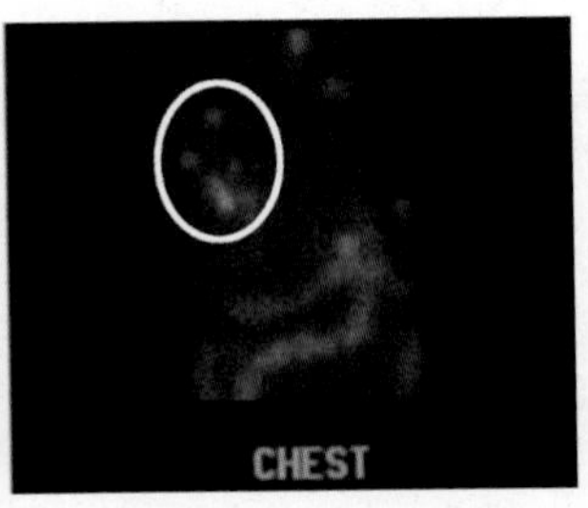

Anterior spot images from a whole-body (WB) scan with and without markers demonstrate multifocal uptake in the thyroid bed, lateral neck (*arrows*), and lung (*circle*). Physiologic activity is seen in the salivary glands, stomach, colon, and bladder.

Differential Diagnosis

- ***Iodine 131 WB scan demonstrating metastatic thyroid cancer:*** Lack of normal bone uptake with physiologic salivary, gastric, intestinal, and bladder uptake makes radioiodine scan of metastatic thyroid cancer most likely.
- *MIBG scan showing metastatic carcinoid:* This has a somewhat similar biodistribution to iodine but typically also has normal myocardial uptake, and the tumor is more often below the diaphragm.
- *Gallium scan showing metastatic melanoma:* This will also have physiologic salivary and bowel activity but in addition should have normal liver, spleen, and bone activity.

Essential Facts

- The incidence of thyroid cancer in a cold nodule is 15 to 20% and probably lower (5%) in regions of the world without iodine deficiency.
- Incidence of cancer in a cold nodule increases under the following circumstances:
  - There has been prior radiation exposure to the head/neck.
  - There is a family history of thyroid cancer.
  - The patient is a child or a person older than 60 years of age.
  - The nodule increases in size with thyroid hormone suppression.
- Papillary and follicular are the most common cancer types and the most iodine-avid. They tend to metastasize regionally in the neck and then distally to the lungs and bones.
- Medullary, anaplastic, and Hürthle cell cancers are less likely to concentrate iodine.
- One treatment algorithm (many variations exist) is shown in table at right.

Procedure	Initial Diagnosis	Follow-up 1 Year Later
Surgery	At the time of diagnosis	Large sites of recurrence should be surgically removed if possible.
Preablation thyroid WB scan with I131 or I123 May or may not be performed based on institutional biases	5–6 wk after thyroidectomy Check thyroid-stimulating hormone (TSH) to ensure > 30 IU.	Two methods: 1. Take patients off Synthroid for 5–6 wk until TSH is > 30 IU. Some prefer higher baseline level. 2. Use recombinant TSH (Thyrogen) to ensure high TSH level.
Ablation	Typically: 1. 100 mCi if limited to thyroid 2. 150 mCi if metastatic Variabilities: some institutions use ~ 30 mCi if thyroid cancer is limited to the thyroid without metastases. A few physicians give 1 Ci for the first and only dose.	If scan is negative, give no I131 therapy. If scan is positive, then give either 150 or 200 mCi based on the initial dose. If scan is negative but thyroglobulin is elevated, consider treatment with 150–200 mCi I131 and/or FDG-PET.

Other Imaging Findings

- Neck US, CT, or MRI can be used to identify regional recurrences (especially enlarged lymph nodes).
- Chest CT can detect pulmonary micrometastases below the level of scintigraphic resolution.
- If a papillary/follicular tumor dedifferentiates and is no longer iodine-avid (iodine scan negative) but the patient has a rising serum thyroglobulin, FDG-PET may identify metabolically active tumor.
- High-grade (e.g., anaplastic) tumors are often hot on FDG-PET, whereas lower-grade papillary and follicular tumors may be cold.
- Medullary thyroid cancers may be positive on MIBG or octreotide scanning.

✓ Pearls & ✗ Pitfalls

✓ For WB scans, if normal skeletal activity is *absent*, the study is probably an OctreoScan, MIBG scan, or iodine 131 WB scan (see "Interpreting Whole-Body Scans").

✓ Papillary and follicular thyroid cancers concentrate iodine, but less than normal thyroid tissue. Hence, they are "cold" on thyroid bed scanning preoperatively but are iodine-avid on WB scans and with iodine therapy.

✓ I123 or I131 may be used for scanning; only I131 can provide therapy (β-emitter).

✗ I131 dosing for pretreatment *scanning* may prevent uptake of subsequent high-dose I131 for therapy because of thyroid tissue "stunning." This leads many to administer < 5 mCi for a diagnostic scan or use I123, although the concept is somewhat controversial.

Case 96

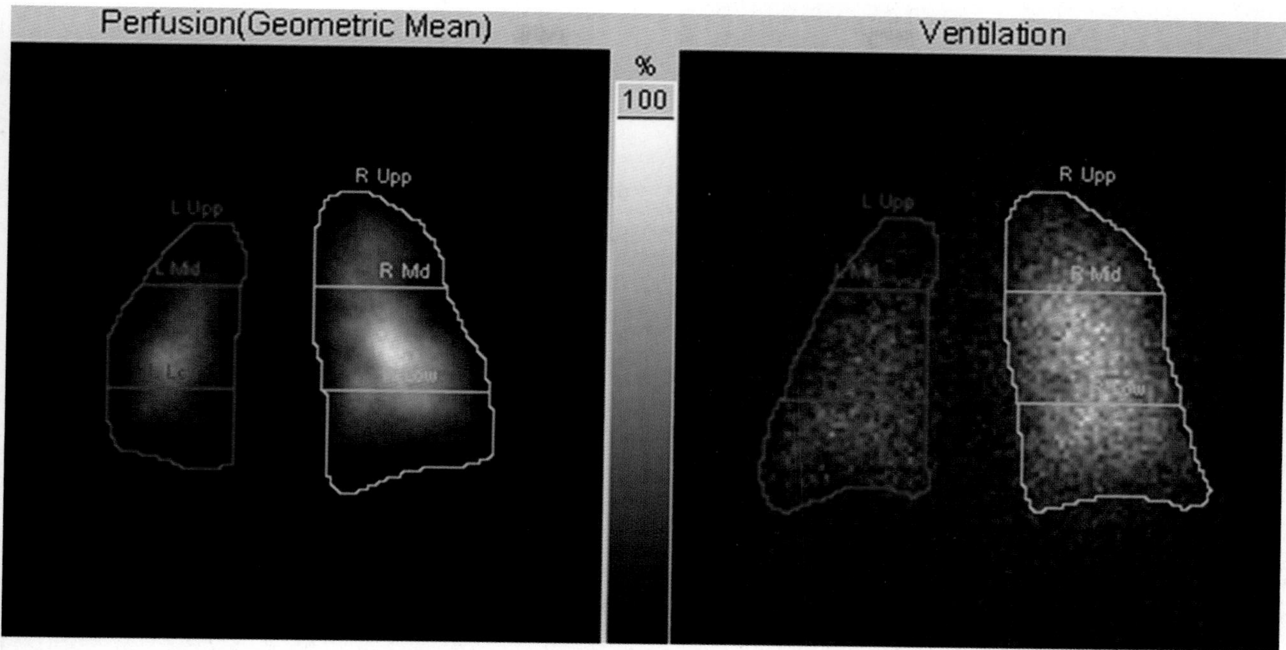

Geometric Mean

(Counts)	Left	Right
Upper	012K	053K
Middle	066K	147K
Lower	024K	064K
Total	102K	264K

(% Ratios)	Left	Right
Upper	3.32	14.49
Middle	18.10	40.06
Lower	6.45	17.58
Total	27.87	72.13

Statistical Table

Perfusion POSTERIOR (Counts)	Left	Right	Ventilation Composite Frame (Counts)	Left	Right
Upper	012K	049K	Upper	002K	008K
Middle	084K	148K	Middle	007K	019K
Lower	043K	076K	Lower	008K	013K
Total	139K	274K	Total	017K	040K

(% Ratios)	Left	Right	(% Ratios)	Left	Right
Upper	3.00	11.91	Upper	3.53	13.75
Middle	20.27	36.00	Middle	12.96	33.80
Lower	10.32	18.51	Lower	13.34	22.61
Total	33.58	66.42	Total	29.84	70.16

Clinical Presentation

A 65-year-old man with left lung cancer presents for evaluation before a left pneumonectomy. His preoperative spirometry revealed a forced expiratory volume in 1 second of 1600 mL.

Imaging Findings

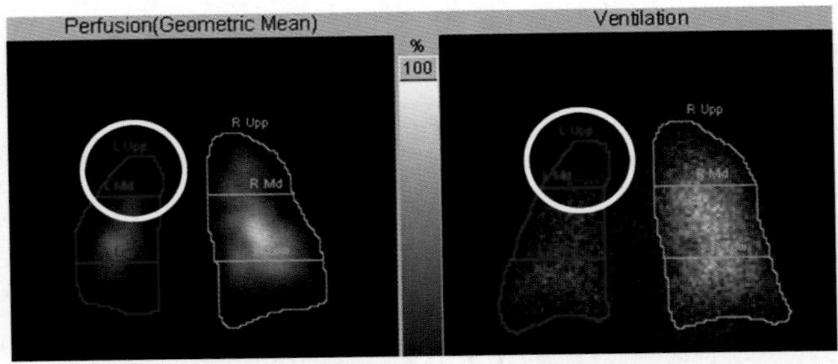

Posterior ventilation and perfusion images from a quantitative lung scan with 4 mCi of Tc99m-MAA and 10 mCi of Xenon 133. A matched ventilation–perfusion (VQ) defect is seen in the left upper lung corresponding to the known cancer on both ventilation and perfusion images (*circles*). A milder relative decrease is seen throughout the remainder of the left lung with a differential lung ventilation of 70% right and 30% left. Differential lung perfusion is 28% left and 72% right based on geometric mean analysis of anterior and posterior views (anterior images not shown).

Differential Diagnosis

- ***Residual forced expiratory volume in 1 second (FEV$_1$) of 1154 mL:*** After a left pneumonectomy, the residual FEV$_1$ in this patient is predicted to be 1154 mL (1600 mL $\times$ 0.7213). This is calculated from the *perfusion* images with use of the geometric mean, which is the standard method recommended by the American College of Chest Physicians (ACCP). A postoperative FEV$_1$ $>$ 800 mL is considered adequate.
- *Residual FEV$_1$ of 1123 mL:* After a left pneumonectomy, residual FEV$_1$ could be predicted to be 1123 mL with the use of split *ventilation* (1600 mL $\times$ 0.7016). However, although the ventilation matches the perfusion values closely, this is not the ACCP recommended method. This is most likely due to the expense and difficulty of performing ventilation imaging when the study was first introduced (data are several decades old).

Essential Facts

- Postsurgical lung function can be evaluated by several methods, including spirometry, quantitative VQ scan, and exercise testing.
- Patients with an FEV$_1$ $<$ 2.0 L should be evaluated with quantitative perfusion lung scan based on the ACCP guidelines.
- Upright anterior and posterior ventilation and perfusion images should be obtained. Three regions of interest are drawn over the upper, middle, and lower lungs. Differential lung function is calculated with use of the geometric mean (square root of the product of the anterior and posterior counts).
- This method can also be used to evaluate and follow lung transplants.
- Studies have shown that even though VQ mismatches may occur within a region of lung, the overall ventilation and perfusion to a lung are very similar. This allows the use of *perfusion* images to predict postoperative FEV$_1$, which is based on spirometry, a test of ventilation.

Other Imaging Findings

- No other imaging modalities are as helpful for this functional evaluation.

✓ Pearls & ✗ Pitfalls

✓ The best correlation with postsurgical FEV$_1$ is obtained by using quantitative SPECT lung scanning. This allows a better analysis of individual lung lobes. However, it is more difficult and time-consuming to perform than planar imaging.

✓ Although ACCP recommends using perfusion images, several studies have shown that ventilation images are a better predictor of postoperative FEV$_1$.

✓ There is no proven benefit to using combined VQ images. Perfusion alone is adequate.

✓ Lung cancers are cold on perfusion imaging (MAA). They are fed by *bronchial* arteries originating from the aorta (oxygenated blood). A perfusion scan demonstrates *pulmonary* arterial distribution (deoxygenated blood).

✗ Postoperative FEV$_1$ as predicted by quantitative VQ scanning tends to underestimate actual postoperative FEV$_1$.

✗ The perfusion tracer should be injected with the patient supine, as regional differences will occur if the patient is injected while upright. Perfusion is dependent on gravity, and increased activity will be seen in the lower lungs if an upright injection is performed (see Case 19).

✗ However, once injected, MAA particles become fixed in location, so scanning can be performed with the patient either supine or upright, preferably in the same position as during ventilation imaging.

Case 97

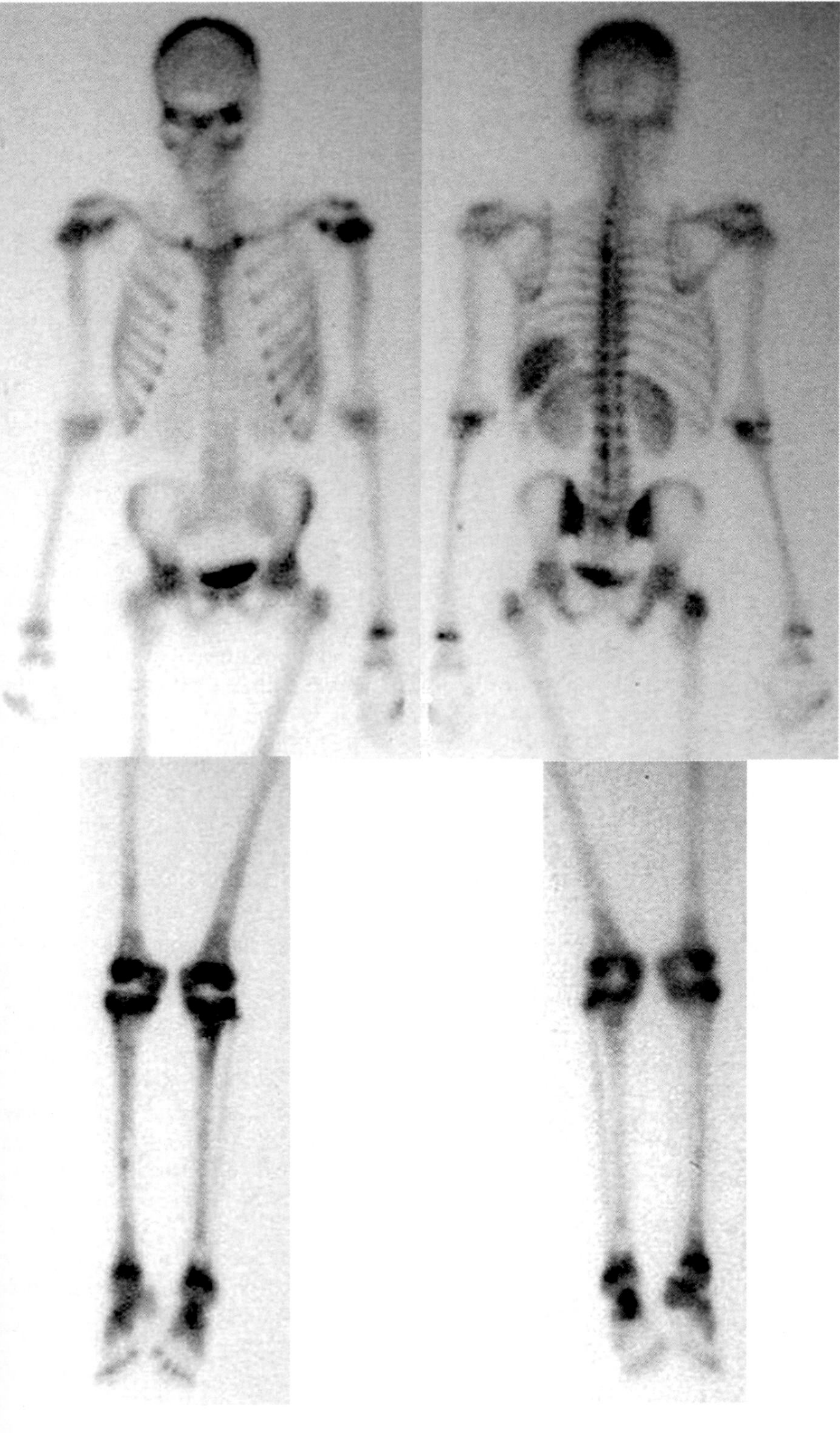

Clinical Presentation

A 14-year-old boy with lower extremity pain.

Imaging Findings

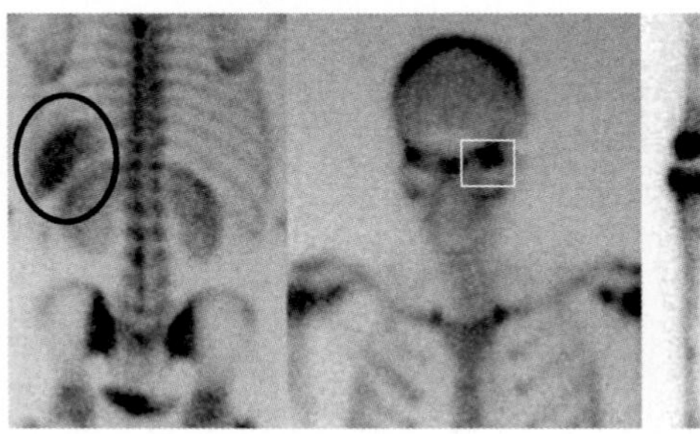
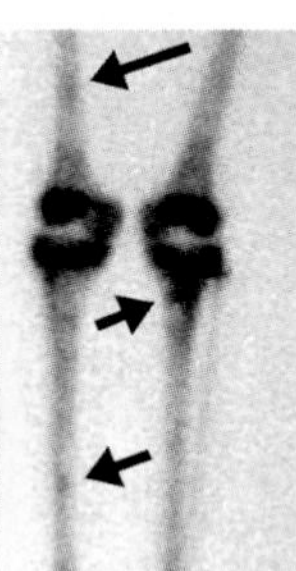

Three-hour–delayed anterior and posterior whole-body bone scan images demonstrate abnormal soft-tissue uptake in the left upper quadrant (*circle*). Also, increased activity is seen around the metaphyses of the knees and ankles and the sphenoid (*square*) that is due to marrow expansion. Other, subtler lesions of increased and *decreased* activity are seen in the extremities (*arrows*).

Differential Diagnosis

- ***Sickle cell disease (SCD):*** Left upper quadrant soft-tissue uptake is consistent with autoinfarction of the spleen. Multifocal bony abnormalities (increased and decreased) are consistent with bony infarcts of various ages. The marrow expansion is also characteristic.
- *Metastatic disease:* This is unlikely as the majority of bone lesions are in the distal skeleton (beyond red marrow). Diffuse splenic activity is also very unlikely.
- *Benign polyostotic bony process (e.g., polyostotic fibrous dysplasia or multiple enchondromas):* Although either one of these benign bony processes could have similar bony appearances, they also do not have an effect on the spleen.

Essential Facts

- SCD is caused by a mutation of the hemoglobin gene that results in deformed, rigid red blood cells.
- SCD is most common in African Americans (1 in 500) and presents in childhood with effects of multiple organ system infarction and infection (bone and soft tissues).
- Severe hemolytic anemia with multiple strokes is also characteristic.
- Frequently, there is increased soft-tissue uptake on bone scan in the left upper quadrant in the region of the spleen secondary to autoinfarction. Subsequent splenic calcification may be seen on CT.
- Anemia leads to marrow expansion with increased skeletal uptake, such as in the metaphyses.
- A significant number of patients with SCD may also have prominent kidneys. This may be due to the inability to concentrate urine.
- Clinical management of SCD includes repeated blood transfusions.

Other Imaging Findings

- Vertebral infarctions with central depressions can result in characteristic "H-shaped" vertebral bodies on radiography or CT.
- MRI can often better delineate the areas of bone infarction as well as the chronicity. MRI or CT can also detect cerebral infarctions, which occur commonly.
- Extramedullary hematopoiesis can be present and detected on CT, often with paraspinal soft-tissue masses.
- On bone scan, acute osseous infarcts will have decreased uptake (on all three bone scan phases if performed), whereas subacute to chronic infarcts can demonstrate increased delayed-phase uptake as bone heals. Such uptake is generally only mildly increased unless there is a superimposed complication (e.g., femoral head collapse), in which case the uptake becomes more pronounced.
- Bone scan can also be hot in osteomyelitis, and Tc99m-SCOL scan can help differentiate. SCOL is cold with infarct but usually normal with infection (although it can occasionally be cold as well). Infarction is more common than infection with SCD.

✓ Pearls & × Pitfalls

- ✓ Splenic uptake plus osseous lesions (increased and/or decreased) is essentially pathognomonic for SCD on bone scan.
- ✓ Soft-tissue infarction elsewhere (e.g., brain, heart, bowel) may also accumulate radiotracer on bone scan.
- ✓ Always look at the patient's age and the distribution of radiopharmaceuticals relative to the axial and appendicular skeleton. Metastatic disease almost always has a much greater number of abnormalities in the axial skeleton and proximal appendicular skeleton, whereas sickle cell and metabolic diseases can commonly have more distal lesions.
- × The splenic uptake in the left upper quadrant can sometimes be misinterpreted as stomach or a prominent left kidney. The spleen is usually lateral to both.
- × If gastric uptake is suspected, look at the neck to see if there is thyroid or salivary uptake (to indicate free pertechnetate; see Case 16).

Case 98

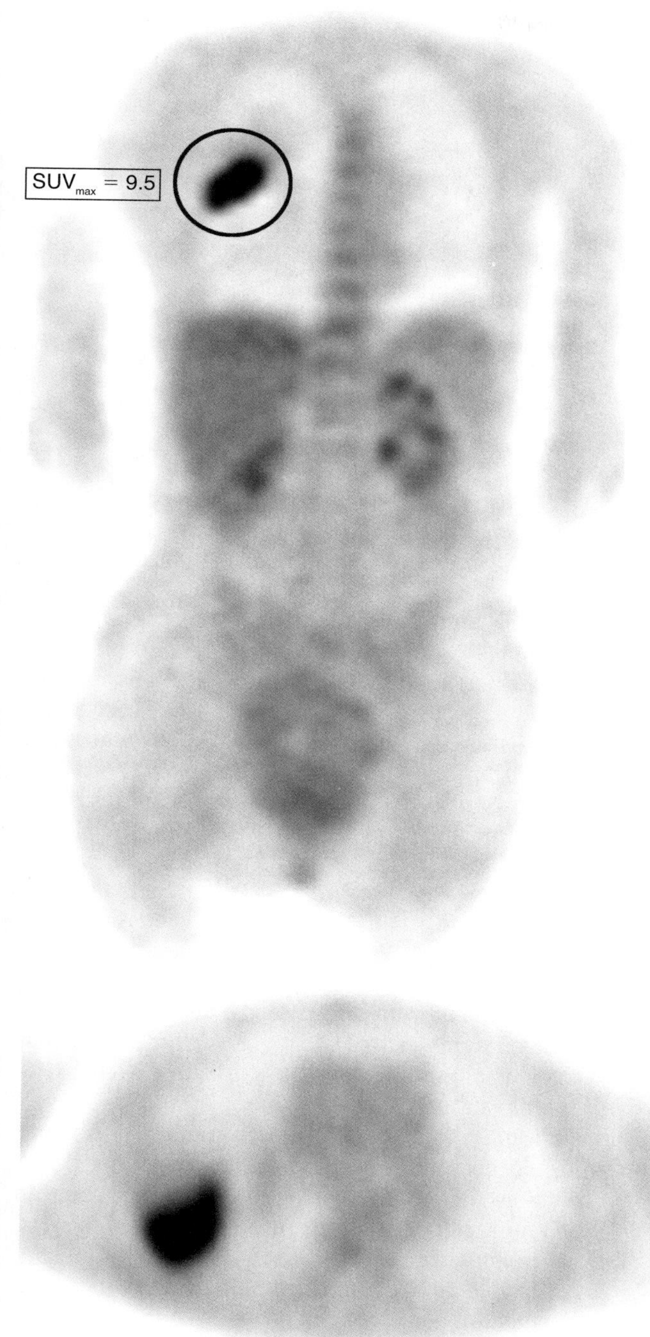

A

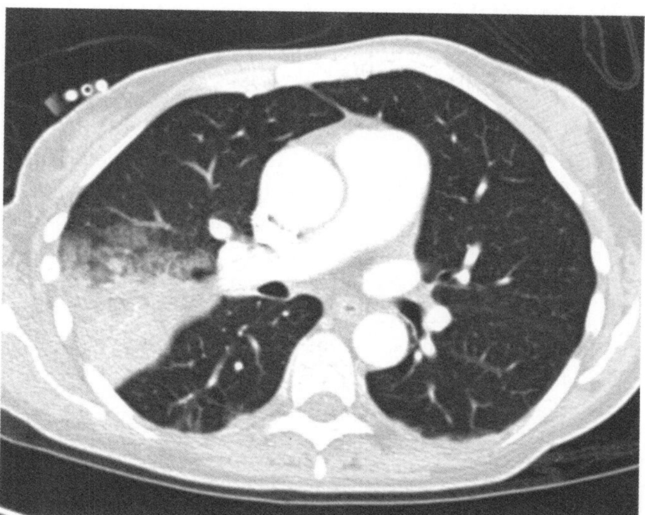

B

Clinical Presentation

A patient presents for colon cancer restaging. The patient reports recent cough and fever.

Imaging Findings

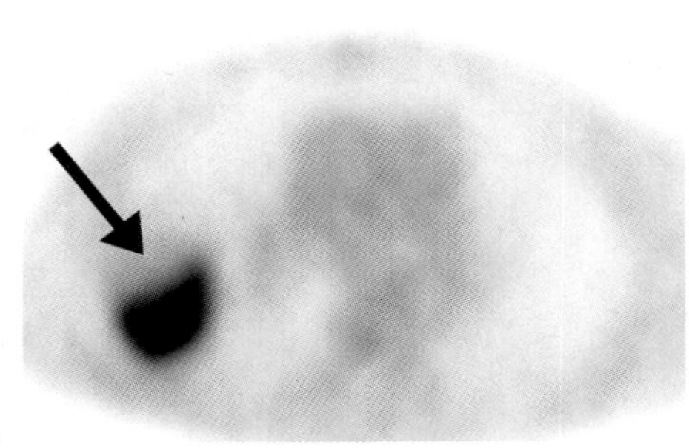

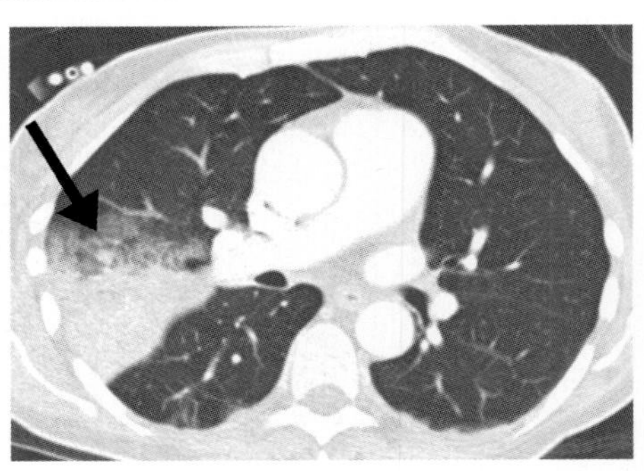

(A) Axial and coronal FDG-PET images demonstrate a markedly hypermetabolic lesion in the right mid lung (*arrow*). **(B)** Corresponding axial CT image demonstrates a wedge-shaped consolidative lesion that is sharply marginated posteriorly with adjacent ground-glass anteriorly (*arrow*).

Differential Diagnosis

- ***Acute pneumonia:*** Segmental consolidation on CT is suggestive of infection, particularly given the history. Active infection will have increased FDG accumulation on PET.
- *Synchronous lung carcinoma:* This is a possible etiology. Follow-up chest radiography or CT should be performed after antibiotic treatment to demonstrate lesion resolution.
- *Colon cancer metastatic to lung:* This will also be hypermetabolic on FDG-PET but is typically more nodular on CT.

Essential Facts

- Hypermetabolic on FDG-PET is often defined as an $SUV_{max} > 2.5$, particularly in the lung. However, it may be more accurately defined as increased above blood pool (e.g., mediastinal) or focally increased above normal portions of an organ (e.g., liver and spleen).
- Increased FDG accumulation indicates hypermetabolism and is present in most malignant processes.
- However, hypermetabolism is also present with most active infectious and inflammatory conditions because of uptake in such processes as activated granulocytes and macrophages.
- Benign neoplasms can also accumulate FDG.

Other Imaging Findings

- Lesion morphology on CT or MRI can add specificity to a hypermetabolic lesion on FDG-PET. Follow-up imaging may also be useful.
- The clinical history should always be considered, as in this case.
- Labeled WBC scintigraphy could confirm the diagnosis of infection in this case.

✓ Pearls & × Pitfalls

✓ SUV_{max} can be quite high (> 10) in some benign processes and indistinguishable from tumor based on SUV alone. Always take the history and CT appearance into account.

✓ Common benign musculoskeletal processes with elevated FDG accumulation include recent fracture, bursal inflammation (especially around hips and shoulders), muscle activation, and "active" degenerative joint disease. Anything that is hot on bone scan can be hot on FDG-PET.

✓ Atherosclerosis of the aorta and larger arteries is an inflammatory process and will accumulate FDG. Localize with the corresponding CT and look for calcium in the arterial wall (although calcification is a later manifestation of the inflammation and does not have to be present).

✓ Besides pneumonia, granulomatous processes such as sarcoid and histoplasmosis can be hot on FDG-PET.

✓ Benign lesions such as adenomas (e.g., adrenal, hepatic, colonic) will sometimes have markedly elevated FDG accumulation.

✓ Ovarian/uterine uptake in a premenopausal woman is more commonly benign (e.g., functional cysts, endometrial menstrual activity, leiomyomas) but can be reimaged after several menstrual cycles if there is concern for tumor.

× Artifactual uptake can also simulate malignancy on attenuation-corrected PET images. When in doubt, always check uncorrected images to confirm that a hypermetabolic process is present (see Case 76).

Case 99

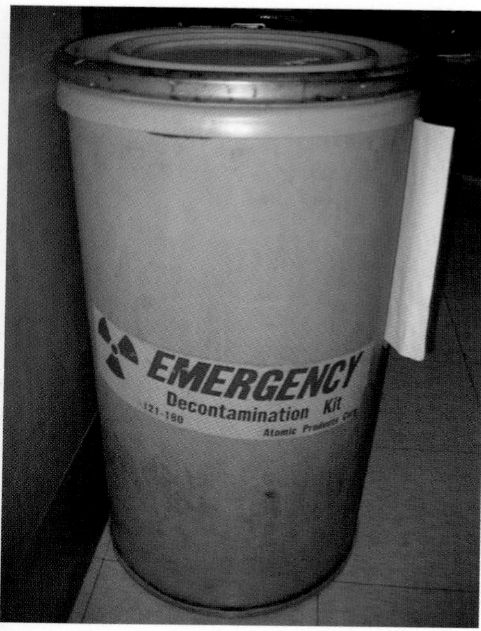

Clinical Presentation

A technologist performing a myocardial perfusion scan spills 25 mCi of Tc99m-MIBI on the floor of the treadmill room. What should be done next?

Differential Diagnosis

Is this a major or a minor spill, and which of the following needs to be done?

- ***Minor spill—prevent the spread of contamination and begin cleanup:*** Correct, see discussion below.
- *Minor spill—get another dose of radiotracer and proceed with the exam:* Incorrect.
- *Major spill—leave the room and notify the Nuclear Regulatory Commission:* Incorrect.

Imaging Findings

- The above example would be considered a minor spill.

Essential Facts

- Threshold levels for major versus minor spill:
  - Tc99m: 100 mCi
  - Tl201: 100 mCi
  - Ga67: 10 mCi
  - In111: 10 mCi
  - I131: 1 mCi
- Before licensed materials are used, a radiation protection plan must be in place that outlines the procedures that will be followed in case of a spill.
- Radiation workers should routinely monitor themselves for contamination before leaving the department or handling radioactive materials.
- All spills should be reported to the radiation safety officer (RSO).

Procedures for a Minor Spill

- Notify personnel that a spill has occurred.
- Cover the spill with absorbent paper to prevent spread.
- Use personnel protection, such as gloves, laboratory coat, and booties. Clean up the spill with absorbent paper and place in a bag marked "Caution: Radioactive Material." Place any contaminated clothing, gloves, etc., in the bag. This will be transferred to a radioactive waste container.
- Monitor the area for any residual contamination, including personnel.
- Notify the RSO.

Procedures for a Major Spill

- Clear the area and evacuate all personnel not involved in the spill.
- Cover the spill with absorbent paper but do not clean the area. Prevent the spread of contamination by limiting the movement of involved personnel.
- Place shielding around the source if possible.
- Close and secure the room. Mark the area with caution signs.
- Notify the RSO.
- Begin the decontamination of involved personnel by removing clothing and washing with soap and water.

Other Imaging Findings

- A spill kit should be maintained in each department consisting of the following:
  - Six pairs of disposable gloves
  - Two disposable laboratory coats
  - Two paper hats
  - Two pairs of shoe covers
  - One roll of absorbent paper with plastic backing
  - Six plastic trash bags with ties
  - Radioactive material labeling tape
  - One marking pen
  - Three radioactive material labeling tags
  - Supplies for 10 wipe samples
  - Clipboard with spills report form and pencil
  - Emergency procedures manual

✓ Pearls & × Pitfalls

✓ If a spill occurs at the end of a day and the room is not needed, the room can be closed off (caution signs must be placed) and decontaminated the next day to allow for decay.

✓ If a xenon gas spill occurs, everyone should leave the room immediately and the door should be closed. The evacuation time in minutes (T) can be calculated based on a derived air concentration (C) for Xenon 133 (10^{-4} μCi/mL), the room volume (V), the activity released (A), and the exhaust rate of the room (Q), with (ln) natural log:

$$T = V/Q \ln (A/[C*V])$$

This should be calculated beforehand for each room in the department where radioactive gases will be used.

× Negative pressure must be maintained in rooms where radioactive gases are used (but is not required for aerosols like DTPA).

× A wipe test cannot be used to detect xenon contamination.

Case 100

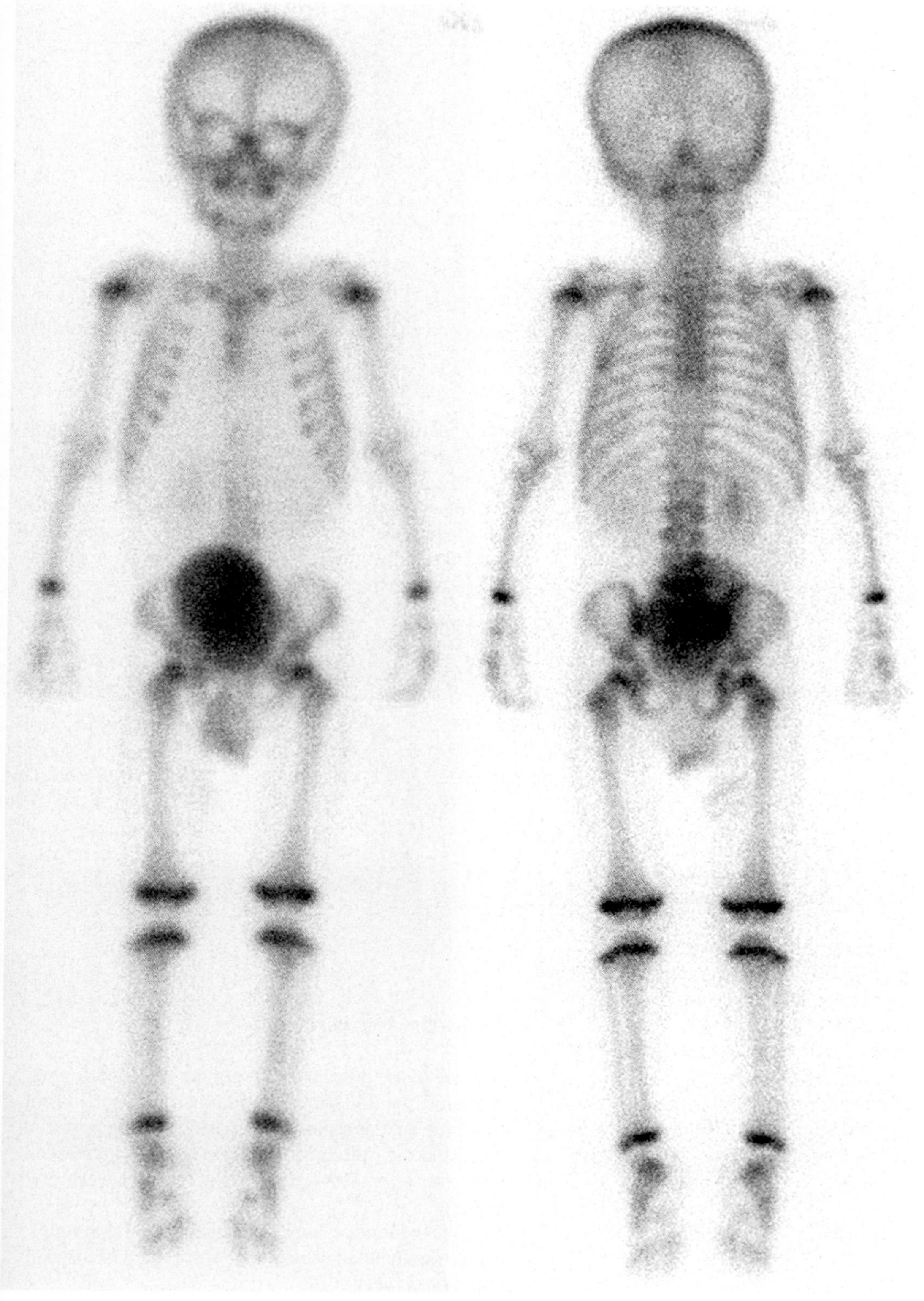

Clinical Presentation

A 3-year-old boy with treated neuroblastoma presents for restaging. What is the etiology of the appearance of the spine?

Imaging Findings

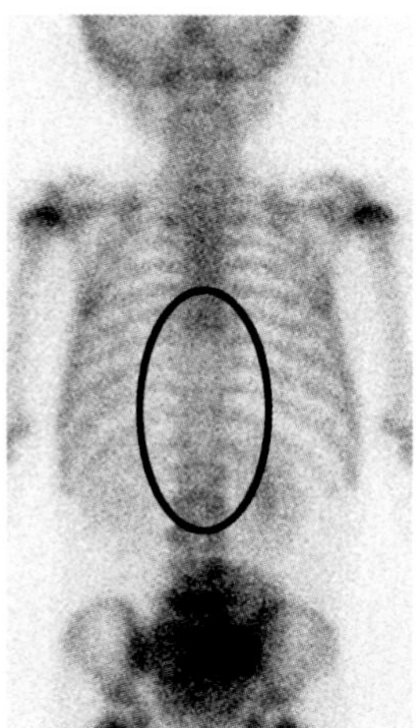

Anterior and posterior whole-body bone scan demonstrates abrupt decrease in radiotracer accumulation in the mid and lower thoracic spine (*circle*).

Differential Diagnosis

- ***Normal prior external beam radiation effect:*** The sharply marginated, diffusely decreased activity at multiple adjacent vertebral levels makes this the most likely etiology.
- *Lytic osseous metastases:* These can have decreased uptake on bone scan (as can myeloma), but the distribution of multiple contiguous levels would be very unusual.
- *Bone infarction:* This can also be decreased, particularly if acute, but it would be very unusual for multiple contiguous levels to be involved.

Essential Facts

- External beam radiation for malignant lesions such as lymphoma, lung cancer, neuroblastoma, and spine metastases can affect subsequent scintigraphy, most notably bone scans.
- A decrease in normal marrow and osteoblastic activity within the radiation port can result in geographic, sharply marginated decreased uptake on bone scan, most commonly affecting the spine.
- This appearance may begin to develop several months following external beam radiation.
- The condition is usually asymptomatic but can be associated with a higher risk for vertebral compression fractures (which would then become increased in uptake).

Other Imaging Findings

- CT will show no change in the bones but can show some radiation-induced changes in the adjacent soft tissues (e.g., pulmonary fibrosis).
- On bone scan, radiation injury to adjacent soft tissues (including portions of the kidneys) can have sharply marginated *increased* uptake.
- MRI can demonstrate a corresponding signal abnormality in affected marrow.
- FDG-PET can demonstrate an analogous decrease in affected marrow metabolism, as in this other patient with prior mediastinal radiation (stimulation of the remainder of the marrow by granulocyte colony–stimulating factor is accentuating the radiation effect; *arrow*):

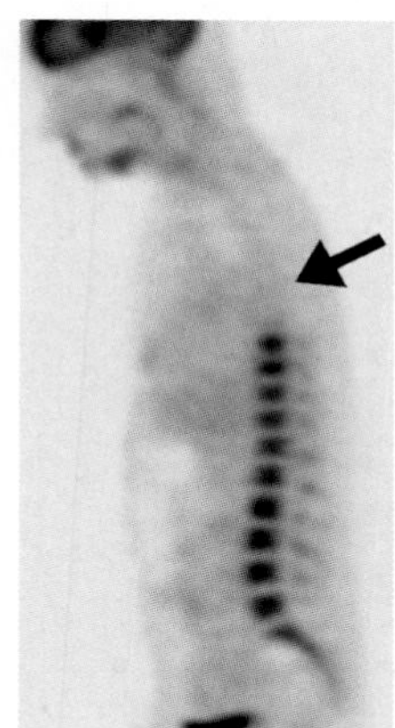

✓ Pearls & ✗ Pitfalls

✓ Because of the normal lordotic/kyphotic curvature of the spine, the mid thoracic and mid sacral portions of the spine appear regionally increased on the posterior view, and the mid lumbar portion appears increased on the anterior view (closer to the respective camera heads).

✗ Metallic orthopedic hardware, including spinal rods, can artifactually make a geographic region of the skeleton appear very cold.

Interpreting Whole-Body Scans

Single organ or targeted scintigraphic studies are immediately apparent, such as lung ventilation–perfusion, renal, thyroid, or HIDA scans. However, when faced with a puzzling whole-body (WB) study, the nerve-wracking situation of "What study am I looking at?" is easily defused using a few simple steps.

The WB bone scan is ubiquitous and therefore easily recognized.

An FDG-PET study is not planar even though the images are frequently previewed as a panoramic coronal MIP.

Almost immediately, the list is contracted to only six common WB studies:

1. Gallium
2. WBC
3. Antibody (such as ProstaScint, Bexxar, and Zevalin)
4. Radioiodine (either I123- or I131-labeled)
5. MIBG (either I123 or I131)
6. OctreoScan (pentetreotide)

Questions to Ask First

Is the normal skeleton visualized?

- If YES, then consider gallium, WBC, and antibody (or bone scan).
- If NO, then consider the "endocrine group" (i.e., radioiodine, MIBG, and OctreoScan).

Is salivary or lacrimal activity present?

- If YES, then consider gallium, radioiodine, and MIBG (or uncommon WB MIBI).

Is myocardial activity present? (left ventricular muscular "horseshoe" as opposed to diffuse blood pool activity within the chamber)

- If YES, then MIBG (or MIBI) (*Note:* obvious myocardial activity will not always be visible on MIBG)

Does the intensity of one or more organs dominate the image?

- If the spleen is dominant, then it is a WBC study.
- If the liver is dominant, then it is an antibody study.
- If the kidneys (parenchyma) and spleen are codominant, then it is a pentetreotide study.

Tracer-Specific Items to Ponder Next

Gallium

- *Key biodistribution:* liver uptake > spleen and bone marrow uptake; also present: bone cortex, salivary/lacrimal glands, and colon
- *Common indications:* tumors (e.g., lymphoma, melanoma), infection (especially pulmonary and spine), inflammation (especially granulomatous/sarcoidosis), and fever of unknown origin
- *Mechanism of localization:* transferrin/lactoferrin binding
- *Pearls:* This is the only study other than the bone scan that demonstrates intense normal growth plates activity in children (both the osseous cortex and the medullary space are gallium-avid).

WBC

- *Key biodistribution:* spleen > liver and bone marrow
- *Common indications:* active infection or inflammation, rarely tumors
- *Mechanism of localization:* WBC migration
- *Pearls:* physiological colonic uptake but only with Tc99m label (after several hours), never with In111 label

Antibody (ProstaScint, Bexxar, Zevalin, etc.)

- *Key biodistribution (all antibody scans appear similar):* Liver, bowel, blood pool (i.e., cardiac chambers, spleen, great vessels), bone marrow. Most intense is diffuse liver uptake that increases the longer the delay (as it clears/decreases blood pool activity over time). Liver typically appears more intense on 5-day delay ProstaScint than 2-day delay Zevalin, for example.
- *Common indications:* soft-tissue metastases from prostate cancer as well as other cancer imaging and therapy (e.g., lymphoma)
- *Mechanism of localization:* cancer-specific antigen binding
- *Pearls:* If liver is the dominant, most intense normal organ, the exam is likely an antibody scan. Can acquire simultaneous Tc99m RBC image to distinguish blood pool (e.g., with ProstaScint).

Radioiodine WB Scan

- *Key biodistribution:* not much to look at: mild salivary, stomach, bladder, sometimes neck "star" (septal penetration artifact), no normal skeleton, occasionally mild homogeneous liver
- *Common indications:* differentiated thyroid cancer (papillary, follicular, and mixed) prior to remnant ablation and occasionally metastatic surveillance
- *Mechanism of localization:* organification in functional thyroid tissue as iodine is a thyroid hormone precursor
- *Pearls:* appears similar to the MIBG study but abnormal uptake is typically localized above the diaphragm (e.g., in the neck, thorax); I123 administration preferred over I131 in some facilities (no risk of "thyroid stunning," less radiation, possibly more sensitive images but somewhat controversial and more expensive)

MIBG

- *Key biodistribution:* not much to look at: mild visualization of salivary, liver, spleen, occasionally myocardial, bladder, but no normal skeleton

- *Common indications:* neuroendocrine tumors especially of the adrenal glands (e.g., pheochromocytoma or neuroblastoma)
- *Mechanism of localization:* Guanethidine analog (hormonal synthesis precursor)
- *Pearls:* appears similar to a radioiodine scan but abnormal uptake is typically localized below the diaphragm; I123 MIBG images better than I131 MIBG; with either, block thyroid (with free cold iodine like potassium iodide)—but still may see thyroid faintly

Pentetreotide (OctreoScan)

- *Key biodistribution:* intense renal cortical (not just collecting system) and splenic activity; milder liver and bowel activity, but no normal skeletal visualization
- *Common indications:* most neuroendocrine tumors
- *Mechanism of localization:* somatostatin analog
- *Pearls:* generally superior to MIBG for neuroendocrine imaging except for adrenal lesions (e.g., pheochromocytoma, neuroblastoma), which can be obscured by intense adjacent renal cortical activity

The following are usually targeted body imaging agents, but they may occasionally be used to obtain WB images.

Sulfur Colloid

- *Key biodistribution:* liver ≥ spleen and bone marrow
- *Common indications:* less common WB scan but may be used to map normal marrow in conjunction with WBC scan for prosthetic joint evaluation (more specifically targeted abdominal indications include assessing for focal nodular hyperplasia in the liver or colloid shift)
- *Mechanism of localization:* reticuloendothelial system uptake
- *Pearls:* similar appearance to WBC but spleen not as intense

Sestamibi (MIBI) or Tetrofosmin

- *Key biodistribution:* salivary, myocardial, liver, biliary, and bowel
- *Common indications:* Uncommon WB scan but can be used for nonspecific tumors or infection/inflammation, similar to FDG-PET
- *Mechanism of localization:* mitochondrial binding
- *Pearls:* More targeted MIBI imaging for myocardial perfusion, parathyroid adenoma evaluation, and scintimammography. Has been used for WB restaging of dedifferentiated (more aggressive) thyroid cancers that are no longer iodine-avid (replaced by FDG-PET for this indication).

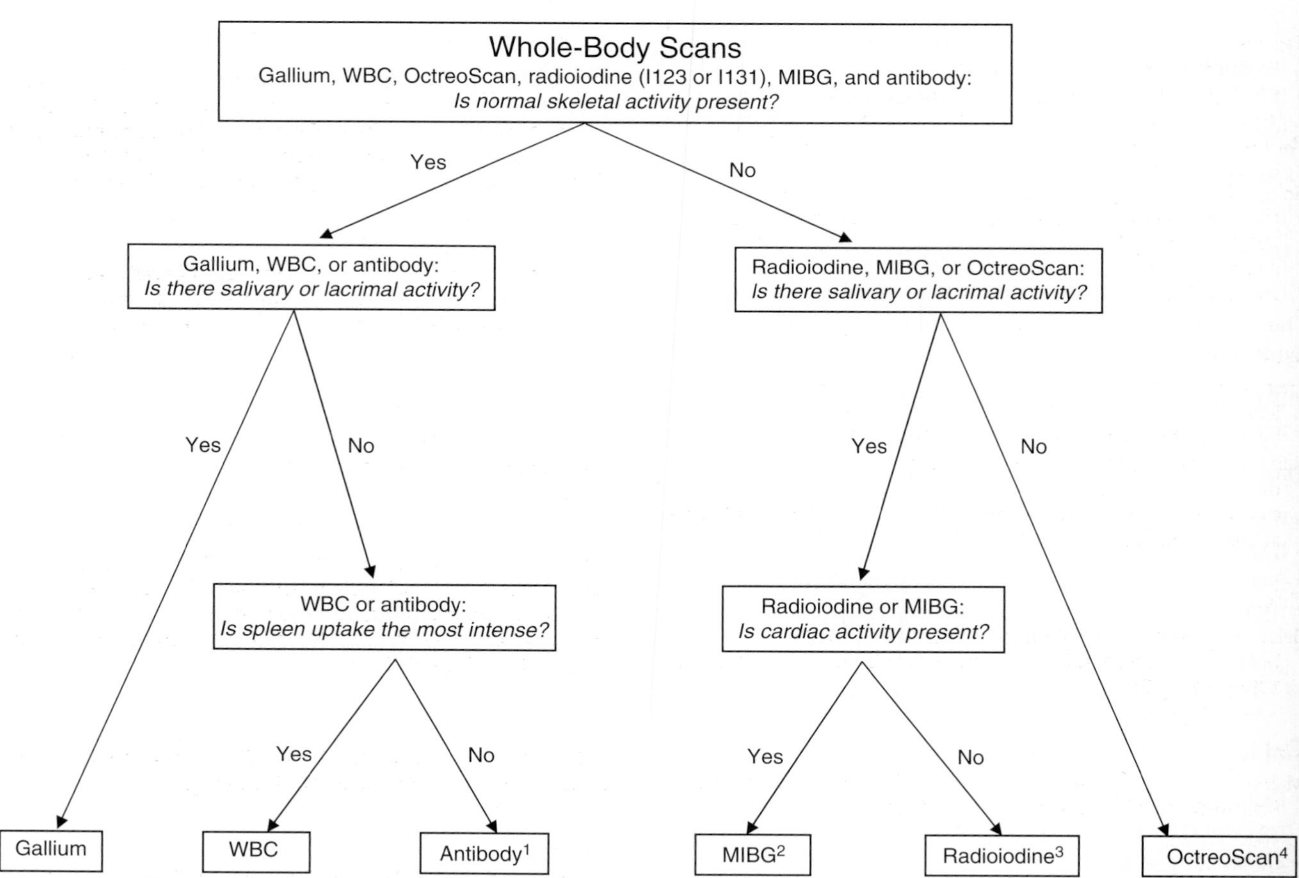

1. With antibody studies, blood pool and renal uptake is usually visible.
2. With MIBG, abnormal activity is more commonly seen below the diaphragm.
3. With radioiodine, abnormal activity is more commonly seen below the diaphragm.
4. With OctreoScan, spleen and renal parenchyma demonstrate the most intense normal activity.

Further Readings

Case 1

Kim DW, Kim CG, Park SA, Jung SA, Yang SH. Metabolic super scan in F-FDG PET/CT imaging. J Korean Med Sci 2010;25(8):1256–1257

Case 2

Okosieme OE, Chan D, Price SA, Lazarus JH, Premawardhana LD. The utility of radioiodine uptake and thyroid scintigraphy in the diagnosis and management of hyperthyroidism. Clin Endocrinol (Oxf) 2010;72(1):122–127

Case 3

Siegel JA. Nuclear Regulatory Commission Regulation of Nuclear Medicine. Guide for Diagnostic Nuclear Medicine and Radiopharmaceutical Therapy. Reston, VA: Society of Nuclear Medicine; 2004

Case 4

Panegyres PK, Rogers JM, McCarthy M, Campbell A, Wu JS. Fluorodeoxyglucose-positron emission tomography in the differential diagnosis of early-onset dementia: a prospective, community-based study. BMC Neurol 2009;9:41

Case 5

Elsässer A, Schlepper M, Klövekorn WP, et al. Hibernating myocardium: an incomplete adaptation to ischemia. Circulation 1997;96(9): 2920–2931

Pagano D, Bonser RS, Townend JN, Ordoubadi F, Lorenzoni R, Camici PG. Predictive value of dobutamine echocardiography and positron emission tomography in identifying hibernating myocardium in patients with postischaemic heart failure. Heart 1998;79(3):281–288

Rahimtoola SH. The hibernating myocardium. Am Heart J 1989; 117(1):211–221

Sciagrà R, Bisi G, Santoro GM, et al. Comparison of baseline-nitrate technetium-99m sestamibi with rest-redistribution thallium-201 tomography in detecting viable hibernating myocardium and predicting postrevascularization recovery. J Am Coll Cardiol 1997;30(2):384–391

Case 6

Lindholm P, Minn H, Leskinen-Kallio S, Bergman J, Ruotsalainen U, Joensuu H. Influence of the blood glucose concentration on FDG uptake in cancer—a PET study. J Nucl Med 1993;34(1):1–6

Rabkin Z, Israel O, Keidar Z. Do hyperglycemia and diabetes affect the incidence of false-negative 18F-FDG PET/CT studies in patients evaluated for infection or inflammation and cancer? A Comparative analysis. J Nucl Med 2010;51(7):1015–1020

Case 7

Bekerman C, Nayak SM. Gallium imaging. In: Henkin RE, Boles MA, Dillehay GL, et al., eds. Nuclear Medicine. St Louis, MO: Mosby, 1996: 1597–1618

Case 8

Malik AA, Wani KA, Khaja AR; Shams-ul-Bari. Meckel's diverticulum-Revisited. Saudi J Gastroenterol 2010;16(1):3–7

Case 9

Sostman HD, Stein PD, Gottschalk A, Matta F, Hull R, Goodman L. Acute pulmonary embolism: sensitivity and specificity of ventilation-perfusion scintigraphy in PIOPED II study. Radiology 2008;246(3):941–946

Case 10

Weissmann HS, Badia J, Sugarman LA, Kluger L, Rosenblatt R, Freeman LM. Spectrum of 99m-Tc-IDA cholescintigraphic patterns in acute cholecystitis. Radiology 1981;138(1):167–175

Case 11

Björgvinsson E, Majd M, Eggli KD. Diagnosis of acute pyelonephritis in children: comparison of sonography and 99mTc-DMSA scintigraphy. AJR Am J Roentgenol 1991;157(3):539–543

Case 12

Intenzo CM, Jabbour S, Lin HC, et al. Scintigraphic imaging of body neuroendocrine tumors. Radiographics 2007;27(5):1355–1369

Case 13

Wu J-Y, Shih J-Y. Leg pains, clubbing of digits and lung mass: what is your call? CMAJ 2008;178(4):395–396

Case 14

Thomas DL, Bartel T, Menda Y, Howe J, Graham MM, Juweid ME. Single photon emission computed tomography (SPECT) should be routinely performed for the detection of parathyroid abnormalities utilizing technetium-99m sestamibi parathyroid scintigraphy. Clin Nucl Med 2009;34(10):651–655

Case 15

Cooper DS, Doherty GM, Haugen BR, et al; American Thyroid Association (ATA) Guidelines Taskforce on Thyroid Nodules and Differentiated Thyroid Cancer. Revised American Thyroid Association management guidelines for patients with thyroid nodules and differentiated thyroid cancer. Thyroid 2009;19(11):1167–1214

Case 16

Kim JH, Shin JH, Yoon HK, et al. Angiographically negative acute arterial upper and lower gastrointestinal bleeding: incidence, predictive factors, and clinical outcomes. Korean J Radiol 2009;10(4):384–390

Case 17

Colina M, La Corte R, De Leonardis F, Trotta F. Paget's disease of bone: a review. Rheumatol Int 2008;28(11):1069–1075

Case 18

Wijdicks EFM, Varelas PN, Gronseth GS, Greer DM; American Academy of Neurology. Evidence-based guideline update: determining brain death in adults: report of the Quality Standards Subcommittee of the American Academy of Neurology. Neurology 2010;74(23):1911–1918

Case 19

Stein PD, Freeman LM, Sostman HD, et al. SPECT in acute pulmonary embolism. J Nucl Med 2009;50(12):1999–2007

Case 20

Donohoe KJ, Maurer AH, Ziessman HA, Urbain JL, Royal HD, Martin-Comin J; Society for Nuclear Medicine; American Neurogastroenterology and Motility Society. Procedure guideline for adult solid-meal gastric-emptying study 3.0. J Nucl Med Technol 2009;37(3):196–200

Case 21

Luk WH, Woo YH, Au-Yeung AW, Chan JC. Imaging in pediatric urinary tract infection: a 9-year local experience. AJR Am J Roentgenol 2009;192(5):1253–1260

Case 22

Zukotynski K, Grant FD, Curtis C, Micheli L, Treves ST. Skeletal scintigraphy in pediatric sports medicine. AJR Am J Roentgenol 2010;195(5):1212–1219

Case 23

Eng CY, Quraishi MS, Bradley PJ. Management of Thyroid nodules in adult patients. Head Neck Oncol 2010;2:11

Mazzaferri EL. Management of a solitary thyroid nodule. N Engl J Med 1993;328(8):553–559

Case 24

Ziessman H, O'Malley JP, Thrall JH. Nuclear Medicine: the Requisites. 3rd ed. Philadelphia: Elsevier, Mosby: 2006

Case 25

Filippi L, Uccioli L, Giurato L, Schillaci O. Diabetic foot infection: usefulness of SPECT/CT for 99mTc-HMPAO-labeled leukocyte imaging. J Nucl Med 2009;50(7):1042–1046

Case 26

Horvat AG, Kovac V, Strojan P. Radiotherapy in palliative treatment of painful bone metastases. Radiol Oncol 2009;43(4):213–224

Liepe K, Kotzerke J. A comparative study of 188Re-HEDP, 186Re-HEDP, 153Sm-EDTMP and 89Sr in the treatment of painful skeletal metastases. Nucl Med Commun 2007;28(8):623–630

Case 27

Freeman LM, Blaufox MD, eds. Orthopedic nuclear medicine (part I). Semin Nucl Med 1997;27(4):307–389

Love C, Marwin SE, Palestro CJ. Nuclear medicine and the infected joint replacement. Semin Nucl Med 2009;39(1):66–78

Case 28

Lyders EM, Whitlow CT, Baker MD, Morris PP. Imaging and treatment of sacral insufficiency fractures. AJNR Am J Neuroradiol 2010;31(2):201–210

Case 29

Fletcher JW, Kymes SM, Gould M, et al; VA SNAP Cooperative Studies Group. A comparison of the diagnostic accuracy of 18F-FDG PET and CT in the characterization of solitary pulmonary nodules. J Nucl Med 2008;49(2):179–185

Case 30

Eisner R, Churchwell A, Noever T, et al. Quantitative analysis of the tomographic thallium-201 myocardial bullseye display: critical role of correcting for patient motion. J Nucl Med 1988;29(1):91–97

Friedman J, Berman DS, Van Train K, et al. Patient motion in thallium-201 myocardial SPECT imaging. An easily identified frequent source of artifactual defect. Clin Nucl Med 1988;13(5):321–324

Friedman J, Van Train K, Maddahi J, et al. "Upward creep" of the heart: a frequent source of false-positive reversible defects during thallium-201 stress-redistribution SPECT. J Nucl Med 1989;30(10):1718–1722

Case 31

Hosono M, Machida K, Honda N, et al. Quantitative lung perfusion scintigraphy and detection of intrapulmonary shunt in liver cirrhosis. Ann Nucl Med 2002;16(8):577–581

Sugiyama M, Sakahara H, Igarashi T, Takahashi M. Scintigraphic evaluation of small pulmonary right-to-left shunt and therapeutic effect in pulmonary arteriovenous malformation. Clin Nucl Med 2001;26(9):757–760

Case 32

Kirchner PT, Siegel BA, Graham S. Nuclear Medicine: Self-Study Program II: Instrumentation. Reston, VA: Society of Nuclear Medicine; 1996

Case 33

Johnson PT, Horton KM, Fishman EK. How not to miss or mischaracterize a renal cell carcinoma: protocols, pearls, and pitfalls. AJR Am J Roentgenol 2010;194(4):W307-15

Tofe AJ, Francis MD, Harvey WJ. Correlation of neoplasms with incidence and localization of skeletal metastases: an analysis of 1,355 diphosphonate bone scans. J Nucl Med 1975;16(11):986–989

Case 34

Vanneste J, Augustijn P, Davies GAG, Dirven C, Tan WF. Normal-pressure hydrocephalus: is cisternography still useful in selecting patients for a shunt? Arch Neurol 1992;49:336–370

Case 35

Dubovsky EV, Russell CD. Radionuclide evaluation of renal transplants. Semin Nucl Med 1988;18(3):181–198

Case 36

Bomeli SR, LeBeau SO, Ferris RL. Evaluation of a thyroid nodule. Otolaryngol Clin North Am 2010;43(2):229–238, vii

Case 37

Sharp SE, Shulkin BL, Gelfand MJ, Salisbury S, Furman WL. 123I-MIBG scintigraphy and 18F-FDG PET in neuroblastoma. J Nucl Med 2009;50(8):1237–1243

Case 38

Knopp MV, Bischoff H, Rimac A, Oberdorfer F, van Kaick G. Bone marrow uptake of fluorine-18-fluorodeoxyglucose following treatment with hematopoietic growth factors: initial evaluation. Nucl Med Biol 1996;23(6):845–849

Shreve PD, Anzai Y, Wahl RL. Pitfalls in oncologic diagnosis with FDG PET imaging: physiologic and benign variants. Radiographics 1999;19(1):61–77, quiz 150–151

Case 39

Bekerman C, Hoffer PB, Bitran JD, Gupta RG. Gallium-67 citrate imaging studies of the lung. Semin Nucl Med 1980;10(3): 286–301

Gupta SM, Sziklas JJ, Spencer RP, Rosenberg R. Significance of diffuse pulmonary uptake in radiogallium scans: concise communication. J Nucl Med 1980;21(4):328–332

Case 40

National Council on Radiation Protection and Measurements. Report No. 54: Medical Radiation of Pregnant and Potentially Pregnant Women. NRC 10 CFR 20.1208

United States Nuclear Regulatory Commission. NRC 10 CFR 20.1208 Dose equivalent to an embryo/fetus. http://www.nrc.gov/reading-rm/doc-collections/cfr/part020/part020-1208.html. Accessed February 4, 2011

Case 41

Intenzo CM, Jabbour S, Lin HC, et al. Scintigraphic imaging of body neuroendocrine tumors. Radiographics 2007;27(5):1355–1369

Case 42

Galbraith RM, Lavallee ME. Medial tibial stress syndrome: conservative treatment options. Curr Rev Musculoskelet Med 2009;2(3):127–133

Moran DS, Evans RK, Hadad E. Imaging of lower extremity stress fracture injuries. Sports Med 2008;38(4):345–356

Story J, Cymet TC. Shin splints: painful to have and to treat. Compr Ther 2006;32(3):192–195

Case 43

Siegel, Jeffry A. Guide for Diagnostic Nuclear Medicine and Radiopharmaceutical Therapy. Reston, VA: Society of Nuclear Medicine; 2004

Case 44

Mettler FA Jr, Huda W, Yoshizumi TT, Mahesh M. Effective doses in radiology and diagnostic nuclear medicine: a catalog. Radiology 2008;248(1):254–263

Parker MS, Hui FK, Camacho MA, Chung JK, Broga DW, Sethi NN. Female breast radiation exposure during CT pulmonary angiography. AJR Am J Roentgenol 2005;185(5):1228–1233

Stein PD, Fowler SE, Goodman LR, et al; PIOPED II Investigators. Multidetector computed tomography for acute pulmonary embolism. N Engl J Med 2006;354(22):2317–2327

Stein PD, Gottschalk A, Sostman HD, et al. Methods of Prospective Investigation of Pulmonary Embolism Diagnosis III (PIOPED III). Semin Nucl Med 2008;38(6):462–470

Strashun AM. A reduced role of V/Q scintigraphy in the diagnosis of acute pulmonary embolism. J Nucl Med 2007;48(9):1405–1407

Case 45

Rocco TP, Dilsizian V, Fischman AJ, Strauss HW. Evaluation of ventricular function in patients with coronary artery disease. J Nucl Med 1989;30(7):1149–1165

Case 46

Conway JJ. "Well-tempered" diuresis renography: its historical development, physiological and technical pitfalls, and standardized technique protocol. Semin Nucl Med 1992;22(2):74–84

Case 47

Bellah RD, Summerville DA, Treves ST, Micheli LJ. Low-back pain in adolescent athletes: detection of stress injury to the pars interarticularis with SPECT. Radiology 1991;180(2):509–512

Rodriguez DP, Poussaint TY. Imaging of back pain in children. AJNR Am J Neuroradiol 2010;31(5):787–802

Case 48

De Leon OA, Blend MJ, Jobe TH, Ponton M, Gaviria M. Application of ictal brain SPECT for differentiating epileptic from nonepileptic seizures. J Neuropsychiatry Clin Neurosci 1997;9:99–101

Duncan R, Patterson J, Roberts R, Hadley DM, Bone I. Ictal/postictal SPECT in the pre-surgical localisation of complex partial seizures. J Neurol Neurosurg Psychiatry 1993;56(2):141–148

Grünwald F, Menzel C, Pavics L, et al. Ictal and interictal brain SPECT imaging in epilepsy using technetium-99m-ECD. J Nucl Med 1994;35(12):1896–1901

Case 49

Siegel JA. Nuclear Regulatory Commission Regulation of Nuclear Medicine. Guide for Diagnostic Nuclear Medicine and Radiopharmaceutical Therapy. Reston, VA: Society of Nuclear Medicine; 2004

Case 50

Bekerman C, Nayak SM. Gallium imaging. In: Henkin RE, Boles MA, Dillehay GL, et al, eds. Nuclear medicine. St Louis, Mo: Mosby, 1996; 1597–1618

Case 51

Derin H, Yetkin E, Ozkilic H, Ozekli K, Yaman C. Detection of splenosis by radionuclide scanning. Br J Radiol 1987;60(717):873–875

Case 52

Castaigne C, Martin P, Blocklet D. Lung, gastric, and soft tissue uptake of Tc-99m MDP and Ga-67 citrate associated with hypercalcemia. Clin Nucl Med 2003;28(6):467–471

Hirose Y, Tachibana J, Sugai S, Konda S, Hayabe T, Konishi F. Metastatic calcification in the stomach demonstrated by a bone scan in Bence Jones lambda myeloma. Jpn J Med 1987;26(1):72–75

Licata AA, Farnand B, Gangemi R, Breckenridge R. Symmetrical bone scan in a patient with acute hypercalcemia. Arch Intern Med 1983;143(9):1779–1780

Case 53

Buchpiguel CA, Alavi JB, Alavi A, Kenyon LC. PET versus SPECT in distinguishing radiation necrosis from tumor recurrence in the brain. J Nucl Med 1995;36(1):159–164

Kosuda S, Fujii H, Aoki S, et al. Reassessment of quantitative thallium-201 brain SPECT for miscellaneous brain tumors. Ann Nucl Med 1993;7(4):257–263

Case 54

Johnson K, Alton HM, Chapman S. Evaluation of mebrofenin hepatoscintigraphy in neonatal-onset jaundice. Pediatr Radiol 1998;28(12):937–941

Poddar U, Bhattacharya A, Thapa BR, Mittal BR, Singh K. Ursodeoxycholic acid-augmented hepatobiliary scintigraphy in the evaluation of neonatal jaundice. J Nucl Med 2004;45(9):1488–1492

Case 55

Nielsen KR, Blake LM, Mark JB, DeCampli W, McDougall IR. Localization of bronchopleural fistula using ventilation scintigraphy. J Nucl Med 1994;35(5):867–869

Seo H, Kim TJ, Jin KN, Lee KW. Multi-detector row computed tomographic evaluation of bronchopleural fistula: correlation with clinical, bronchoscopic, and surgical findings. J Comput Assist Tomogr 2010;34(1):13–18

Skorodin MS, Gergans GA, Zvetina JR, Siever JR. Xenon-133 evidence of bronchopleural fistula healing during treatment of mixed aspergillus and tuberculous empyema. J Nucl Med 1982;23(8):688–689

Case 56

Reid JR, Wheeler SF. Hyperthyroidism: diagnosis and treatment. Am Fam Physician 2005;72(4):623–630

Case 57

Luk WH, Au-Yeung AWS, Yang MK. Diagnostic value of SPECT versus SPECT/CT in femoral avascular necrosis: preliminary results. Nucl Med Commun 2010;31(11):958–961

Mitchell DG, Rao VM, Dalinka MK, et al. Femoral head avascular necrosis: correlation of MR imaging, radiographic staging, radionuclide imaging, and clinical findings. Radiology 1987;162(3):709–715

Case 58

Cypess AM, Lehman S, Williams G, et al. Identification and importance of brown adipose tissue in adult humans. N Engl J Med 2009;360(15):1509–1517

Yeung HW, Grewal RK, Gonen M, Schöder H, Larson SM. Patterns of (18)F-FDG uptake in adipose tissue and muscle: a potential source of false-positives for PET. J Nucl Med 2003;44(11):1789–1796

Case 59

Basu S, Zhuang H, Torigian DA, Rosenbaum J, Chen W, Alavi A. Functional imaging of inflammatory diseases using nuclear medicine techniques. Semin Nucl Med 2009;39(2):124–145

Becker W, Fischbach W, Reiners C, Börner W. Three-phase white blood cell scan: diagnostic validity in abdominal inflammatory diseases. J Nucl Med 1986;27(7):1109–1115

Case 60

Boubaker A, Prior JO, Meuwly JY, Bischof-Delaloye A. Radionuclide investigations of the urinary tract in the era of multimodality imaging. J Nucl Med 2006;47(11):1819–1836

Case 61

Taillefer R, Boucher Y, Potvin C, Lambert R. Detection and localization of parathyroid adenomas in patients with hyperparathyroidism using a single radionuclide imaging procedure with technetium-99m-sestamibi (double-phase study). J Nucl Med 1992;33(10):1801–1807

Case 62

Coleman RE, Rubens RD, Fogelman I. Reappraisal of the baseline bone scan in breast cancer. J Nucl Med 1988;29(6):1045–1049

Even-Sapir E, Metser U, Mishani E, Lievshitz G, Lerman H, Leibovitch I. The detection of bone metastases in patients with high-risk prostate cancer: 99mTc-MDP Planar bone scintigraphy, single- and multi-field-of-view SPECT, 18F-fluoride PET, and 18F-fluoride PET/CT. J Nucl Med 2006;47(2):287–297

Min J-W, Um SW, Yim JJ, et al. The role of whole-body FDG PET/CT, Tc99m MDP bone scintigraphy, and serum alkaline phosphatase in detecting bone metastasis in patients with newly diagnosed lung cancer. J Korean Med Sci 2009;24(2):275–280

Takenaka D, Ohno Y, Matsumoto K, et al. Detection of bone metastases in non-small cell lung cancer patients: comparison of whole-body diffusion-weighted imaging (DWI), whole-body MR imaging without and with DWI, whole-body FDG-PET/CT, and bone scintigraphy. J Magn Reson Imaging 2009;30(2):298–308

Case 63

Roberts KE, Hamele-Bena D, Saqi A, Stein CA, Cole RP. Pulmonary tumor embolism: a review of the literature. Am J Med 2003;115(3):228–232

Sostman HD, Brown M, Toole A, Bobrow S, Gottschalk A. Perfusion scan in pulmonary vascular/lymphangitic carcinomatosis: the segmental contour pattern. AJR Am J Roentgenol 1981;137(5):1072–1074

Case 64

Garai I, Varga J, Szomják E, et al. Quantitative assessment of blood flow reserve using 99mTc-HMPAO in carotid stenosis. Eur J Nucl Med Mol Imaging 2002;29(2):216–220

Hoeffner EG, Case I, Jain R, et al. Cerebral perfusion CT: technique and clinical applications. Radiology 2004;231(3):632–644

Hosoda K, Kawaguchi T, Shibata Y, et al. Cerebral vasoreactivity and internal carotid artery flow help to identify patients at risk for hyperperfusion after carotid endarterectomy. Stroke 2001;32(7):1567–1573

Ogasawara K, Yukawa H, Kobayashi M, et al. Prediction and monitoring of cerebral hyperperfusion after carotid endarterectomy by using single-photon emission computerized tomography scanning. J Neurosurg 2003;99(3):504–510

Case 65

Crawford ES, Guarasci DT, Larson SA. A survey of thyroid gland scintigraphy. J Nucl Med Technol 2009;37(3):173–178

Williams JD, Sclafani AP, Slupchinskij O, Douge C. Evaluation and management of the lingual thyroid gland. Ann Otol Rhinol Laryngol 1996;105(4):312–316

Case 66

Williams KA, Hill KA, Sheridan CM. Noncardiac findings on dual-isotope myocardial perfusion SPECT. J Nucl Cardiol 2003; 10(4):395–402

Case 67

Gotthardt M, Bleeker-Rovers CP, Boerman OC, Oyen WJ. Imaging of inflammation by PET, conventional scintigraphy, and other imaging techniques. J Nucl Med 2010;51(12):1937–1949

Case 68

Siegel JA. Nuclear Regulatory Commission Regulation of Nuclear Medicine. Guide for Diagnostic Nuclear Medicine and Radiopharmaceutical Therapy. Reston, VA: Society of Nuclear Medicine; 2004

Howe DB, Beardsley SR, Bakhsh SR. Consolidated Guidance About Materials Licenses: Program-Specific Guidance About Medical Use Licenses (NUREG-1556, Volume 9, Revision 2, Appendix P. Washington, DC: U.S. Nuclear Regulatory Commission; 2008. http://www.nrc.gov/reading-rm/doc-collections/nuregs/staff/sr1556/v9/r2. Accessed February 4, 2011

Case 69

Ziessman HA, Silverman PM, Patterson J, et al. Improved detection of small cavernous hemangiomas of the liver with high-resolution three-headed SPECT. J Nucl Med 1991;32(11):2086–2091

Case 70

Sugawara Y, Fisher SJ, Zasadny KR, Kison PV, Baker LH, Wahl RL. Preclinical and clinical studies of bone marrow uptake of fluorine-1-fluorodeoxyglucose with or without granulocyte colony-stimulating factor during chemotherapy. J Clin Oncol 1998;16(1):173–180

Sugawara Y, Zasadny KR, Kison PV, Baker LH, Wahl RL. Splenic fluorodeoxyglucose uptake increased by granulocyte colony-stimulating factor therapy: PET imaging results. J Nucl Med 1999;40(9): 1456–1462

Weiler-Sagie M, Bushelev O, Epelbaum R, et al. (18)F-FDG avidity in lymphoma readdressed: a study of 766 patients. J Nucl Med 2010;51(1):25–30

Yamane T, Daimaru O, Ito S, et al. Decreased 18F-FDG uptake 1 day after initiation of chemotherapy for malignant lymphomas. J Nucl Med 2004;45(11):1838–1842

Case 71

Biersack HJ, Thelen M, Torres JF, et al. Focal nodular hyperplasia of the liver as established by Tc99m-sulfur colloid and HIDA scintigraphy. Radiology 1980;137:187–190

Case 72

Brown ML, O'Connor MK, Hung JC, Hayostek RJ. Technical aspects of bone scintigraphy. Radiol Clin North Am 1993;31(4): 721–730

Case 73

Dworkin HJ, Meier DA, Kaplan M. Advances in the management of patients with thyroid disease. Semin Nucl Med 1995;25(3):205–220

Kusić Z, Becker DV, Saenger EL, et al. Comparison of technetium-99m and iodine-123 imaging of thyroid nodules: correlation with pathologic findings. J Nucl Med 1990;31(4):393–399

Case 74

Conway JJ. "Well-tempered" diuresis renography: its historical development, physiological and technical pitfalls, and standardized technique protocol. Semin Nucl Med 1992;22(2):74–84

Case 75

Anderson DR, Kahn SR, Rodger MA, et al. Computed tomographic pulmonary angiography vs ventilation-perfusion lung scanning in patients with suspected pulmonary embolism: a randomized controlled trial. JAMA 2007;298(23):2743–2753

Miniati M, Sostman HD, Gottschalk A, Monti S, Pistolesi M. Perfusion lung scintigraphy for the diagnosis of pulmonary embolism: a reappraisal and review of the Prospective Investigative Study of Acute Pulmonary Embolism Diagnosis methods. Semin Nucl Med 2008;38(6):450–461

Stein PD, Woodard PK, Weg JG, et al; PIOPED II investigators. Diagnostic pathways in acute pulmonary embolism: recommendations of the PIOPED II investigators. Am J Med 2006;119(12):1048–1055

Case 76

Halpern BS, Dahlbom M, Waldherr C, et al. Cardiac pacemakers and central venous lines can induce focal artifacts on CT-corrected PET images. J Nucl Med 2004;45(2):290–293

Case 77

Gordon L, Schabel SI, Holland RD, Cooper JF. 99mTc-methylene diphosphonate accumulation in ascitic fluid due to neoplasm. Radiology 1981;139(3):699–702

McDevitt GR Jr, Heironimus JD, Toney MO, Billingsley JL. Diffuse abdominal uptake of technetium-99m-methylene diphosphonate in a patient on continuous ambulatory dialysis during bone scintigraphy. J Nucl Med 1992;33(11):2052–2054

Rutherford GC, Green DJ, O'Connor AR. Accumulation of Tc-99m MDP by omental tumor in metastatic cecal cancer. Clin Nucl Med 2006;31(10):655–657

Case 78

Harbert JC, Eckelman WC, Neumann RD. Nuclear Medicine Diagnosis and Therapy. New York, NY: Thieme; 1996

Case 79

Brown KA. Prognostic value of thallium-201 myocardial perfusion imaging. A diagnostic tool comes of age. Circulation 1991;83(2):363–381

Case 80

Alazraki NP, Eshima D, Eshima LA, et al. Lymphoscintigraphy, the sentinel node concept, and the intraoperative gamma probe in melanoma, breast cancer, and other potential cancers. Semin Nucl Med 1997;27(1):55–67

Gulec SA, Moffat FL, Carroll RG, et al. Sentinel lymph node localization in early breast cancer. J Nucl Med 1998;39(8):1388–1393

Yudd AP, Kempf JS, Goydos JS, Stahl TJ, Feinstein RS. Use of sentinel node lymphoscintigraphy in malignant melanoma. Radiographics 1999;19(2):343–353, discussion 354–356

Case 81

Davenport MS, Brown RK, Frey KA. Utility of delayed whole-body bone scintigraphy after directed three-phase scintigraphy. AJR Am J Roentgenol 2009;193(2):338–342

Greyson ND, Tepperman PS. Three-phase bone studies in hemiplegia with reflex sympathetic dystrophy and the effect of disuse. J Nucl Med 1984;25(4):423–429

Leitha T. Role of mineralisation in the uptake of bone-seeking tracers. Eur J Nucl Med Mol Imaging 1996;23(3):256–262

Tondeur M, Sand A, Ham H. Interobserver reproducibility in the interpretation of bone scans from patients suspected of having reflex sympathetic dystrophy. Clin Nucl Med 2005;30(1):4–10

Veldman PH, Reynen HM, Arntz IE, Goris RJ. Signs and symptoms of reflex sympathetic dystrophy: prospective study of 829 patients. Lancet 1993;342(8878):1012–1016

Case 82

Ashburn WL, Harbert JC, Briner WH, Di Chiro G. Cerebrospinal fluid rhinorrhea studied with the gamma scintillation camera. J Nucl Med 1968;9(10):523–529

Di Chiro G, Ommaya AK, Ashburn WL, Briner WH. Isotope cisternography in the diagnosis and follow-up of cerebrospinal fluid rhinorrhea. J Neurosurg 1968;28(6):522–529

Stone JA, Castillo M, Neelon B, Mukherji SK. Evaluation of CSF leaks: high-resolution CT compared with contrast-enhanced CT and radionuclide cisternography. AJNR Am J Neuroradiol 1999;20(4):706–712

Case 83

Kuligowska E, Schlesinger A, Miller KB, Lee VW, Grosso D. Bilomas: a new approach to the diagnosis and treatment. Gastrointest Radiol 1983;8(3):237–243

Case 84

Ghobrial I, Witzig T. Radioimmunotherapy: a new treatment modality for B-cell non-Hodgkin's lymphoma. Oncology (Williston Park) 2004;18(5):623–630, discussion 633–634, 637–638, 640

Gisselbrecht C, Vose J, Nademanee A, Gianni AM, Nagler A. Radioimmunotherapy for stem cell transplantation in non-Hodgkin's lymphoma: in pursuit of a complete response. Oncologist 2009;14(Suppl 2):41–51

Plosker GL, Figgitt DP. Rituximab: a review of its use in non-Hodgkin's lymphoma and chronic lymphocytic leukaemia. Drugs 2003;63(8):803–843

Case 85

Kleinman PL, Kleinman PK, Savageau JA. Suspected infant abuse: radiographic skeletal survey practices in pediatric health care facilities. Radiology 2004;233(2):477–485

Mandelstam SA, Cook D, Fitzgerald M, Ditchfield MR. Complementary use of radiological skeletal survey and bone scintigraphy in detection of bony injuries in suspected child abuse. Arch Dis Child 2003;88(5):387–390, discussion 387–390

Section on Radiology; American Academy of Pediatrics. Diagnostic imaging of child abuse. Pediatrics 2009;123(5):1430–1435

Case 86

Ellis RJ, Zhou EH, Fu P, et al. Single photon emission computerized tomography with capromab pendetide plus computerized tomography image set co-registration independently predicts biochemical failure. J Urol 2008;179(5):1768–1773, discussion 1773–1774

Ellis RJ, Zhou H, Kim EY, et al. Biochemical disease-free survival rates following definitive low-dose-rate prostate brachytherapy with dose escalation to biologic target volumes identified with SPECT/CT capromab pendetide. Brachytherapy 2007;6(1):16–25

Haseman MK, Rosenthal SA, Polascik TJ. Capromab Pendetide imaging of prostate cancer. Cancer Biother Radiopharm 2000;15(2):131–140

Kumar R, Zhuang H, Alavi A. PET in the management of urologic malignancies. Radiol Clin North Am 2004;42(6):1141–1153, ix

Proaño JM, Sodee DB, Resnick MI, Einstein DB. The impact of a negative (111)indium-capromab pendetide scan before salvage radiotherapy. J Urol 2006;175(5):1668–1672

Case 87

Cohade C, Osman M, Leal J, Wahl RL. Direct comparison of (18)F-FDG PET and PET/CT in patients with colorectal carcinoma. J Nucl Med 2003;44(11):1797–1803

Rohren EM, Turkington TG, Coleman RE. Clinical applications of PET in oncology. Radiology 2004;231(2):305–332

Case 88

Rothstein RD. The role of scintigraphy in the management of inflammatory bowel disease. J Nucl Med 1991;32(5):856–859

Society of Nuclear Medicine procedure guideline for 99mTc-exametazime (HMPAO)-labeled leukocyte scintigraphy for suspected infection/inflammation. Version 3.0, approved June 2, 2004. http://interactive.snm.org/docs/HMPAO_v3.pdf. Accessed February 4, 2011

Case 89

Bozkurt MF, Uğur O. Intra-arterial Tc-99m MDP injection mimicking reflex sympathetic dystrophy. Clin Nucl Med 2001;26(2):154–156

Loutfi I, Collier BD, Mohammed AM. Nonosseous abnormalities on bone scans. J Nucl Med Technol 2003;31(3):149–153, quiz 154–156

Case 90

Titton RL, Gervais DA, Hahn PF, Harisinghani MG, Arellano RS, Mueller PR. Urine leaks and urinomas: diagnosis and imaging-guided intervention. Radiographics 2003;23(5):1133–1147

Case 91

Brink I, Reinhardt MJ, Hoegerle S, Altehoefer C, Moser E, Nitzsche EU. Increased metabolic activity in the thymus gland studied with 18F-FDG PET: age dependency and frequency after chemotherapy. J Nucl Med 2001;42(4):591–595

Ferdinand B, Gupta P, Kramer EL. Spectrum of thymic uptake at 18F-FDG PET. Radiographics 2004;24(6):1611–1616

Case 92

Howarth DM. The role of nuclear medicine in the detection of acute gastrointestinal bleeding. Semin Nucl Med 2006;36(2): 133–146

Case 93

Grames GM, Jansen C, Carlsen EN, Davidson TR. The abnormal bone scan in intracranial lesions. Radiology 1975;115(1): 129–134

Suzuki A, Togawa T, Kuyama J, et al. Extraosseous accumulation of 99mTc phosphonate complexes in primary brain tumor evaluated with SPECT. Ann Nucl Med 2002;16(7):495–498

Case 94

Germano G, Kavanagh PB, Berman DS. An automatic approach to the analysis, quantitation and review of perfusion and function from myocardial perfusion SPECT images. Int J Card Imaging 1997;13(4):337–346

Udelson JE, Beshansky JR, Ballin DS, et al. Myocardial perfusion imaging for evaluation and triage of patients with suspected acute cardiac ischemia: a randomized controlled trial. JAMA 2002;288(21):2693–2700

Case 95

Dworkin HJ, Meier DA, Kaplan M. Advances in the management of patients with thyroid disease. Semin Nucl Med 1995;25(3):205–220

Puxeddu E, Filetti S. The 2009 American Thyroid Association Guidelines for management of thyroid nodules and differentiated thyroid cancer: progress on the road from consensus- to evidence-based practice. Thyroid 2009;19(11):1145–1147

Case 96

Boysen PG, Block AJ, Olsen GN, Moulder PV, Harris JO, Rawitscher RE. Prospective evaluation for pneumonectomy using the 99mtechnetium quantitative perfusion lung scan. Chest 1977;72(4):422–425

Win T, Tasker AD, Groves AM, et al. Ventilation-perfusion scintigraphy to predict postoperative pulmonary function in lung cancer patients undergoing pneumonectomy. AJR Am J Roentgenol 2006;187(5):1260–1265

Case 97

Kim HC, Alavi A, Russell MO, Schwartz E. Differentiation of bone and bone marrow infarcts from osteomyelitis in sickle cell disorders. Clin Nucl Med 1989;14(4):249–254

Rao S, Solomon N, Miller S, Dunn E. Scintigraphic differentiation of bone infarction from osteomyelitis in children with sickle cell disease. J Pediatr 1985;107(5):685–688

Case 98

Asad S, Aquino SL, Piyavisetpat N, Fischman AJ. False-positive FDG positron emission tomography uptake in nonmalignant chest abnormalities. AJR Am J Roentgenol 2004;182(4):983–989

Pauls S, et al. Clinical Value of Combined Positron Emission Tomography/Computed Tomography Imaging in the Interpretation of 2-Deoxy-2-[F-18]fluoro-d -glucose–Positron Emission Tomography Studies in Cancer Patients. Mol Imaging Biol 2008;10:121–128

Case 99

Siegel JA. Nuclear Regulatory Commission Regulation of Nuclear Medicine. Guide for Diagnostic Nuclear Medicine and Radiopharmaceutical Therapy. Reston, VA: Society of Nuclear Medicine; 2004

Case 100

Gundlapalli S, Ojha B, Mountz JM. Granulocyte colony-stimulating factor: confounding F-18 FDG uptake in outpatient positron emission tomographic facilities for patients receiving ongoing treatment of lymphoma. Clin Nucl Med 2002;27(2):140–141

Vogel CL, Schoenfelder J, Shemano I, Hayes DF, Gams RA. Worsening bone scan in the evaluation of antitumor response during hormonal therapy of breast cancer. J Clin Oncol 1995;13(5):1123–1128

Index

Note: Locators refer to case number. Locators in **boldface** indicate primary diagnosis or main discussion.

A

Abscess, pelvic, **27**
AC. *See* Attenuation correction (AC)
Acute tubular necrosis (ATN), **74**
AD. *See* Alzheimer dementia (AD)
Adenoma(s)
  parathyroid
    ectopic, **61**
    multiple, 14
  thyroid
    functioning ("warm nodule"), 23
    hyperfunctioning, **23**, 65
      benign, 72
    hypofunctioning, 36
    multiple, 14
    toxic hyperfunctioning ("hot nodule"), **23**
Adenopathy
  benign reactive, 87
  mediastinal, compressing pulmonary vessels, 44
Adipose tissue, brown. *See* Brown fat
Alzheimer dementia (AD), **4**
Angiosarcoma, 69
Antithyroid medications, 78
Aortic aneurysm, 16
Aortic regurgitation, 45
Arachnoid cyst, 82
Arthritis, 89
  inflammatory, 81
  septic, 57
Artifact(s)
  breast attenuation, 79, 94
  colloid formation, 37
  diaphragmatic creep, 94
  diaphragm attenuation, **30**
  free pertechnetate, **16**, 52
  of PET attenuation correction (AC), **76**
  of upright Tc99m-MAA injection, **19**
  urinary contamination, 60
Ascites, malignant, **77**
Aspiration, 75
Asthma, 19
Attenuation correction (AC), for positron emission tomography, artifact of, **76**
Avascular necrosis (AVN), acute, **57**
AVN (avascular necrosis), acute, **57**

B

BAT (brown adipose tissue). *See* Brown fat
Bexxar therapy, **84**
Biliary atresia, **54**
Biliary leak, **83**
Biodistribution, altered, 6, 38
Bleeding. *See also* Hemorrhage
  gastric, 16
  gastrointestinal, 88, 92
  small-bowel, 92
Body badge, 3
Bone infarct, 100
  acute, 33
Bone marrow
  benign stimulation, **38**
  normal packing, 27
Bone metastasis, 22, 47, **77**, 85
  gallium scan showing, 25
Bony process, benign polyostotic, 97
Bowel. *See also* Gastrointestinal *entries;* Small bowel
  inflammation of. *See also* Inflammatory bowel disease (IBD)
    PET scan of, 76
  metastasis to, PET scan of, 76
  necrosis, 77
  physiologic intraluminal excretion in, WBC scan and, 59
Brain, tracer uptake in, **93**
Brain death, **18**
Breast attenuation artifact, 79
  shifting, 94
Breast cancer
  axillary regional metastases, lymphoscintigraphy of, 80

Breast cancer *(continued)*
sentinel nodes in
emission-only lymphoscintigraphy of, 80
emission/transmission lymphoscintigraphy of, **80**
Bronchopleural fistula, persistent right, **55**
Brown adipose tissue (BAT). *See* Brown fat
Brown fat hypermetabolism, 6, **58**

C

Cancer. *See also specific cancer*
thoracic, **66**
Carcinoid, metastatic, MIBG scan of, 95
Cardiomyopathy, ischemic, **45**
Cavernous hemangioma, **69**
CDE. *See* Committed dose equivalent (CDE)
CEDE. *See* Committed effective dose equivalent (CEDE)
Cellulitis, **27**, 67
Central nervous system (CNS). *See also* Brain
infection, 48, 53
Cerebral infarct. *See also* Multi-infarct dementia (MID)
right hemispheric, 64
Cerebral vascular blood flow reserve, diminished, **64**
Cerebrospinal fluid (CSF) leak, 34
anterior, **82**
Cerebrovascular disease, 18
Chemical purity, 24
Chemotherapy, cardiotoxicity, 45
Child abuse, **85**
Cholecystitis
acalculous, 10
acute, **10**
chronic, 10
Cholestasis, intrahepatic, 54
Chronic obstructive pulmonary disease (COPD), 19, 55
CNS. *See* Brain; Central nervous system (CNS)
Collimator, damaged, 32
Colloid cyst, of thyroid, 36
Colloid formation artifact, 37
Colon cancer. *See also* Colorectal cancer
metastatic to lung, 98
with synchronous lung cancer, 98
Colonic hemorrhage, active, **92**
Colorectal cancer. *See also* Colon cancer
metastases, non-FDG–avid, **87**
Committed dose equivalent (CDE), 3
Committed effective dose equivalent (CEDE), 3
Communicating hydrocephalus, obstructing, **34**
COPD. *See* Chronic obstructive pulmonary disease (COPD)
Coronary artery disease, **79**, **94**. *See also* Myocardial infarction; Myocardial ischemia; Myocardium, hibernating
Craniotomy defect(s), 93
Crystal, cracked, 32
CSF. *See* Cerebrospinal fluid (CSF) leak
Cyst(s)
arachnoid, 82
colloid, of thyroid, 36
duplication, ectopic gastric mucosa in, 8
renal upper pole, large, 35

D

DDE. *See* Deep dose equivalent (DDE)
Deep dose equivalent (DDE), 3
Diabetic foot, 67
Diaphragmatic creep artifact, 94
Diaphragm attenuation artifact, **30**
Diffuse skeletal metastases, **1**
Duplication cyst, ectopic gastric mucosa in, 8

E

Electronic dosimeter, 3
Enchondromas, multiple, 97
Exercise, recent, 6
External beam radiation, normal spinal effects, **100**

F

Fatty liver, xenon retention in, 9, 55
FEV_1. *See* Forced expiratory volume in 1 second (FEV_1)
Fibrous dysplasia, polyostotic, 97
Fistula(s), urinary enteric, 90
FNH. *See* Focal nodular hyperplasia (FNH)

Focal nodular hyperplasia (FNH), 51, 69, **71**
Forced expiratory volume in 1 second (FEV_1), residual
of 1123 mL, 96
of 1154 mL, **96**
Fracture(s), 67. *See also* Stress fracture
hip, gallium scan of, 25
sacral insufficiency, **28**

G

Gallium scan
of bone metastasis, 25
of hip fracture, 25
of lymphoma, **7**, 86
of metastatic melanoma, 41, 95
of osteomyelitis, **25**
of *Pneumocystis* pneumonia, **39**
of sarcoidosis, 7, **50**
Gastric bleed, 16
Gastric emptying, delayed, **20**
Gastric mucosa, ectopic
in duplication cyst, 8
in Meckel diverticulum, **8**
Gastrointestinal bleeding, 88, 92
Gastrostomy tube tract, physiologic WBC accumulation around, **59**
Germ cell tumor, 91
Glioblastoma multiforme, recurrence, **53**
Glioma, low-grade, 48
Goiter
ectopic, 65
toxic nodular, 2
Graves disease, 56
plus indeterminate cold nodule, **2**

H

Head and neck carcinoma, 15
Hemangioma
cavernous, **69**
hepatic, 71
cavernous, **69**
nondamaged RBC scan of, 51
Hemorrhage
colonic, active, **92**
intraperitoneal, active, 83
Hepatic hemangioma, 71
cavernous, **69**
nondamaged RBC scan of, 51
Hepatitis, neonatal, 54
Hibernating myocardium, **5**, 30, 79
Hip fracture, gallium scan of, 25
Hip prosthesis
infected, **27**
loosening, 27
Hip splints, **42**
Hodgkin lymphoma, 15
Hydrocephalus
communicating, obstructing, **34**
normal pressure, 34, 82
Hypercalcemia, **52**
Hyperinsulinemia, altered biodistribution from, **6**
Hyperparathyroidism, 17

I

Indium 111-capromab pendetide. *See* ProstaScint scan
Infection(s), 50, 72. *See also specific infection*
abdominal, 59
active, WBC scan showing, 7
central nervous system, 48, 53
pulmonary, 61
Inflammation of bowel. *See also* Inflammatory bowel disease (IBD)
PET scan of, 76
pulmonary, 61, 66. *See also* Pneumonia; Sarcoidosis
Inflammatory arthritis, 81
Inflammatory bowel disease (IBD), **88**
Insufficiency fracture, sacral, **28**
Intracranial soft-tissue uptake, **93**
Intraperitoneal hemorrhage, active, 83
Iodine 131, for thyroid cancer, **43**
Iodine organification defect, **78**
Iodine 131 scan, of metastatic thyroid cancer, 12, **95**
Iodine 131-tositumomab. *See* Bexxar therapy
Iodine 131 whole-body (WB) scan, of metastatic thyroid cancer, **95**

Ischemic cardiomyopathy, **45**
Islet cell carcinoma, metastatic, **41**

J

Joint(s), neuropathic, 67

K

Kidney(s). *See also* Renal *entries*
compound, with upper pole hydronephrosis, 35
upper pole cyst, large, 35
upper pole infarct and partially contained urinary leak, **35**

L

LDE. *See* Lens dose equivalent (LDE)
Left anterior descending artery disease, **79**, **94**
Lens dose equivalent (LDE), 3
Lewy body dementia, 4
Lingual thyroid, **65**
Liver. *See also* Fatty liver; Focal nodular hyperplasia (FNH)
cavernous hemangioma, **69**
hemangioma, 51, 71
metastasis to, 37
regenerating nodules, 71
Lung(s). *See also* Forced expiratory volume in 1 second (FEV_1); Pulmonary *entries*
right, base, ventilatory retention at, 9
Lung cancer, 75
with ipsilateral hilar metastasis, **29**
synchronous (with colon cancer), 98
Lymphoma(s), 50, 58
FDG-PET demonstrating, **70**
gallium scan showing, **7**, 86
Hodgkin, 15
non-Hodgkin, 58
recurrent, 91
Lymphoproliferative neoplasm. *See also* Lymphoma(s)
secondary, 87
Lymphoscintigraphy
of axillary regional metastases, in breast cancer, 80
emission-only, of sentinel nodes, in breast cancer, 80
emission/transmission, of sentinel nodes, in breast cancer, **80**
Lytic metastasis, **33**, 100

M

MAA. *See* Tc99m MAA
Malignancy. *See also* Cancer; *specific malignancy*
thoracic, **66**
Meckel diverticulum, ectopic gastric mucosa in, **8**
Mediastinum
adenopathy in, compressing pulmonary vessels, 44
benign neoplasm in, 66
tumor in, 61
Medical event, recordable, **49**
Melanoma, metastatic, gallium scan showing, 41, 95
Mesothelioma, peritoneal, 77
Metabolic bone disease, 1
Metabolic disorder, multiple bone lesions associated with, 62
Metabolic superscan, 1
Metastatic disease, 97
bone. *See* Bone metastasis
diffuse
FDG-PET demonstrating, 70
osteoblastic, **62**
skeletal, **1**
gallium scan of, 95
gastrointestinal, PET scan of, 76
hepatic, 37
iodine-131 whole-body scan of, **95**
lytic, **33**
osseous, 100
MIBG scan of, 95
non-FDG–avid, **87**
octreotide scan showing, 12
osseous, lytic, 100
pelvic, 28
ProstaScint scan of, **86**
skeletal, 17
diffuse, **1**

skull involvement in, 93
thyroid cancer, **95**
Metastatic superscan, **1**
Metastron. *See* Strontium 89 (Metastron)
MIBG scan
of metastatic carcinoid, 95
of metastatic neuroblastoma, **12**, 41
MID. *See* Multi-infarct dementia (MID)
Multi-infarct dementia (MID), 4
Myeloma, 33
Myocardial infarction, 5
inferior, 30
left anterior descending artery, **79**
Myocardial ischemia
peri-infarct, **79**
reversible, **94**
stress-induced reversible, 5
Myocardium, hibernating, **5**, 30, 79
Myositis, 6, 58

N

Neoplasm(s). *See also* Lymphoproliferative neoplasm; Tumor(s); *specific neoplasm*
mediastinal, benign, 66
Neuroblastoma
metastatic, **12**, 41
primary, **37**
Neuropathic joint, 67
Nonaccidental trauma, **85**
Non-Hodgkin lymphoma, 58
Normal pressure hydrocephalus (NPH), 34, 82
Nuclear study, recent prior, 31

O

OctreoScan, of metastatic islet cell carcinoma, **41**
Octreotide scan, of metastatic tumor, 12
Organification defect, **78**
Osseous metastases. *See* Bone metastasis; Metastatic disease
Osseous tumor, widespread, 38
Osteoarthropathy, hypertrophic, **13**, 42
Osteoblastic metastases, diffuse, **62**
Osteoid osteoma, 47, **72**
Osteomyelitis, **67**, 81
gallium scan showing, **25**
polyostotic, 85

P

Package(s), radioactive, labeling and handling, **68**
Paget disease, 13, **17**
multifocal, 1, 62
Parathyroid adenoma(s)
ectopic, **61**
multiple, 14
Parathyroid hyperplasia, with supernumerary gland, **14**
Pars interarticularis, fracture, **47**
PCP. *See Pneumocystis* pneumonia (PCP)
Pelvic abscess, **27**
Pentetriotide. *See* OctreoScan
Peritoneal mesothelioma, 77
Pertechnetate, free, 31
artifact caused by, **16**, 52
PET
attenuation correction (AC), artifact of, **76**
[^{18}F] FDG
of diffuse metastatic disease, 70
of lymphoma, **70**
of sarcoidosis, 70
of non-FDG–avid metastases, **87**
Phosphate 32, 26
Photomultiplier tube, faulty, **32**
Pleural fluid, in fissures, 63
Pneumocystis pneumonia (PCP), gallium scan showing, **39**
Pneumonia, 75
acute, **98**
Pneumocystis (PCP), gallium scan of, **39**
Pocket ion chamber, 3
Pregnancy, occupational exposure during, **40**
ProstaScint scan, 84
of metastatic disease, **86**
of tortuous abdominal vessels, 86
Pseudomembranous colitis, 88

Pulmonary embolism
high probability for, 19, **44**
intermediate probability for, 9
with evidence of pulmonary infarction, **75**
low probability for, **9**
Pulmonary infarction, **75**
Pulmonary infection/inflammation, 61. *See also* Pneumonia
Pulmonary inflammatory process, 66. *See also* Sarcoidosis
Pulmonary vasculitis, 44
Pyelonephritis, acute, **11**, 46

Q

Quadramet. *See* Samarium 153 (Quadramet)

R

Radial artery injection, of radiopharmaceutical, **89**
Radiation
annual exposure limits, 3
annual occupational dose limits, 3
committed dose equivalent (CDE), 3
committed effective dose equivalent (CEDE), 3
deep dose equivalent (DDE), 3
dose equivalent to embryo/fetus, 40
lens dose equivalent (LDE), 3
occupational exposure, during pregnancy, **40**
shallow dose equivalent (SDE), 3
total effective dose equivalent (TEDE), 3
Radiation necrosis, 53
Radioactive White I, Yellow II, or Yellow III label(s), **68**
Radiochemical purity, 24
Radioiodine. *See* Iodine 131
Radionuclide purity, 24
Radiopharmaceutical
inadvertent radial artery injection of, **89**
spills, **99**
Radiotracer, infiltrated dose, 18
RBC scan
heat-damaged, showing splenosis, **51**
nondamaged, of hepatic hemangioma, 51
Recordable event, **49**
Reflex sympathetic dystrophy (RSD), **81**, 89
Renal collecting system, upper, dilated but nonobstructed, **21**
Renal disease, chronic medical, 46, 74
Renal obstruction, 74
current, 21
Renal pelvis, ectopic, 8
Renal scarring, chronic, 11
Renal tumor, 11
Renovascular hypertension (RVH), **46**
Right coronary artery disease, **94**
Right hemispheric infarct, 64
Right-to-left shunt, **31**
Ring badge, 3
RSD. *See* Reflex sympathetic dystrophy (RSD)
RVH. *See* Renovascular hypertension (RVH)

S

Sacral insufficiency fracture, **28**
Sacroiliitis, 28
Safety
labeling and handling of radioactive packages for, **68**
major spills and, 99
minor spills and, **99**
monitoring badges and, 3
Samarium 153 (Quadramet), **26**
Sarcoidosis, 29, 39, **50**
FDG-PET demonstrating, 70
gallium scan showing, 7, **50**
SCD. *See* Sickle cell disease (SCD)
SCOL scan, of hepatic focal nodular hyperplasia, 51
SDE. *See* Shallow dose equivalent (SDE)
Seizure, right cerebral (ictal and interictal appearance), 64
Seizure focus, interictal, **48**
Shallow dose equivalent (SDE), 3
Shin splints, 13, 22, **42**
Sickle cell disease (SCD), **97**
Skeletal metastases, 17. *See* Bone metastasis Metastatic disease
diffuse, **1**

Skull metastasis, 93
Small bowel
bleed in, 92
perforation, 83
Soft tissue
intracranial, radiotracer uptake, **93**
mucinous metastases to, 52
Solitary pulmonary nodule (SPN), hypermetabolic, 29
Spill(s) (radiotracer)
major, 99
minor, **99**
Spine, normal effects of external beam radiation in, **100**
Splenic infarct, **16**
Splenosis, RBC scan showing, **51**
SPN. *See* Solitary pulmonary nodule (SPN)
Stress fracture, **22**, 72
Strontium 89 (Metastron), 26

T

Tc99m-labeled radiotracer, concurrently present, from recent prior study, 31
Tc99m MAA, injection, upright, artifact of, **19**
Tc99m MAG3, physiologic biliary excretion of, 90
TEDE. *See* Total effective dose equivalent (TEDE)
Thymic hyperplasia, benign, **91**
Thyroid adenoma(s)
functioning ("warm nodule"), 23
hyperfunctioning, 65
benign, 72
hypofunctioning, 36
multiple, 14
toxic hyperfunctioning ("hot nodule"), **23**
Thyroid cancer, 23, **36**
dedifferentiated, metastatic, **15**
iodine 131 for, **43**
metastatic
dedifferentiated, **15**
iodine 131 scan showing, 12
whole-body scan showing, **95**
remnant ablation, **43**
Thyroid gland
benign colloid nodule, 72
colloid cyst, 36
discordant nodule indeterminate for malignancy, **72**
lingual, **65**
Thyroiditis, 78
focal, 2
subacute, **56**
Thyroid nodule(s)
benign colloid, 72
discordant, indeterminate for malignancy, **72**
"hot," **23**
indeterminate cold, Graves disease and, **2**
"warm," 23
Thyroid scan, organification defect, **78**
Thyrotoxicosis factitia, 56
TM. *See* Tumor microemboli (TM)
Total effective dose equivalent (TEDE), 3
Toxic nodular goiter, 2
Trauma, nonaccidental, **85**
Tuberculosis (TB), 29
Tumor(s), 57. *See also* Neoplasm(s); *specific tumor*
chest, 50
Ga67-avid, 39
mediastinal, 61
recurrence, **53**
renal, 11
vascular intraperitoneal, 92
Tumor microemboli (TM), **63**

U

Urinary contamination artifact, 60
Urinary enteric fistula, 90
Urinary leak, **35**, 60, **90**

V

Vascular intraperitoneal tumor(s), 92
Vasculitis, pulmonary, 44
Venous stasis, 42
Venous thromboembolic disease, high probability for, 63
Venous thrombosis, 42

Ventilation. *See* Forced expiratory volume in 1 second (FEV_1)
Vesicoureteric reflux, **60**
  chronic, 21

W

WB scan. *See* Whole-body (WB) scan
WBC scan
  and physiologic intraluminal excretion in bowel, 59
  and physiologic WBC accumulation around gastrostomy tube tract, 59
  showing active infection, 7
White I radiation label, 68
Whole-body (WB) scan, iodine 131, of metastatic thyroid cancer, **95**

X

Xenon
  retention in fatty liver, 9, 55
  ventilatory retention at right lung base, 9

Y

Yellow III radiation label, 68
Yellow II radiation label, **68**
Yttrium 90-ibritumomab tiuxetan. *See* Zevalin therapy

Z

Zevalin therapy, 84